The Psychology of Reproduction 3

Current Issues in Infancy and Parenthood

Current Issues in Infancy and Parenthood

Edited by

Catherine A. Niven RGN, BSc, PhD
Professor of Nursing and Midwifery Studies
University of Stirling

and

Anne Walker BSc, PhD
Senior Research Fellow
Health Services Research Unit
University of Aberdeen

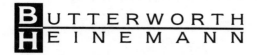

OXFORD BOSTON JOHANNESBURG MELBOURNE NEW DELHI SINGAPORE

Butterworth-Heinemann
Linacre House, Jordan Hill, Oxford OX2 8DP
225 Wildwood Avenue, Woburn, MA 01801-2041
A division of Reed Educational and Professional Publishing Ltd

R A member of the Reed Elsevier plc group

First published 1998

© Reed Educational and Professional Publishing Ltd 1998

British Library Cataloguing in Publication Data
A catalogue record for this book is available from the British Library

Library of Congress Cataloguing in Publication Data
A catalogue record for this book is available from the Library of Congress

ISBN 0 7506 2442 6

Typeset by Keyword Publishing Services Ltd.
Printed and bound in Great Britain by Biddles Ltd, Guildford and King's Lynn

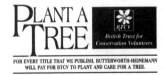

Contents

Series preface

Sex, gender, adolescence, menstruation, pregnancy, childbirth, parenthood – these experiences are linked by their relationship to human reproduction. Reproductive experiences and behaviours can be divided into four broad categories. First, there are those concerned with the activity of reproduction: pregnancy and childbirth, for instance. Second are those to do with the potential for reproduction: puberty, menstruation and the menopause, for example. Going through puberty or having menstrual periods does not in itself constitute reproduction, but people who do not experience these things usually are not able to experience active reproduction either. What might be considered the prototypical reproductive activity, heterosexual sexual inter-course, does not fit neatly into either of these categories. In the late twentieth century, and perhaps for many centuries, only a minority of sexual acts are concerned with reproduction. The creation of another human being is only one of the many reasons for engaging in sexual activity of whatever type, so sex might be better considered as an activity with reproductive potential, rather than a reproductive act. A third category of activities and experiences are those concerned with fertility control: the things we do and decisions we make to control whether or not we have children. A fourth category is concerned with the consequences of reproductive activity: pre-natal develop-ment, parenthood and parent–child relationships. These four elements of reproduction form a large part of many people's lives.

Reproduction is fundamental to human life. If we were all to decide tomor-row not to reproduce, then there would simply be no more people. How often we reproduce has economic and social implications for all areas of a society. The effects of the post-war 'baby boom' on education policy, employment possibilities and the care of older people can be clearly seen in our own society, for example. On a more global scale, the human population explosion has devastating environmental effects and significant qualitative costs for those humans who are produced, in terms of inadequacy of resources. Most govern-ments attempt to control the reproductive activity of their people – either discouraging or limiting reproduction in a variety of ways, or promoting reproduction for religious or political reasons (Fathalla 1992). Restrictive methods of control may range from the provision of family planning services and the discouragement of parenthood outside marriage to enforced steriliza-tion programmes. Governments may encourage (or enforce) parenthood by not providing contraceptive information and/or access to abortion, by not educating women or encouraging women to be economically independent (hence promoting motherhood as the only choice). Clearly, reproduction is important for societies.

Reproduction is also a concern for individuals. Most people will have children at some time in their lives and are concerned about when to conceive children and how many children to have. Individuals, like governments, may be influenced by political, religious or economic factors in the desire to have children or remain child-free. Other more individual factors are involved though, such as a sense of identity as a parent, a need for 'immortality', pressure from potential grandparents, a desire to consolidate a relationship or a wish to be closely involved with a child from its earliest moments (see Walker and McNeill, 1991). Our society clearly sees the ability and desire to have children as 'normal' – writers in newspapers and magazines express sympathy for people who are unable to have children, and much money is spent on technologies to assist conception for the involuntarily childless. Choosing to remain child-free, by contrast, is less likely to be viewed positively, and women especially who decide not to have children may be seen as 'selfish' or 'unnatural' (Matlin, 1993).

Societies and cultures have not only controlled how many children people may have, but also the circumstances in which children may be conceived (e.g. only within marriage) and in which they are born (e.g. in hospital). In the late twentieth century control of conception has extended from the ability to prevent pregnancy (which has always been practised to some extent), to the ability, through technology, to enable conception in circumstances which would previously have prevented it. At present, the technology is far from perfect and many people who attempt to conceive using the new reproductive technologies are disappointed. However, the capacity for control both of conception and of gestation are present, with alarming moral and ethical implications, especially for women (Rowland, 1992; Chadwick, 1992).

Pictures of parents holding a longed-for baby whose conception was only possible through modern technology are emotive and heart-warming. Few of us could fail to be moved by them. They imply though that reproduction is a purely mechanical process, involving only the chance, or planned, meeting of sperm and egg. Of course, the physiological and mechanical processes involved in becoming pregnant, sustaining pregnancy and giving birth are important if we want to understand human reproduction. But as we have seen, reproduction has meaning both for individual men and women, and for society. Reproduction is not just a physical event. It also has psychological and social implications.

So, what is the 'psychology of reproduction'? From its earliest beginnings, psychologists have concerned themselves with some aspects of the reproductive process. Heterosexual sex and the development of gender identity have been of particular interest to researchers. Child development, both before and after birth, has also attracted attention. Few attempts have been made, however, to draw this research together as a coherent discipline. The establishment of the Society for Reproductive and Infant Psychology (SRIP) in the early 1980s, and its journal, the *Journal of Reproductive and Infant Psychology* (JRIP) in 1983, acknowledged the growth of psychological research in areas relating to reproduction and the likely further growth in these areas resulting from the development of 'new reproductive technologies'. In the first editorial of the journal, Christopher Macy outlines the scope of reproductive and infant psychology as follows:

> pregnancy and infancy . . . might be regarded as central concerns within the field of reproduction. . . . But in order to understand women's experience of pregnancy we need to understand why women become pregnant. . . . We must look at the social value systems surrounding childbearing and childrearing, and equally at the psychological parameters associated with childlessness and infertility. . . . We take the view that psychological aspects of contraception and termination also fall squarely in our field as do many aspects of the psychology of women.

We would add to this by suggesting that many aspects of the 'psychology of men' fall into the remit of reproductive psychology too. The cultural tendency to see reproduction as 'women's work' has resulted in a neglect of men's experiences of puberty, fertility, contraception, sexuality, fatherhood and so on. The emphasis on women in this series of books should not be taken to imply that we consider reproduction only to be women's concern.

Reproductive issues have been approached from a variety of perspectives within psychology. The chief areas of interest have lain within clinical psychology and developmental psychology. Hence, the research which falls into the scope of reproductive psychology is dominated by 'problem-focused' studies and/or studies of infants and small children, rather than investigations of normative experiences. Not surprisingly, there is more to be said about reproductive activities and consequences than there is about reproductive potential and fertility control. Reproductive issues have attracted interest from a variety of other disciplines and epistemological movements too, which have influenced the approach of psychologists. The largest influence is that of the biomedical sciences. Since psychology has adopted similar research methods, and has often been concerned with similar research questions, biomedical themes have had a significant impact. This impact is shown in the concern of psychologists with psychiatric indices and labels of distress (e.g. post-natal depression) or with the psychological factors which predict distress, rather than understanding the experiences of people who are not distressed. Some psychologists have made important steps towards redressing this imbalance, however. For example, Myra Hunter's longitudinal studies of women going through the menopause (see Chapter 4, volume 1) have challenged the assumption from clinical studies that the menopause is necessarily a time of emotional turmoil and psychological dysfunction.

In addition to an emphasis on 'problems' such as post-natal depression, infertility, etc., the biomedical influence has also endorsed a positivist, hypothesis-testing approach within psychology. This approach usually requires measurement of experiences, and psychologists have played a role in developing a number of inventories and tools for quantifying distress or psychological state. Scores on such measures can be correlated with other factors in epidemiological surveys or used to evaluate interventions in treatment trials. Randomized controlled trials and measurement of experiences are clearly important in the appropriate context. However, the exclusivity of this approach in psychology has been criticized (e.g. Hollway, 1989; Potter and Wetherell, 1987). The emphasis on the use of existing measures can reduce the sensitivity of research to the specific experiences of participants in a particular study, and assumes that quantification of experiences such as depression, joy, anxiety or pain is meaningful as well as functional. For these reasons, many researchers are turning towards qualitative or postmodernist approaches within psychology. In addition, a hypothesis-testing approach can encourage reductionism, that is the tendency to see the factor evaluated as the only important one. For example, if we test the hypothesis that anxiety management techniques reduce the intensity of pain during labour, and find them to be effective, then we (or others) may be tempted to infer that anxiety is the only important factor in labour pain. Clearly in this case that is a ridiculous conclusion. In other circumstances, though, the involvement of multiple factors may not be so apparent. The inadequacy of single-factor biomedical models to explain many modern health-related experiences has resulted in the development of biopsychosocial approaches to health and illness (e.g. Engel, 1977) and the birth of the new sub-discipline of health psychology. A biopsychosocial influence can be seen clearly in many of the chapters of this series, with reproductive psychologists avoiding reductionism by explicitly placing their work within a multi-factored framework (e.g. Ussher, 1992; Hunter, 1994). The influence of the biomedical approach and its emphasis on problems, quantification and reductionism will also be seen throughout this series.

A second influence is feminism and feminist theory. As we have already said, reproduction has historically been seen as the defining characteristic of womankind. The view of woman as a womb-container has had profound implications as many feminist writers have pointed out (e.g. Martin, 1989; Ussher, 1989). To attribute experiences such as premenstrual syndrome, post-natal depression, depression in middle age, emotionality in pregnancy, and so on, simply to the biological or psychological consequences of the female reproductive system is to ignore the effects of a patriarchal culture on women. Many feminist writers have described the inherent gender bias in modern societies which influences women's positions within heterosexual relationships, our earning capacity and the expectations held about the unpaid work we will do (e.g. Oakley, 1993). Women on average are poorer than men, whether employed or not. Women are more likely to be the recipients of domestic violence and sexual abuse. Women are more likely to care for children, ageing relatives or other dependent family members. In these circumstances it is at best misogynist to attribute distress solely to biological circumstances, or to attempt to adapt women's biology to enable us to cope with intolerable situations. So, feminist critiques are demanding the contextualization of women's reproductive experiences. A further impact of feminism in social science has been the questioning of power relationships within the research process and the critique of science itself as a patriarchal institution (see Harding, 1991). Medicine has been deconstructed as an instrument of social control – especially of women (see Ehrenreich and English, 1978; Showalter, 1987). Psychology too can be a powerful social control mechanism. The implications of this critique for the processes of doing research and reporting findings are far reaching. The interpretation of research as a political activity raises questions about who is doing the research, why they are doing it, who is paying for it and what the perceived benefits are. Many feminists are struggling to develop research methodologies which do not reinforce the imbalance of power between 'researcher' and 'researched', and which offer benefits for research participants in terms of empowerment, for example (see Neilson, 1990). These approaches have as yet had little influence on mainstream psychology, but the concern of reproductive psychology with the psychology of women means that they are having more of an impact here.

The purpose of this series of three books is to bring together the disparate strands of research and theory which can be called reproductive psychology. In our own work with undergraduate psychology, nursing and midwifery students, we have often felt the need for a single source of reference which could allow students to see the breadth and scope of psychological approaches to human reproduction. Our original intention was to bring these together in a single volume. The number of topics to be covered and the vigour of current research activity surprised us though, and we soon realized that a single volume would be inadequate to encompass it all. So, we have solicited contributions from currently active researchers for a three-volume series. The subject matter of each volume reflects the categories within reproductive psychology which we outlined at the beginning of this introduction. The first volume is concerned with reproductive potential and fertility control, the second with reproductive activity – conception, pregnancy and birth – and the third with the consequences of reproduction – early development, parenting and so on. There is no particular beginning or end to this series, although we have arranged the contributions in what seems to us to be a logical order. The circularity of human reproduction is apparent though; once the child has been born then she or he begins the process of gender identity and the development of their own reproductive potential, and so on. Like the seasons of the year, reproduction has no particular beginning or end. It is a continuous process, influencing all of our lives whether we are reproductively active or not. We hope that, like us, you will find the psychology of human reproduction, despite its inadequacies and omissions, a fascinating topic and that you will learn something of personal as well as academic interest from these books.

Catherine A. Niven
Anne Walker
1995

References

Chadwick, R. (ed.) (1992). *Ethics, Reproduction and Genetic Control.* Revised edn. London: Routledge.

Ehrenreich, B. and English, D. (1978). *For Her Own Good: A Hundred Years of Experts' Advice to Women.* New York: Anchor Doubleday.

Engel, G. L. (1977). The need for a new medical model. *Science,* **196**, 129–36.

Fathalla, M. F. (1992). Society and reproductive life. In *Reproductive Life: Advances in Psychosomatic Obstetrics and Gynaecology* (K. Wijma and B. von Schoultz, eds) Carnforth: Parthenon.

Harding, S. (1991). *Whose Science? Whose Knowledge?* Milton Keynes: Open University Press.

Hollway, W. (1989). *Subjectivity and Method in Psychology: Gender, Meaning and Science.* London: Sage.

Hunter, M. (1994). *Counselling in Obstetrics and Gynaecology.* Leicester: BPS Books.

Macy, C. (1983). The Society for Reproductive and Infant Psychology: a statement of aims. *Journal of Reproductive and Infant Psychology*, **1** (1) 1–4.

Martin, E. (1989). *The Woman in the Body*. Milton Keynes: Open University Press.

Matlin, M. (1993). *The Psychology of Women*. 2nd edn. New York: Harcourt Brace Jovanovich.

Nielson, J. M. (ed.) (1990). *Feminist Research Methods*. Boulder, CO: Westview Press.

Oakley, A. (1993). *Essays on Women, Medicine and Health*. Edinburgh: Edinburgh University Press.

Potter, J. and Wetherell, M. (1987). *Discourse and Social Psychology*. London: Sage.

Rowland, R. (1992). *Living Laboratories: Women and Reproductive Technology*. London: Lime Tree.

Showalter, E. (1987). *The Female Malady*. London: Virago.

Ussher, J. (1989). *The Psychology of the Female Body*. London: Routledge.

Ussher, J. (1992). Research and theory related to female reproduction: Implications for clinical psychology. *British Journal of Clinical Psychology*, **31**, 129–51.

Walker, A. and McNeill, E. (eds) (1991). Family planning and reproductive decisions. *Journal of Reproductive and Infant Psychology*, Theme Issue, **9** (4).

Preface to Volume 3

In the third and final volume of this series, we are concerned with the consequences of reproductive activity – and particularly the experiences of both parents and infants in the early years of a baby's life. Of all the areas we have covered in the series, infant development is the one which has received most research attention. It would simply be impossible to include all aspects of infancy and parenthood research to any depth in a volume of this size. So we have not attempted here to produce a comprehensive text. Instead, we have focused on those areas which are currently of most interest for practitioners, either because they are particularly topical or newsworthy or because new theoretical or empirical insights are emerging. The major aim of this book is to bring the experiences of infants and their parents together in one volume, to emphasize that childbirth is a significant psychological event for mothers and fathers, as well as the starting point of a new developmental story.

As with all the areas which have concerned us in this series, early infancy is a time during which physiological, social, cultural and psychological factors interact, for both babies and parents. As a result of this, no two experiences are identical, and each new cohort of babies and their carers adapt to different circumstances. In westernized cultures, changes in health care, medical technology, working patterns, housing, family structure and mobility, for example, mean that the experiences of parents and infants in the late 1990s are very different from those in the 1950s or 1960s. One of the goals of research in this area has been to understand the psychological implications of these changes, and this research is well represented in this book in chapters about parents and their babies after assisted conception (Chapter 2), changing family patterns (Chapter 3), age and parenting (Chapter 4), post-partum experiences (Chapter 5), differing forms of childcare (Chapter 9) and care for premature or ill babies (Chapter 13).

Change may be a significant feature of this period of life, but continuity across generations remains. The majority of infants develop into adults, and the majority of adults adapt to their infants, in developmental sequences which show consistency over generations despite the social milieu – and one of the goals of developmental psychology is to understand these sequences. A new baby is always a little awe-inspiring, and questions about how such an (apparently) helpless and inarticulate 'scrap of humanity' becomes a talking, thinking, emotionally and socially competent adult, have an enduring fascination in psychology. From a philosophical perspective, infants are of interest because their abilities and capacities provide a test for questions about the origins and nature of human cognition and self-consciousness (Bermudez, Marcel and Eilan, 1995). These questions are far from being purely academic, for apart from their intrinsic interest the answers to them have implications for the care of young babies – a perennial concern and source of controversy in all cultures and societies. So the psychology of infancy has a relatively long history and is a well established research area represented in a large number of developmental psychology texts. The current issues we have chosen to focus on in relation to infants are feeding (Chapter 10), sleeping (Chapter 11), parent–infant interaction (Chapter 8), early sex roles (Chapter 7) and pain in infancy (Chapter 12). These are areas in which new theoretical ideas and empirical developments have significantly broadened our understanding in recent years, as well as being areas which are of critical concern for many health care practitioners who work with young children.

Developmental psychology has focused almost entirely on the changing abilities and experiences of the child. Parents have received relatively little attention, and when they have been considered, it is usually in relation to the child's needs. Becoming a parent is a developmental process for adults too, however, and an experience which is attracting more research interest in its own right (e.g. Phoenix, Woollett and Lloyd, 1991; Marsiglio, 1995). In many ways, parental experiences are more immediately affected by cultural and technological changes than are those of infants, and, in the first half of the book, we have focused on the psychological impact of particular types of change. For example: changes in health care after childbirth and their impact on post-partum experiences (Chapter 5), varying family circumstances (Chapter 3), parenting after assisted conception (Chapter 2), and the experience of 'young' (under 20) and 'older' (over 35) mothers (Chapter 4). The way in which a society constructs motherhood and fatherhood is clearly of significance here – providing parents with an internalized 'gold standard' for mothering or fathering (Chapter 1). Physiological changes and more immediate social circumstances also have an impact though, especially on the well-being of mothers (Chapter 6).

The book begins by considering the social construction of motherhood and fatherhood (Chapter 1) and then moves on to discuss mothering and fathering in relation to infant development (Chapters 2 and 3), and parental experience (Chapters 4, 5 and 6). The next chapters investigate the interaction and developing relationship between infants, their parents and carers (Chapters 7, 8 and 9). Attention then moves more specifically to infants, and especially the development of eating (Chapter 10) and sleeping (Chapter 11) patterns. In the final two chapters, the particular health care needs of babies are considered in relation to their experiences of pain (Chapter 12) and neonatal intensive care (Chapter 13). Taken together, these chapters provide a synthesis of the key issues and themes which have arisen throughout the series.

Catherine A. Niven
Anne Walker
1997

References

Bermudez, J. L., Marcel, A. and Eilan, N. (eds) (1995). *The Body and the Self*. Cambridge, Mass: MIT Press.

Marsiglio, W. (ed.) (1995). *Fatherhood: Contemporary Theory, Research and Social Policy*. Thousand Oaks, CA: Sage.

Phoenix, A., Woollett, A. and Lloyd, E. (eds) (1991). *Motherhood: Meanings, Practices and Ideologies*. London: Sage.

Acknowledgements

The existence of these books owes a great deal to the Society for Reproductive and Infant Psychology (SRIP). Most of the authors are members of SRIP, and it is through the activities of the society that we have become aware of their work. At a more personal level, SRIP has enabled each of us to develop our research interests and discuss our research findings in a supportive and friendly atmosphere. Many SRIP members, past and present, have influenced our thinking and encouraged us to continue to work in this area. Particular thanks are due to the founder members of the society, and editors of the *Journal of Reproductive and Infant Psychology* (now published by Carfax), whose vision and commitment have made the editing of these books possible.

Thanks are also due to the authors of the chapters who responded to our editorial demands with good humour and speed, and to Susan Devlin, Myriam Brearley and Helen Reece at Butterworth-Heinemann for their patience and efficiency.

Contributors

Julia C. Berryman, BSc, PhD, AFBPsS, CPsychol
Julia Berryman is a Senior Lecturer in Psychology at the University of Leicester. She completed her first degree at the University of Aberdeen and her PhD at Leicester University. She has researched and published widely on developmental psychology, sex and gender, parenthood and parenting. She set up the Parenthood Research Group at Leicester University and has investigated a variety of aspects of parenthood, recently completing a longitudinal study of women of all ages, designed to highlight the effects of age and parity on women's experience of motherhood – the Leicester Motherhood Project. Currently she is carrying out a research project entitled Later Motherhood: Psychological Health and Adjustment in the Children.

Robert Drewett, DPhil
Robert Drewett is a Senior Lecturer in Psychology at the University of Durham. He is a member of the College of Paediatrics and Child Health, and of the Society for Reproductive and Infant Psychology, of which he was the Chairman until 1996. His principal research interests are in human lactation, in infant feeding behaviour, growth and development and in non-organic failure to thrive, and he has carried out research projects in these areas in the UK, South-East Asia and East Africa. He also works on social aspects of learning disabilities.

Sandra A. Elliott, BSc, MPhil, PhD, CPsychol, AFBPsS
Sandra Elliott began her research into post-natal depression in 1977. This research, combined with her experience of setting up and managing the primary care therapy service in Maidstone, has enabled her to set up the trainer training programme with Janice Gerrard (manager of the Stoke-on-Trent Parent and Baby Day Unit) at the University of Keele Perinatal Mental Health Unit, where she holds a post as Honorary Senior Clinical Lecturer. She is currently Senior Lecturer at the University of Greenwich, where she teaches clinical psychology to final year psychology undergraduates, and Chartered Clinical Psychologist at the Maudsley Hospital.

Sheila Glenn, BSc, PhD, AFBPsS, CPsychol
Sheila Glenn is Head of Research and Professor of Applied Developmental Psychology at the School of Health, Liverpool John Moores University.

She has published widely in the area of infancy and disability, and is currently involved in a number of research projects including: studies of the pain expression in prematurely born infants, neonates following surgical procedures and infants with disabilities; the environment in the Neonatal Intensive Care Unit; the development of mastery motivation in infants with Down's syndrome; transition to adult life of young people with Down's syndrome; information needs of parents with infants with severe disabilities.

Maureen F. Horgan, BA(Hons), RSCN, RGN, SCM, Cert PE

Maureen Horgan trained and worked as a paediatric nurse developing a particular interest in neonatal care. Her clinical work led her to develop a role as a research nurse looking at assessing pain in non-ventilated neonates. This work is ongoing and forms the basis of her higher degree study. She is presently Senior Lecturer in Nursing (Children's) in the School of Health, Liverpool John Moores University. Her teaching interests include pain assessment and management.

Charlie Lewis BA, MA, PhD

Charlie Lewis is Reader in Social Development at the Department of Psychology, Lancaster University. His research examines both family relationships and the development of social–cognitive skills in childhood. His central focus of attention has been on the role of the father in family relationships. This has made early gender development an issue to which he has returned many times.

Rhoda Martin, BSc(Hons)

Rhoda Martin is completing her PhD by research on the emotional expressions of premature babies of varying gestational age in medical, caregiving and social situations over time. Currently based in the Department of Midwifery Studies at the University of Central Lancashire, she is also interested in caregivers' perceptions of the abilities and potentialities of premature and full-term neonates, and how this affects their care. Other areas of research and clinical interest include aspects of communication and its therapeutic applications in pregnancy and babies exposed to drugs *in utero*.

Catherine A. McMahon, BPhysiotheraphy(Hons), BA(Hons) (Pschy)

Catherine McMahon is a Research Psychologist who is currently completing a doctorate. Her research involves a longitudinal follow-up of IVF parents and their children at Royal North Shore Hospital in Sydney, Australia. Families have been assessed at 30 weeks of pregnancy, 4 months post partum and 12 months post partum and assessment focuses on the psychological adjustment of the parents and the quality of the parent–child relationship.

Edward C. Melhuish, BSc, PhD

Edward Melhuish is Professor of Human Development at the School of Education, University of Wales, Cardiff. He has carried out extensive research in the areas of early social development, parent–child relationships, family and non-family influences on child development, and day care. His research has often involved data collection in several countries and making use of international comparisons. He is currently involved in a large scale longitudinal study of the effects of different forms of preschool education and care.

David Messer, Bsc, PhD

David Messer has had an interest in children's sleeping which began after the birth of his first son! He is a co-editor of *Infant Crying, Feeding and Sleeping* (with Ian St James Roberts and Gillian Harris; Harvester Wheatsheaf, 1993) and is currently engaged in a longitudinal study of sleeping during the preschool years which has been funded by WellBeing and the NHS Research Executive. David also has had a long standing interest in early development and communication and has written a text on this subject for advanced undergraduates (*The Development of Communication*, Wiley, 1994).

Paula Nicolson, BSc, MSc, PhD

Paula Nicolson is a Senior Lecturer in Health Psychology at the University of Sheffield where she lectures to undergraduate medical students. Her research interests are in reproductive health – particularly sexuality and post-natal depression. She is also researching gender in organizations. Her two latest books, both published by Routledge, are: *Gender, Power and Organisation: a Psychological Perspective* (1996) and *Post-natal Depression: Science, Psychology and the Transition to Motherhood*.

Carol Parker, BSc(Hons)

Carol Parker originally trained as a nurse and then went on to work in Child Health Clinics with health visitors and developed an interest in infant well-being. As a mature student she studied for a psychology degree which she achieved in 1992. Her final year project was a study of infant sleep patterns. Since graduating she has worked with Professor David Messer on a much larger study of infant sleep patterns and is now working towards a PhD.

Karen Thorpe, BEd, DipPsych, MA, PhD, CPsychol

Karen Thorpe is a Research Fellow in Psychology at the University of Bristol Institute of Child Health. Since 1989 she has vorked on the Avon Longitudinal Study of Pregnancy and Childhood – a study which follows families from early pregnancy through the first seven years of their child's life. Her major areas of interest are the emotional well-being of mothers, particularly the impact of the childcare burden, patterns of family interaction, twins and later motherhood.

Judy A. Ungerer, BA, PhD

Judy Ungerer is a Senior Lecturer in the School of Behavioural Sciences at Macquarie University. She received her BA from the University of California at Berkeley and her PhD from Harvard University. She did post-doctoral research in clinical child psychology at the University of California at Los Angeles before moving to Australia. Her current research interests include the study of families in the transition to parenthood and the emotional development of their young children.

Jo Warin, BA, MA, PGCE

After a career as a drama teacher Jo Warin completed a masters in education at Lancaster University. She was then employed by the Unit for Applied Research at University College of St Martin's, Lancaster. She is currently completing PhD research at Lancaster University on the development of gender identity in young children.

David White, BSc, PhD

David White is Professor of Psychology at Staffordshire University. He was previously head of the AIDS Research Unit at the University of East London. He publishes in the areas of developmental psychology and health psychology with a particular interest in the family and health. His recent research activities include an investigation of the experiences of drug dependent women, including their experiences as mothers and their experience of risk, including risks to parenting.

Kate C. Windridge, BSc, PGCertEd, PhD

Kate Windridge is a Research Fellow with the Parenthood Research Group at Leicester University. She obtained her BSc in psychology, music and philosophy at Leicester University and spent some time teaching and playing the bass guitar before studying for a post-graduate teaching qualification, followed by a PhD in developmental psychology. Since then she has spent over ten years teaching psychology and carrying out research in university and hospital settings, and she has published widely. Currently she is working on the Leicester Mother and Child Project. She the mother of two daughters.

Dieter Wolke, PhD, DiplPsych, CPsychol, AFBPsS

Professor Dieter Wolke has specialized in research on the development of medically and socially at-risk children. He has studied and worked both in Germany and England at the Institute of Child Health in London (1986–90) and the University of Munich Children's Hospital (1990–95). He is currently Professor of Psychology (Research) at the University of Hertfordshire, and heads a newly established international research group. He is also Honorary Director of Psychology of the Bavarian-Finnish Longitudinal Study at the University of Munich, co-directing a multi-disciplinary longitudinal study of nearly 10,000 at-risk children in two countries. He has published widely in leading medical and psychology journals and books.

Anne Woollett, PhD

Anne Woollett is a Professor in the Department of Psychology, University of East London and past Chair of the Psychology of Women Section of the British Psychological Society. Her research interests include women's experiences of motherhood; reproductive health, including childbirth and infertility, and the ideas and experiences of women bringing up children in a multi-ethnic community. With Ann Phoenix and Eva Lloyd she edited *Motherhood: Meanings, Practices and Ideologies* (Sage, 1991) and co-authored with David White *Families: A Context for Development* (Falmer, 1992).

Peter Wright, MA, DPhil, CPsychol

Peter Wright is a Senior Lecturer in Psychology at the University of Edinburgh and a founder member of the Edinburgh Centre for Research in Child Development. He has published extensively on the development of feeding during infancy and is currently working on the prevention of injuries in childhood. He is a Fellow of the British Psychological Society, a beekeeper of long standing and an enthusiastic opera singer.

Bridget Young, BA(Hons)

Bridget Young is currently a Lecturer in Health Psychology in the Department of Epidemiology at the University of Leicester. Her research interests are in infant and child health, especially feeding in young children, growth during early childhood and parental behaviour in relation to the feeding of children. She is currently writing up a longitudinal research project carried out while at the University of Durham on the prediction of weight gain during infancy from measures of feeding behaviour.

M. Suzanne Zeedyk, PhD

Suzanne Zeedyk is a Lecturer in Developmental Psychology and completed her PhD at Yale University in the USA. Having first come to Scotland a decade ago and fallen in love with the countryside, her current post at the University of Dundee has allowed her to put down permanent roots. Her research interests focus on epistemological issues of science and psychology, and her work on parent–child relationships reflects this by seeking to give a greater voice to the experiences of others. Epistemological interests are also displayed in her work on the intersection of psychology and law, and she is currently co-authoring a text on this topic, to be published by Routledge, which considers the relation of the two disciplines from a feminist perspective.

The social construction of motherhood and fatherhood

Anne Woollett and Paula Nicolson

What does it mean to be a 'good' father or a 'good' mother in western societies? Are these ideas changing and what implications do they have for individuals, researchers and policy makers? In the opening chapter of the book, Anne Woollett and Paula Nicolson set the scene by considering the social construction of motherhood and fatherhood – that is, the cultural beliefs and ideologies about how mothers and fathers should behave and what being a mother or father means. They show how pervasive these ideas are and how much they impact on both individual experience and scientific approaches to parenthood. The issues raised in this chapter appear again throughout the book, but especially in Chapters 2, 3, 4 and 7.

Introduction

Despite cultural and demographic changes, it is still the case that most men and women become parents at least once in their lives (Graham, 1993). The desire to have children is closely related to the way parenthood is socially constructed around ideologies of family life and gender roles (Chodorow, 1978; Woollett, 1995). Women are viewed as having children because it asserts their 'natural' femininity (Woollett, 1995); men because it affirms their potency (Owens, 1982); and both sexes because they believe that parenthood gives them a stake in the next generation.

Expectations and ideologies about parenthood are widely articulated in public accounts of parenting, ranging from those in the media (such as magazines, childcare manuals and soap operas) which are readily available to parents, and in government reports which inform health, social and educational policy (e.g. Phoenix and Woollett, 1991; New and David, 1985). These ideologies are often related to ideas and beliefs about children and their 'needs' and about what it is to be a 'good' or effective parent derived from empirical research (Woodhead, 1991). Scientific and popular constructions of parenting draw on some beliefs and value systems more than others.

But where do beliefs about children's needs and prescriptions of good parenting come from? Medical and psychological scientists have set out to establish parenting rules and norms. However, some researchers, for example Nsamenang (1992), Ogbu (1981), Greenfield and Cocking (1994) question the generalizability and universality of scientific constructions of parenthood because of the limited constituency of parents on which they are drawn. The ideas and values of white, US, middle class parents (and researchers and policy makers) inform beliefs about parenthood more than those from poor families, from ethnic minority communities in the US or Europe, and from the Third World (White and Woollett, 1992; Phoenix and Woollett, 1991; Nsamenang, 1992).

Even within this limited framework, the ways in which parenting is construed are often contradictory. Parenthood is idealized and romanticized with parenting presented as a highly valued and satisfying experience for individual men and women. However, there is also increased awareness that being a parent, particularly for women for whom it remains the major responsibility, is depressing (S. Lewis, 1995) and that depressed parents do not make the best ones (Downey and Coyne, 1990).

At the same time the support services parents need to provide effective parenting are often not available because parenting is viewed as the responsibility of parents as individuals rather than the wider society (New and David, 1985; Scarr and Dunn, 1987). In what follows we examine and compare the social construction of motherhood and fatherhood and discuss their implications for women and men.

The social construction of motherhood

Motherhood is *socially constructed* in a number of diverse and overlapping ways. Beliefs and ideologies of motherhood impact upon women's lives, whether or not they become mothers (Woollett, 1995; Glenn, 1994). Motherhood prescribes women's identities, pre-defines their role in the family and the workplace, and this in turn reinforces what are seen to be feminine qualities. In this sense the social construction of motherhood is equally about the social construction of womanhood/femininity. The everyday experience of mothering itself (from the transition to motherhood through to the experience of mothering older children and adolescents) is important to understanding the social construction of motherhood. Norms and 'facts' about motherhood are drawn from empirical data about the practice of mothering, although the relationship between beliefs and norms and empirical data are complex and often contradictory (Singer, 1992; Riley, 1983). The norms and 'facts' about motherhood inform everyday understandings about how mothers 'should' behave and what being a mother means (Nicolson, 1993).

Beliefs and ideologies of motherhood

Motherhood is construed as *an essential and central component of adult identity for all women*. Being a mother is closely linked to women's sense of themselves as a woman. Becoming a mother provides 'the' way to be recognized as having a proper adult female identity (Woollett, 1991; Nicolson, 1993; Ussher, 1989). In contrast, without motherhood, a woman's identity is tenuous: infertile women are portrayed as 'desperate' and childless women as missing out on 'the most meaningful, significant and emotionally satisfying' experience (Weaver and Ussher, 1997; Wetherell, 1995).

Motherhood is *compulsory, expected and mandatory* (Weaver and Ussher, 1997; Phoenix, Woollett and Lloyd, 1991; Wetherell, 1995). This can be seen in women's accounts of motherhood as being inevitable – 'always wanted to have children' – and as the 'natural thing to do'. In this way women are seen as driven by a need to have children/become mothers. The view that *motherhood is natural* is linked to ideas about 'instincts' to explain why women want to be mothers and why mothers (rather than fathers) are best suited to take responsibility for children.

The 'natural' and 'instinctive' themes in the social construction of motherhood are linked to the biological and physical nature of pregnancy and childbirth (Marshall, 1991). These (and women's hormonal changes post partum) are used to explain women's developing attachment to their infants. Such explanations fail to address the close relationships mothers develop with children with whom they have no biological/physical links, as is the case with adopted children, children born as a result of the use of reproductive technologies who do not share their parents' genes or are not 'born' to their mothers, and step-children. In these cases the lack of biological links has not prevented mothers from establishing warm, close relationships with their children or being 'good/normal' mothers (Golombok, Cook, Bish and Murray, 1995).

Because motherhood is seen as 'natural', mothers are expected to experience *motherhood as overwhelming love* and to be child-centred and sensitive (see Woollett and Phoenix, 1991; 1996). 'Good/normal' mothers are always available to give their children love, time and attention, they are calm, patient and in control of their own emotions, and hence able to put children first (Wearing, 1984).

The practice of motherhood in everyday life

Motherhood (and especially the initial transition to motherhood) brings substantial changes in women's lives as they take responsibility for children and care for them on a day-to-day basis. While mothers often experience great pleasure in looking after their children and their feelings of closeness, they also find the relentless and repetitive nature of looking after small children and the associated housework tedious and depressing (see Chapters 2 and 3) (Boulton, 1983; Oakley, 1979). The nature of mothering often contrasts sharply with women's expectations about motherhood and is experienced as loss of freedom and identity (Boulton, 1983; Ussher, 1989; Nicolson, 1993; Thompson and Walker, 1989). Motherhood involves substantial changes in women's economic and employment status and hence in their identities and social relations (Lewis, 1991; Westwood and Bhachu, 1988). For women bringing up children with a partner, becoming a mother involves changes in their relationship with their partner and the negotiation of new roles and responsibilities (Wetherell, 1995; Thompson and Walker, 1989). Frequently women's activities and their relationships with the wider social networks also change: links with the wider family may increase whereas engagement in non-parenting activities is reduced.

The meanings and satisfactions of motherhood for women vary considerably, often related to women's motivations for becoming mothers, their experiences as mothers and the situations in which they become mothers (Nicolson, 1993; Phoenix, Woollett and Lloyd, 1991). There is, however, often little or no acknowledgement of the limited constituency from which ideas are derived or the limited range of women for whom they are relevant. Diversity in the form of age ('young', 'old' mothers), women's marital position (single, cohabiting, married), social class, 'race' and ethnicity is increasingly acknowledged. However, this is done to define 'non- optimal' or 'bad' mothering rather than to examine the experiences of women who mother in diverse situations or to incorporate these into constructions of 'good/normal' mothering (Phoenix, 1991; Phoenix and Woollett, 1991; Nicolson, 1993; Woollett and Phoenix, 1997).

Science and the practice of motherhood

However, in spite of constructions of motherhood and mother love as 'natural', there are clear prescriptions about how women should mother, based often on ideas drawn from psychiatry and developmental psychology. One such prescription is that mothers should have educational goals: mothers are exhorted to turn every activity into a learning situation (Woollett and Phoenix, 1996). Walkerdine and Lucey (1989), however, argue that this view of 'good/normal' mothering, while constructed as representing motherhood in general, is espoused by middle class mothers more than working class mothers. As a result constructions of mothering based on the ideas and experiences of middle class mothers are held to be universal, and key aspects of the mothering of working class women are omitted from constructions of mothering or viewed as 'bad/deviant'.

Constructions of motherhood as 'natural' discourage women from questioning or resisting those constructions. Any problems they experience are explained not in terms of the inappropriateness of the constructions of motherhood or the lack of applicability to their circumstances but in terms of individual problems or pathology. Mothers are encouraged to feel guilty if they fail to live up to the ideas of 'good' mothering (Wetherell, 1995). The natural quality of motherhood is contrasted with women's other choices, such as choosing to remain childless (Morrell, 1994; Ireland, 1993) or opting to combine motherhood with employment, etc. (Lewis, 1991).

'Good/normal' mothering as constructed in psychological accounts carries with it personal and psychological costs for women. To provide 'good' mothering, women are required to subordinate their own needs, ambitions and identities to those of their children. Mothers acknowledge these costs, drawing on themes of *motherhood as self-sacrifice*. They refer frequently to the hard and relentless work of motherhood, of being tied and of lack of freedom and spontaneity (things highly valued in individualistic societies) (Boulton, 1983; Weaver and Ussher, 1997). The hard work of motherhood is compensated for by women's love for their child and the sense that 'it was all worth it'. In this way mothering is rendered invisible and the belief that motherhood is easy is reinforced (Graham, 1993; Marshall, 1991).

Motherhood is also construed as *ultimate fulfilment*, and as providing women with valuable and important roles because of the impact mothers are considered to have on their children and their development. Motherhood provides women with an opportunity to make their mark by being a 'good' mother who brings up 'good' and successful children (Woollett and Phoenix, 1996; Wetherell, 1995). This is reinforced by assumptions about mothers being 'the' influence on their children's lives. This appears to put mothers in a powerful position but also means that they are viewed as individually to blame if their children's needs are not met or their children 'go wrong' (Urwin, 1985; Glenn, 1994). At the same time the impact and responsibility of fathers, other family and non-family childcare is played down (Chodorow and Contratto, 1982; Nicolson, 1993).

Mothers who do not wish to/cannot engage in exclusive mothering or want to maintain relationships and identities beyond their mothering role (e.g. through employment) are seen as neglecting or providing non-optimal environments for their children's development. Issues such as poverty, the availability of adequate housing, and the problems encountered by women who are trying to mother in poor physical or family circumstances are either omitted from analyses of what is required for the upbringing of 'good' or 'healthy' children or they are viewed as less critical for children's development than, for example, whether mothers engage in educative play or one-to-one language games (New and David, 1985; Huston, McLoyd and Coll, 1994).

When motherhood is viewed as *ultimate fulfilment* it is assumed that it is women's main and only substantial role. Mothers who engage in paid employment outside the home and other non-parenting activities often talk about 'fitting' these around mothering and hence minimize their failure to comply with this aspect of the social construction of motherhood. In contrast fathers talk in terms of fitting parenting around employment (Brannen, Dodd, Oakley and Story, 1994). The context of other experiences and relationships within which women bring up children is increasingly recognized, although in doing so women are given responsibility for balancing their relationships with their child with that with a partner (Marshall, 1991; Wetherell, 1995; Thompson and Walker, 1989).

One impact of construing motherhood as ultimate satisfaction is that women find it difficult to express reservations about mothering and concerns about loss of a separate identity. Hence when they discuss the hard work and the problems they experience as mothers, women's accounts are invariably modified by statements such as 'I wouldn't be without them', as if reassuring themselves (and others) of their compliance with the norms of 'good mothering' (Weaver and Ussher, 1997; Marshall, 1991).

Social construction of fatherhood

In contrast to the compulsory nature of motherhood, fatherhood is construed as *optional*. While men are seen as gaining emotional satisfaction from fatherhood as well as identity and status (and a proof of their heterosexuality in a homophobic world), they are able to retain a positive identity of themselves as men without becoming a father. Terms such as 'childless' and 'barren' do not denigrate men as they do women (Nicolson, 1993; Busfield, 1987).

While fatherhood is seen as desirable, and many men expect to become fathers, it is less often construed in terms of biology and instincts in the way that motherhood is. Men who do not become fathers are not seen as resisting their biology or their instincts. When socio-biological theories talk about fatherhood it is in terms of the imperative to ensure continuity or dominance of a man's genes. Television soap operas and British Government practice, as exemplified through the Child Support Agency, links men's responsibility for providing financially for a child with being the child's biological father.

Men's involvement in fathering is viewed positively: fathers are expected to be present at the birth of their children and to 'help' with childcare. Fathers' main engagement in childcare, however, is through play: fathers' play (and especially their play directed at boys) is more active and physical than is that of mothers, which is more verbal, educational and responsive to the child. Fathers are seen to influence their children's development by providing them with a less child-centred and predictable experience of play and hence as preparing them for the world beyond the family (Edley and Wetherell, 1995; White and Woollett, 1992).

Fathers are less involved than mothers in the more arduous and continuous (but less exciting) tasks of parenting which require parents to respond to their children's needs (Lewis and O'Brien, 1987; Marsiglio, 1995). As a result mothers are a more constant presence in children's lives as they provide care and comfort, in contrast to fathers whose presence and behaviour require less time and energy and are less predictable. Because fathers rarely combine play with other household or childcare routines they can make their play interesting and exciting. Fathers are rarely alone with children, and hence their involvement is more visible than is that of mothers, who tend to manage and monitor fathers' involvement with their children, 'rescuing' them if children become too excited or too fractious (Clarke-Stewart, 1978; C. Lewis, 1995).

Fathers' involvement and participation is also limited compared with mothers because they are expected to obtain validation of their masculinity through the public and employment domains rather than through family/ fathering and the private sphere. However, as Edley and Wetherell (1995) argue, this may be more the case for middle class than for working class men. By and large, working class (and unemployed) men obtain less validation and sense of their identity from work and once they are at home their work impinges less on their family roles and responsibilities. There are also cultural differences: in the UK fathers are expected to return to work promptly after the birth of a child, in contrast with most other European countries where fathers can take paternity leave. Ideas about fatherhood are rooted in constructions of masculinity: fathers need to balance being 'unemotional' and 'in control' with their emotional and practical commitment to their children (Edley and Wetherell, 1995). This reinforces their role as 'helper' with childcare and their engagement only in certain aspects of childcare such as play rather than in feeding or bathing, which are often considered to lie more within the 'women's sphere'.

In contrast to constructions of motherhood which stress the compulsory nature of motherhood for *all* women, diversity in men's commitment to parenting is acknowledged within the context of 'good/normal' fatherhood. Fathers' involvement may vary considerably (in terms of their physical and emotional commitment and the centrality of fatherhood to their lives and identities) and still be considered as 'good' fathers. As a result, social constructions of 'poor' or 'deviant' fathers are much less developed (and are found largely in accounts of domestic violence and child abuse) (White and Woollett, 1992).

A number of styles of fathering have been identified. Two are discussed here to examine the constructions of fatherhood which underlie them (Russell, 1983; Wetherell, 1995). The first style is often labelled *traditional or breadwinner*: such fathers are seen as spending time at home and playing with children but as taking only minimal responsibility for the day-to-day care of children, and as being more involved with sons than daughters. Their impact on children and their development is seen largely in terms of their encouragement of gendered roles and behaviour such as the expression of emotion. Their impact is considered to be largely indirect, through the material context they provide for mothering. There is little discussion of the appropriateness of this model for fathers (and mothers) who, because of structural factors such as unemployment or racism, are unable to act as breadwinners, or the extent to which such a construction of fatherhood militates against a more equitable distribution of tasks in families where women are employed (Bjornberg, 1995; Wetherell, 1995).

A second kind of father identified in research is the *non-traditional highly participant father*, often known as the 'new man'. This kind of father shares childcare with the mother and is highly involved with his children, even though mothers usually retain overall responsibility. Underlying this construction of fatherhood is the assumption that parenting is not gendered and that fathers can parent as sensitively and effectively as mothers, given the opportunity and commitment. It is often considered that this 'new man' style of fathering is increasing, in response to women's greater participation in the work force as well as men's preferences. However, evidence suggests that while men and women are more committed to fathers' equal participation in childcare, levels of participation have not increased substantially and the 'new man' is largely a media myth (Wetherell, 1995; Marsiglio, 1995; Bjornberg, 1995).

However, media images of the 'new man' reflect increasing expectations of involvement, especially as the numbers of mothers in the work force have increased. Fathers and mothers increasingly expect fathers to be involved in childcare. While mothers' expectations are fairly low, their accounts of fathers' participation indicates that when fathers do not take their 'fair share' of childcare, issues about equity are a concern and a potential source of tension (Backett, 1987; Croghan, 1991).

Relations between motherhood and fatherhood

Mothers and fathers do not operate independently of one another. Mothers' evaluations of fathers' involvement relate to their expectations and their sense of whether fathers' contribution is 'fair' or reasonable (Backett, 1987; Ruble, Fleming, Hackel et al., 1988; Thompson and Walker, 1989; Pleck, 1985). Middle class fathers express a greater commitment to shared parenting prior to becoming fathers than working class fathers. However they are no more likely to be involved in childcare. This is often explained in terms of 'need' to keep careers or outside activities going (Nicolson, 1990; 1993). As a result the gap between middle class men's commitment and their involvement is greater and middle class mothers feel more 'let down' (Thompson and Walker, 1989; Ruble, Fleming, Hackel et al., 1988; Croghan, 1991).

In contrast fathers are less influenced by the division of family labour and do not express concern about the inequity of the division of family work in the majority of families where mothers do more than their fair share. Nor is there a relationship between fathers' participation, their personal and marital well-being and the extent of women's employment outside the home (Thompson and Walker, 1989).

Fathers are able to opt in and out of parenting and to decide which parenting tasks they engage in much more than mothers. This power differential is also reflected in the different levels of commitment required of mothers and fathers. Women's commitment to parenting (at the level of what they do and how they feel) is seen as obligatory and hence any evidence of a total lack of commitment is construed as 'bad' or 'unnatural' mothering whereas fathers may contribute little without being considered as other than 'good/normal' fathers.

Changing ideas about parenthood

The social construction of motherhood and fatherhood has changed somewhat in line with demographic changes. These include changes in family composition, such as a reduction in family size, in the older age at which women have their first child, and in the reduction in traditional two parent families in which fathers are employed outside the home and mothers are engaged full-time in childcare. Women are central to many families, their activities and experiences, and with the increasing instability of families, mother-centred and mother-headed families are likely to increase. Mothers of young children are increasingly in paid employment outside the home and hence have greater need for and expectations of 'help' with childcare. The stability of families have also changed with the result that an increasing number of children are brought up in women-headed families, or in families with step-fathers and step-brothers and sisters (White and Woollett, 1992; Brannen and O'Brien, 1995).

Expectations of fathers' involvement have changed, although as has been argued, in spite of media interest in the 'new man' and a commitment to 'sharing the caring', there is little evidence of substantial changes in fathers' involvement or a more equitable division of childcare and family work (Croghan, 1991; Wetherell, 1995). With their increasing involvement in paid work outside the home, women's roles have changed more than those of men. There are some changes in young women's expectations and ideas about parenting. They argue, for example, that it is important for them to be financially independent, reflecting a sense that men cannot be relied on to provide financially for women and children (Wetherell, 1995). So in spite of an increased commitment amongst men to fathering, the instability of families and high unemployment rates means that women are also aware that, however committed men may be, women cannot count on their commitment (financially and practically) (Sharpe, 1994).

Most of the research on fatherhood is conducted in intact two parent families, in spite of comparatively high levels of family breakdown in Europe and North America. There is little information about the involvement of men/fathers in families headed by women and especially the extent to which fathers remain involved in childcare when they leave families (in spite of the emphasis on the value of fathers for their children of pressure groups such as Families Need Fathers in the UK). Concerns about fathers' involvement largely focus on their financial support. Fathers' absence may bring benefits to mothers in terms, for example, of regaining control of money and time, and not having to negotiate with reluctant fathers about their involvement and financial support (Graham, 1993; Kier and Lewis, 1995).

There have been few attempts to identify the key features of fatherhood. Fathers can be construed in terms of providing an 'extra pair of hands' and hence as supplementing what mothers do, but not in a specifically gendered way. On the other hand, fathers are sometimes construed in terms of having a distinct and gendered role to play in parenting. This view is based on research which suggests that fathers parent in somewhat different ways than mothers do, and especially that they are sensitive to, and reinforce, gendered roles. According to this view fathers' masculinity and the provision for children of gendered experience is an important aspect of what they bring to parenting (White and Woollett, 1992).

Motherhood and fatherhood are all too frequently theorized in universal terms, without sufficient recognition of diversity in the circumstances and characteristics of men and women and how these influence parenting and expectations of mothers and fathers. Aspects of diversity which it is important to address are social class, and 'race' and ethnicity. While all parents, whatever their race and ethnicity and their social class, are concerned to parent and bring up children well, parents differ somewhat in how they construe parenting and, for example, how involved they expect fathers to be. They also differ somewhat in the qualities they consider important to encourage in children, and the ways they consider appropriate or effective for encouraging those qualities (Goodnow and Collins, 1990; Greenfield and Cocking, 1994; Wetherell, 1995; White and Woollett, 1992; Mayall, 1990).

Fathers' involvement and constructions of fatherhood vary considerably depending on their personal preferences and motivations (a result of their greater power and hence their ability to opt in or out of parenting). Some differences in the expectations and involvement of middle class and working class fathers have been discussed. Sometimes it is argued that fathers from black and ethnic minority families are less involved. While the majority of black children are brought up in 'traditional' two parent families, somewhat more black (than white and especially Asian) women bring up their children on their own. In these families it is assumed that because fathers are not living with children they are less available and less involved. In families which originated from the Indian subcontinent, fathers are sometimes also considered to be less involved but for different reasons. Asian families are assumed to be characterized by traditional gender roles and childcare to be construed as 'women's work', and fathers are thereby discouraged from becoming involved. There is, however, little evidence of differences in involvement or expectations of the involvement of black and ethnic minority fathers (Wetherell, 1995; Greenfield and Cocking, 1994; Woollett and Dosanjh-Matwala, 1990; Graham, 1993). However, while acknowledging diversity, it is important to recognize that mothers are not the passive carriers of culture, and that ideas and expectations about motherhood and fatherhood are changing and being challenged by women (Brah, 1992; Woollett, Marshall, Nicolson et al., 1994; Glenn, 1994).

The ways in which mothering and fathering are practised depends to some extent on the wider family (Bronfenbrenner, 1986). In nuclear families, fathers are more involved, either because women receive less help from other family members or because men and women who are more committed to fathers' participation choose to live in nuclear rather than extended families (Woollett, 1995; Bhachu, 1988).

Conclusions

Fatherhood and motherhood are both viewed as important and meaningful experiences for the individuals involved and their development. Parenting is seen increasingly as a form of personal growth and achievement for both men and women, although the meanings associated with fatherhood and motherhood are somewhat different: motherhood provides women with the means to achieve adult status and fatherhood allows men access to their emotionality.

The social constructions of fatherhood differ from those of motherhood in a number of significant ways. This means that to discuss parenting and parenthood as gender-free activities and identities is, as Busfield (1987) suggests, to ignore some important distinctions. While motherhood is construed as compulsory for *all* women, and as essentially similar for *all* women, fatherhood is optional and men are able to opt in to fatherhood to a greater or lesser extent within current definitions of 'good/normal' fathering. While fatherhood provides men with a sense of validation and satisfaction, it is not as closely tied to their identities as men in the ways that motherhood is tied to women's identity. In spite of the emergence of the 'new man', acceptable levels of fathers' involvement and responsibility for childcare (and the blame when children do not turn out 'right') is less than is the case for mothers (Glenn, 1994; Woollett and Phoenix, 1996).

Applications

1. Ideologies and the realities of parenthood
There are strongly held ideas and beliefs about motherhood which are used to regulate women: to determine what they 'ought' to do and feel, and to 'blame' them if they do not mother 'properly'. However, we need to consider how appropriate these ideas and beliefs are, for mothers and for children.

2. Fathers' involvement
Ideas about fathers' involvement have changed, with men now expected (and expecting) to be highly involved with their children and in childcare. However, fatherhood is still largely optional and there are a variety of models of 'good' fathering.

3. Avoiding stereotyping
Constructions of motherhood and fatherhood pay insufficient attention to the context (social, economic, cultural, historical) in which people bring up children.

Further reading

Brannen, J. and O'Brien, M. (eds) (1995). *Childhood and Parenthood*. London: Institute of Education.

Marsiglio, W. (ed.) (1995). *Fatherhood: Contemporary Theory, Research and Social Policy*. London: Sage.

Glenn, E. N., Chang, G. and Rennie Forcey, L. (eds) (1994). *Mothering. Ideology, Experience, and Agency*. New York: Routledge.

Phoenix, A., Woollett, A. and Lloyd, E. (1991). *Motherhood: Meanings, Practices and Ideologies*. London: Sage.

Thompson, L. and Walker, A. J. (1989). Gender in families: women and men in marriage, work, and parenthood. *Journal of Marriage and the Family*, **51**, 845–71.

References

Backett, K. (1987). The negotiation of fatherhood. In *Reassessing Fatherhood: New Observations on Fathers* (C. Lewis and M. O'Brien, eds). London: Tavistock.

Bhachu, P. (1988). Apni marzi kardhi. Home and work: Sikh women in Britain. In *Enterprising Women: Ethnicity, Economy and Gender Relations* (S. Westwood and P. Bhachu, eds). London: Routledge.

Bjornberg, U. (1995). Family orientation among men: fatherhood and partnership in the process of change. In *Childhood and Parenthood* (J. Brannen and M. O'Brien, eds). London: Institute of Education.

Boulton, G. M. (1983). *On Being a Mother: A Study of Women with Preschool Children*. London: Tavistock.

Brah, A. (1992). Women of South Asian origin in Britain: issues and concerns. In *Racism and Anti-Racism: Inequalities, Opportunities and Policies* (P. Braham, A. Rattansi and R. Skellington, eds). London: Sage.

Brannen, J. and O'Brien, M. (eds) (1995). *Childhood and Parenthood*. London: Institute of Education.

Brannen, J., Dodd, K., Oakley, A. and Story, P. (1994). *Young People, Health and Family Life*. Buckingham: Open University Press.

Bronfenbrenner, U. (1986). Ecology of the family as a context for human development. *Developmental Psychology*, **22**, 723–42.

Busfield, J. (1987). Parenting and parenthood. In *Social Change and Life Course* (G. Cohen, ed.). London: Tavistock.

Chodorow, N. (1978). *The Reproduction of Mothering: Psychoanalysis and the Sociology of Gender*. Berkeley: University of California Press.

Chodorow, N. and Contratto, S. (1982). The fantasy of the perfect mother. In *Rethinking the Family* (B. Thorne and M. Yalom, eds). London: Longman.

Clarke-Stewart, K. A. (1978). And daddy makes three: the father's impact on mother and young child. *Child Development*, **49**, 466–78.

Croghan, R. (1991). First time mothers' accounts of inequality in the division of labour. *Feminism and Psychology*, **1**, 221–46.

Downey, G. and Coyne, J. C. (1990). Children of depressed parents: an integrative review. *Psychological Bulletin*, **108**, 50–76.

Edley, N. and Wetherell, M. (1995). *Men in Perspective: Practice, Power and Identity*. Hemel Hempstead: Prentice Hall/Harvester Wheatsheaf.

Glenn, E. N. (1994). Social constructions of mothering. In *Mothering, Ideology, Experience, and Agency* (E. N. Glenn, G. Chang and L. Rennie Forcey, eds). New York: Routledge.

Golombok, S., Cook, R., Bish, A. and Murray, C. (1995). Families created by the new reproductive technologies: quality of parenting and social and emotional development of the children. *Child Development*, **64**, 285–98.

Goodnow, J. J. and Collins, W. A. (1990). *Development According to Parents: The Nature, Sources and Consequences of Parents' Ideas*. Hove and London: LEA.

Graham, H. (1993). *Hardship and Health in Women's Lives*. London: Harvester Wheatsheaf.

Greenfield, P. M. and Cocking, R. R. (1994). *Cross-Cultural Roots of Minority Child Development*. Hillsdale, NJ: Lawrence Erlbaum Associates.

Huston, A. C., McLoyd, V. C. and Coll, C. G. (1994). Children and poverty: issues in contemporary research. *Child Development*, **65**, 275–82.

Ireland, M. S. (1993). *Reconceiving Women: Separating Motherhood from Female Identity*. New York: Guildford Press.

Kier, C. and Lewis, C. (1995). Family dissolution: mothers' accounts. In *Childhood and Parenthood* (J. Brannen and M. O'Brien, eds). London: Institute of Education.

Lewis, C. (1995). Fathers' perspectives on the family. Paper presented at Society for Reproductive and Infant Psychology, University of Leicester, September 1995.

Lewis, C. and O'Brien, M. (1987). *Reassessing Fatherhood: New Observations on Fathers*. London: Tavistock.

Lewis, S. (1991). Motherhood and employment: the impact of social and organisational values. In *Motherhood: Meanings, Practices and Ideologies* (A. Phoenix, A. Woollett and E. Lloyd, eds). London: Sage.

Lewis, S. (1995). A search for meaning: making sense of depression. *Journal of Mental Health*, **4**, 369–82.

Marshall, H. (1991). The social construction of motherhood: an analysis of childcare and parenting manuals. In *Motherhood: Meanings, Practices and Ideologies* (A. Phoenix, A. Woollett and E. Lloyd, eds). London: Sage.

Marsiglio, W. (ed.) (1995). *Fatherhood: Contemporary Theory, Research and Social Policy*. London: Sage.

Mayall, B. (1990). A joy or a hassle: child health care in a multi-ethnic society. *Children and Society*, **4**, 197–224.

Morrell, C. M. (1994). *Unwomanly Conduct: The Challenges of Intentional Childlessness*. London: Routledge.

New, C. and David, M. (1985). *For the Children's Sake: Making Childcare More than Women's Business*. Penguin: Harmondsworth.

Nicolson, P. (1990). A brief report of women's expectations of men's behaviour in the transition to parenthood: contradictions and conflicts for counselling psychology practice. *Counselling Psychology Quarterly*, **3**, 4, 353–61.

Nicolson, P. (1993). The social construction of motherhood. In *Introducing Women's Studies, Feminist Theory and Culture* (D. Richardson and V. Robinson, eds). London: Macmillan.

Nsamenang, A. B. (1992). *Human Development in Cultural Context*. Newbury Park: Sage.

Ogbu, J. U. (1981). Origins of human competence: a cultural ecological perspective. *Child Development*, **52**, 413–29.

Owens, D. J. (1982). The desire to father: reproductive ideologies and involuntarily childless men. In *The Father Figure* (L. McKee and M. O'Brien, eds). London: Tavistock.

Phoenix, A. (1991). *Young Mothers?* Cambridge: Polity.

Phoenix, A. and Woollett, A. (1991). Motherhood: social construction, politics and psychology. In *Motherhood: Meanings, Practices and Ideologies* (A. Phoenix, A. Woollett and E. Lloyd, eds). London: Sage.

Phoenix, A., Woollett, A. and Lloyd, E. (eds) (1991). *Motherhood: Meanings, Practices and Ideologies*. London: Sage.

Pleck, J. H. (1985). *Working Wives/Working Husbands*. Beverly Hills: Sage.

Riley, D. (1983). *War in the Nursery*. London: Virago.

Ruble, D. N., Fleming, A. S., Hackel, L. S. and Stangor, C. (1988). Changes in the marital relationship during the transition to first time motherhood: effects of violated expectations concerning division of household labor. *Journal of Personality and Social Psychology*, **55**, 78–87.

Russell, G. (1983). *The Changing Role of Fathers*. Milton Keynes: Open University Press.

Scarr, S. and Dunn, J. (1987). *Mother Care/Other Care*. Harmondsworth: Penguin.

Sharpe, S. (1994). *Just Like a Girl: How Girls Learn to be Women: From the Seventies to the Nineties* (2nd edn). Harmondsworth: Penguin.

Singer, E. (1992). *Child-care and the Psychology of Development*. London: Routledge.

Thompson, L. and Walker, A. J. (1989). Gender in families: women and men in marriage, work, and parenthood. *Journal of Marriage and the Family*, **51**, 845–71.

Urwin, C. (1985). Constructing motherhood. In *Language, Gender and Childhood* (C. Steedman, C. Urwin and V. Walkerdine, eds). London: Routledge and Kegan Paul.

Ussher, J. M. (1989). *The Psychology of the Female Body*. London: Routledge.

Walkerdine, V. and Lucey, H. (1989). *Democracy in the Kitchen: Regulating Mothers and Socialising Daughters*. London: Virago.

Wearing, B. (1984). *The Ideology of Motherhood*. Sydney: Allen and Unwin.

Weaver, J. and Ussher, J. (1997). How motherhood changes life: a discourse analytic study with mothers of young children. *Journal of Reproductive and Infant Psychology*, **15**, 51–68.

Westwood, S. and Bhachu, P. (eds) (1988). *Enterprising Women: Ethnicity, Economy and Gender Relations*. London: Routledge.

Weatherell, M. (1995). Social structure, ideology and family dynamics: the case of parenting. In *Understanding the Family* (J. Muncie, M. Wetherell, R. Dallos and A. Cochrane, eds). London: Sage.

White, D. and Woollett, A. (1992). *Families: A Context for Development*. Basingstoke: Falmer Press.

Woodhead, M. (1991). Psychology and the cultural construction of 'children's needs'. In *Growing Up in a Changing Society* (M. Woodhead, P. Light and R. Carr, eds). London: Routledge.

Woollett, A. (1991). Having children: accounts of childless women and women with reproductive problems. In *Motherhood: Meanings, Practices and Ideologies*. (A. Phoenix, A. Woollett and E. Lloyd, eds). London: Sage.

Woollett, A. (1995). Questioning motherhood as a model for women's lives and development. Invited address: BPS Psychology of Women Section Annual Conference, University of Leeds: July.

Woollett, A. and Dosanjh-Matwala, N. (1990). Asian women's experiences of childbirth in East End: the support of fathers and female relatives. *Journal of Reproductive and Infant Psychology*, **8**, 11–22.

Woollett, A., Marshall, H., Nicolson, P. and Dosanjh-Matwala, N. (1994). Asian women's ethnic identity: the impact of gender and context in the accounts of women bringing up children in East London. *Feminism and Psychology*, **4**, 119–32.

Woollett, A. and Phoenix, A. (1991). Psychological views of mothering. In *Motherhood: Meanings, Practices and Ideologies* (A. Phoenix, A. Woollett and E. Lloyd, eds). London: Sage.

Woollett, A. and Phoenix, A. (1996). Motherhood as pedagogy: contrasting feminist and development psychology accounts. In *Feminisms and Pedagogies of Everyday Life* (C. Luke, ed.). New York: SUNY Press.

Woollett, A. and Phoenix, A. (1997). Deconstructing developmental psychology accounts of mothering. *Feminism and Psychology*, **7**, 275–282.

2

Parenting and infant development following conception by reproductive technology

Catherine A. McMahon and Judy A. Ungerer

The new reproductive technologies have raised a range of ethical and scientific questions about parenthood, parenting and infant development. In Volume 2, Edelmann and Connolly considered psychological aspects of the process of assisted conception. In this chapter, McMahon and Ungerer are concerned about the consequences when it is successful. Are IVF babies over protected and idealized? How do parents adjust to the presence of a baby after the stress of infertility treatment and pregnancy? Do IVF parents worry about being 'good' mothers and fathers more than parents who conceived more easily? How does the publicity and controversy around reproductive technology impact on IVF families? Do artificially conceived children differ from other children in their emotional or cognitive development?

Introduction

The world's first assisted reproductive technology (ART) child was born in Britain in 1978. Although use of assisted reproduction technology was limited during the early 1980s, by the end of the decade a World Collaborative Report (1991) indicated that more than 40,000 children had been born worldwide as a result of ART. By 1995 approximately 33,000 IVF babies were being born worldwide each year (ART world reports 1995). The rapid development of the technology over a twenty year period has been accompanied by changing perceptions of ART from a controversial (miraculous) experimental procedure to an accepted and relatively commonplace treatment for infertile couples. However, the rate of development of the technology has made it difficult for health professionals working clinically and in research to keep pace. As a result, the social consequences of the technology for families, particularly the psychological well-being of the parents experiencing the intervention and the physical and emotional development of their children, are only beginning to be explored.

Findings of research to date suggest that overall adjustment of ART parents is not significantly different from that of other parents, and their children do not differ on either cognitive or social-emotional indices of development (Colpin, Demyttenaere and Vandemeulebroecke, 1995; Golombok, Cook, Bish et al., 1995). While these findings are encouraging, they do not tell the whole story. Although overall adjustment may be good, there is a lack of research which aims to understand the experience of pregnancy and parenthood after infertility and ART from the perspective of the parents who have 'lived' it. Our current research indicates that the transition to parenthood may not be completely smooth, and that these parents may have particular concerns and fears as they conceive, bear and raise their children.

Furthermore, even though the majority of parents may adjust well, for some the process is more complicated. Parents who are not genetically related to their child, parents of twins or triplets, parents whose baby is born prematurely, or parents with differing experiences of treatment failure and reproductive loss may have specific difficulties at different stages of parenthood. In addition, some parents, vulnerable anyway because of life history factors or poor marital or social support, may be particularly troubled by the unique stresses of infertility and ART during the transition to parenthood. The challenging task for health professionals is to remain alert and sensitive to the needs of those ART families whose adjustment is likely to be problematic while at the same time avoiding unhelpful, pejorative and stereotyped labelling of the group as a whole.

The purpose of this chapter is to review the literature on ART families to provide both a 'big picture' and a focus on specific issues which will assist health professionals who work with these families. The chapter will survey clinical writings and empirical research in four main areas: the experience of pregnancy, the post-partum adjustment of parents, the parent–child relationship and child development. Where empirical data exist, we will provide an overview of how ART parents and children are functioning in each of these areas compared with other families. We will then examine in more detail ways in which unique features of the ART context may interfere with or enhance the adjustment to parenthood for some families, drawing on clinical observations and comments by ART parents themselves in order to provide a more comprehensive picture of their experiences of early parenthood.

A range of psychological and developmental theories have formed the conceptual framework for looking at psychological adjustment at different stages of the infertility and ART experience. Olshansky (1987) has pointed to the benefits of grounded theory methodology in research with infertile families. This approach is rooted in the theoretical perspective of symbolic interactionism (Blumer, 1969) in which the goal of the research is to construct meanings for phenomena within a specific social context. Clinical researchers (Blenner, 1990; Boivin, Takefman, Tulandi et al., 1995; Sandelowski, 1987) working within this framework have described psychological processes of surprise, denial, anger and resolution in response to the diagnosis of infertility, analogous to those outlined in Kubler-Ross' (1975) work on death and dying. Other theorists have proposed models of an 'infertile identity' (Olshansky, 1987) to explore the meaning of infertility to those experiencing it. Some limited theorizing has also been done incorporating these same models into explanations of how couples respond to ART treatment and adjust to pregnancy and parenthood when treatment has been successful.

In the area of parenting after ART, well-documented determinants of adjustment in the transition to parenthood in non-ART contexts have underpinned quantitative and qualitative research. In particular, literature on violated expectations has informed many of the hypotheses about ART parents suggesting that incongruence between high expectations of parental performance and of the child and the reality of early parenthood may constitute a major risk factor in the adjustment of this group of parents. The impact of anxiety on parenting and attachment as manifested in overprotective parenting has also been a recurrent theme. The other major theoretical model invoked to explain positive outcomes has been the notion of psychosocial resilience. In the following discussion, where applicable, reference will be made to the usefulness of existing psychological theories in interpreting experiences of ART parents.

The experience of pregnancy

Anxiety

Very little is known about the experience of pregnancy after ART concep- tion. However, previous research (Beaurepaire, Jones, Thiering et al., 1994; Freeman, Boxer, Rickels et al., 1985; Newton, Hearn and Yuzpe, 1990; Thiering, Beaurepaire, Jones et al., 1993) has demonstrated that couples on IVF treatment have elevated levels of anxiety and depression compared to community norms, and there is concern that these psychological difficul- ties may persist into the pregnancy and post-birth periods (Raoul-Duval, Bertrand-Savais, Letur-Konirsch et al., 1994).

On the basis of clinical case material, it has been suggested that ART parents are likely to experience elevated levels of anxiety during pregnancy due to the juxtaposition of their high psychological investment in having a child and the high-risk status of their pregnancies. However, there is only limited empirical support for this idea. A study by Reading, Chang and Kerin (1989) indicated that IVF mothers did have more concerns than con- trol group women when concerns specific to the pregnancy were assessed. In contrast, global measures of state and trait anxiety have repeatedly failed to demonstrate differences between IVF and control groups.

Furthermore, vulnerability to psychological difficulties during pregnancy may not be uniform in IVF groups but may vary according to differences in the experience of treatment failure. Research evidence indicates that during treatment there are significantly more psychological symptoms in couples who have experienced treatment failure, compared to those who have had only one treatment cycle. Specifically, repeat cycle women have been reported to have higher levels of anxiety (Newton, Hearn and Yuzpe, 1990), depression (Beaurepaire, Jones, Thiering et al., 1994; Litt, Tennen, Affleck et al., 1992), and anger and frustration (Leiblum, Kemmanen and Lane, 1987). Interestingly, Boivin, Takefman, Tulandi et al. (1995) have demonstrated that women who experienced a moderate amount of treatment failure experienced more distress than women experiencing no treatment failure or those experiencing large numbers of failed treatment cycles. There is concern that differences in past experiences of ART treatment and the coping strategies associated with them may have an ongoing effect on psychological adjustment to pregnancy and parenthood.

In our own research we have explored the psychological adjustment of IVF women to their pregnancy by asking a range of specific questions regarding concerns about pregnancy and childbirth as well as using global measures of state and trait anxiety. Recognizing the heterogeneity of the IVF group, we have included analyses which take account of the impact of past experience of treatment failure on anxiety levels in pregnancy. We have also included measures of the extent to which IVF couples may suppress their emotions, as a failure to express feelings may contribute to psychosomatic disorders (Beaurepaire, Jones, Thiering et al., 1994) and may be a manifestation of a tendency to positive self-reporting which has been noted with this group (Halasz, Munro, Saunders et al., 1993).

Our results (McMahon, Ungerer, Beaurepaire et al., 1997) showed that, overall, IVF couples did not differ from other couples on global measures of anxiety. However, when concerns specifically focused around the baby were addressed, the IVF mothers at 30 weeks of pregnancy were significantly more anxious about the well-being of their unborn baby and about damage to the baby during childbirth. There was a tendency for IVF mothers to feel more anxious about the prospect of separating from their baby after it was born and to have a higher tolerance for medical interventions in childbirth associated with a belief that this would make the birth safer for the baby. The anxiety about the well-being of the baby was expressed in the IVF group by delaying telling others the news of their pregnancy which was associated with a persistent fear of pregnancy loss. Many of the IVF mothers reported that they still did not trust that their pregnancy would be viable even when they had progressed to the third trimester.

As one mother in our sample expressed it at 30 weeks of pregnancy, '. . . after the scan I relaxed a little, maybe at about 14 weeks or so, but in the back of my mind, even now I worry that something is going to happen. I think until I actually see the baby, I won't believe it. You just sort of wait for the next disappointment to come along.' Another expressed similar feelings, 'After 28 weeks I thought it will probably be viable in Intensive Care. It's only just now I can get a bit excited and talk about it – when you've had so many disappointments you get good at suppressing those kinds of feelings . . .'

When IVF couples were differentiated in our analyses according to their experience of treatment failure, it was clear that women with a history of two or more treatment cycles were reporting the most concerns, while women who had only one treatment cycle were not different in their reporting of concerns from the controls.

Our results (McMahon, Ungerer, Beaurepaire et al., 1997) also suggest that the anxieties reported by IVF mothers may underestimate the degree of concern actually experienced by these women. The IVF couples in our sample were significantly more likely than the control group to report suppressing their feelings of anxiety, depression and anger during pregnancy. This may reflect a desire by these couples to be seen to be functioning well during pregnancy, but it may have adverse consequences for their adjustment to pregnancy and later parenthood.

Attachment

What are the implications of the presence of specific anxieties for the evolving relationship between ART parents and their child? Clinical observations of IVF mothers during pregnancy present an inconsistent picture. While some clinicians describe a tentative pregnancy characterized by delayed attachment to the fetus in the context of anxiety about its survival (Garner, 1985; Raphael-Leff, 1991; Sandelowski, 1987), others have suggested that elevated anxiety may actually intensify the mother's feelings of attachment to the baby (Greenfeld, Diamond and DeCherney, 1988; Klein, 1989). One mother in our sample who had a bleed at 20 weeks of pregnancy described frequent conversations with her unborn baby, 'Especially when I wasn't sure of what was happening, I would tell it how much I wanted it and liked it – or, you know, if you want me to prove to you how much I want you – I'm in bed for four weeks . . . that sort of thing.'

Increased, and perhaps excessive, attachment to the developing baby may also be fostered by some of the unique aspects of the IVF experience, such as the fact that the parents see the fertilized embryo before it is implanted, and the high psychological investment in the pregnancy (Greenfeld, Diamond and DeCherney, 1988). One father graphically described his earliest encounter with his baby: 'I saw Jan's egg minutes after it was picked up. It is funny looking at not even a new born infant but the basis of life I guess. To know your child before the egg is even fertilised would be a truly intimate thing' (Walters and Singer, 1982, p. 14). It is possible that for both parents this experience may make the pregnancy seem more real to them and facilitate their attachment to their developing baby.

Research studies to date provide no empirical support for suggestions that ART couples have anomalous attachment relationships to their unborn babies. Stanton and Golombok (1993) found no differences between IVF mothers and controls using Cranley's (1981) Maternal Fetal Attachment Scale. However concerns about the reliability and validity of this measure (Condon, 1993) limit the usefulness of this finding. In our own research, we employed a different measure, The Antenatal Bonding Questionnaire (Condon, 1993), but also failed to find any differences in mothers' or fathers' attachment to their unborn babies (McMahon, Ungerer, Beaurepaire et al., 1997). It seems that despite the increased levels of anxiety about the well-being of the baby in the IVF group, this does not necessarily translate into an increased risk for the development of attachment.

Post-partum adjustment of ART parents

Writings on parenting after assisted reproduction have suggested a range of factors that may complicate adjustment to parenthood. These include a heightened risk of post-natal depression and marital discord due to the strain of infertility and participation in assisted reproduction treatment programmes, and difficulties taking on a maternal identity as a consequence of infertility, both of which may be compounded by the presumed unrealistic expectations these couples may have about themselves as parents.

Maternal depression

It has been suggested that previously infertile mothers, and IVF mothers in particular, may be vulnerable to post-natal depression as a consequence of the likelihood of experiencing depression following repeated IVF treatment (Beaurepaire, Jones, Thiering et al., 1994), the stress associated with 'high-risk' pregnancies, and possible unrealistic expectations about motherhood (Garner, 1985). However, the research to date does not support the hypothesis of increased levels of depression in women conceiving by IVF. Indeed, a study by Golombok, Cook, Bish et al. (1995) reported significantly higher levels of anxiety and depression in parents of normally conceived children compared to those who had conceived by assisted reproduction. However, the IVF parents in that study were not assessed until their children were from four to eight years of age, and it may be the early months of parenting that are most problematic for IVF families.

For example, the only prospective study of IVF parents reported to date (Raoul-Duval, Bertrand-Savais, Letur-Konirsch et al., 1994) found a non-significant trend for IVF mothers to report more depressive symptoms in the early post-partum period and at 9 months, but these symptoms had decreased by the time the children were 18 months of age. Interestingly, reported depressive symptoms were associated with a history of a difficult pregnancy, and partner relationship difficulties, suggesting that it may be the interactions between well-documented risk factors in the transition to parenthood and the unique stresses of the ART context which are of clinical significance. However, our prospective study of IVF parents found no differences between IVF and control group mothers on reported depression when the baby was four months old (McMahon, Ungerer, Tennant et al., 1997). More prospective research is needed to explore ways in which ART couples manage the transition to parenthood.

Marital relationship

There have also been suggestions that marital difficulties may occur as a result of the stress of infertility and ART treatment (Cook, Parsons, Mason et al., 1989) which may impact directly on parent–child relationships when the difficulties persist (Cox, Owen, Lewis et al., 1989). In such cases it is possible that poor marital satisfaction may result in the lack of a supportive context for the parenting of the child.

Here again the studies that have assessed marital satisfaction by self-report measures report that marital relationships are as good or better in ART couples as in comparison groups (Golombok, Cook, Bish et al., 1995; Halasz, Munro, Saunders et al., 1993, McMahon, Ungerer, Tennant et al., 1997). Halasz, Munro, Saunders et al. (1993) suggest two possible explanations for the positive marital ratings in IVF groups. Firstly, these ratings may reflect the high level of commitment these couples have to making their marriages work. Furthermore, the demands of participating in IVF treatment may have facilitated the development of emotional expression and a confiding relationship. However, they also acknowledge a possible bias towards positive reporting and a possible inhibition of negative emotion within relationships which may be due to a sensitivity to public scrutiny and an ongoing need to demonstrate suitability as parents. Independent assessments of marital functioning would help to tease out the role of positive self-reporting in ART groups.

In the case of conception by donor insemination, it has been suggested that the alienation of the father from the process of conception and the lack of a genetic relationship between the father and the child may place additional strain on the marital relationship. However, two recent studies (Durna, Bebe, Leader et al., 1995; Golombok, Cook, Bish et al., 1995) which have assessed marital quality (by self-report) after donor insemination have reported positive ratings of marriage satisfaction in this group. In both cases, however, the response rate for participation by donor families was only 60 per cent, raising the possibility that the findings present a more positive view than is, in reality, the case. The major reason for refusal to participate in both studies was believed to be related to concerns about secrecy and a reluctance to have further contact with the fertility clinic for fear of the children finding out about their origins.

Maternal identity

A group of researchers (Blenner, 1990; Dunnington and Glazer, 1991; Olshansky, 1987; Sandelowski, 1987) have approached the study of the impact of previous infertility on mothering from the perspective of symbolic interactionist theory, focusing on the meanings and experiential aspects of human behaviour within the particular ART context. Blenner (1990) has suggested that those women for whom treatment is drawn out may become immersed in an 'infertile identity'. A pilot study by Dunnington and Glazer (1991) examined the hypothesis that as a consequence of this 'infertile identity', previously infertile women might have difficulties in taking on a maternal identity. Their research showed that previously infertile women did, in fact, have lower post-partum maternal identity scores, tended to delay preparation of the home environment, and expressed less self-confidence about their ability to perform mothering tasks than never-infertile women. The authors suggested that these women may have internalized an infertile identity which had the potential to impact negatively on maternal behaviour. However, while the variation in maternal identity between the groups seemed to impact on the mothers' perceptions of their performance in their new role, it did not seem to influence actual maternal behaviours, which were measured by observers blind to history of infertility. Interestingly, in our own research we found similar results. While IVF mothers differed from comparison mothers in reporting lower self-efficacy as a mother at four months post-partum, videotaped observations of maternal sensitivity during mother–child interactions revealed no differences.

This line of research is interesting and further study is needed. In particular, studies which incorporate both self-report measures and independent observations will help to tease out distinctions between maternal perceptions and actual performance. As we will see in the next section, ART mothers' perceptions of themselves may be coloured by context specific expectations they have of themselves, or which they believe the wider community has of them.

Unrealistic expectations

Despite overall positive findings on adjustment to parenting from studies using self-report questionnaire measures, interview and clinical case literature suggest that some ART parents may have expectations of themselves which make the adjustment to parenthood more difficult.

However, empirical research has not so far provided convincing evidence to support or refute this view. It is not yet clear to what extent ART parents do approach parenthood with unrealistic expectations or what impact such expectations might have on their children. In the absence of empirical data, the material discussed here is drawn largely from clinical writings and parents' reports of their own experiences.

Perfect and forever grateful parents

IVF mothers, as forever grateful beneficiaries of the technology, are commonly believed to experience more than the usual level of concern about their performance as parents and may aspire to an idealized notion of what a mother should be. Lesley Brown (Brown and Brown, 1979), the mother of the first IVF child, expressed this in the following way: 'Having a miracle was a lot to live up to. I felt as if the whole world expected me to be a perfect mother . . . It really shocked me once when I shouted at the baby because she was crying . . . it wasn't a question of not loving her. It just seemed as if I didn't deserve her if I behaved like that. There were so many childless women who would have been better mothers if they'd been given the same chance' (p. 180). Feeling guilty about the normal frustrations of early motherhood may be a source of considerable distress for some ART mothers.

Of course, feelings of guilt about being an imperfect mother are common in non-ART mothers, but the intensity of such feelings in the ART context may prevent these mothers from discussing their difficulties and negative feelings. This stoicism may also be accompanied by a reluctance to ask for or accept help. One IVF mother of twins interviewed in our study described her experiences in retrospect when her children were three years old. She reported a delayed onset of depression at about nine months after the birth of her children, 'It took me that long before I could admit it! I'm not enjoying this – how dare I? I wanted this so much. On bad days my husband would yell accusingly, "You said babies would make you happy . . ."' Another, also a mother of twins, who managed to get help at nine weeks rather than nine months, described her experience as follows, 'By the time I got to nine weeks I was desperate. By that stage everyone would say "Oh how is it?" and I'd say "Fine, I can cope, everything's wonderful, they're such good babies" and then they'd walk out and I'd go "arrgh I can't stand it!" . . . In the first six weeks I just didn't exist, then six to ten weeks I was there, but I was sinking fast. I actually believed that because I had such trouble getting pregnant, I didn't have the right to feel angry that I couldn't cope. I didn't have the right because I couldn't do it naturally. I had such trouble and I wanted these babies so much, how dare I say they irritate me. How dare I say I hate it. I just hated it and I felt so guilty about that . . .'

While feelings of gratefulness and stoicism are clearly risk factors for some mothers, for others such feelings may bolster their psychological resources and help contribute to highly motivated extra-caring parenting and 'not taking anything about the experience for granted'. A number of parents in our study have expressed this view. While acknowledging that they may have difficulty owning up to or expressing negative feelings, they believe this gives them a higher tolerance. 'You know how lucky you were to get them and you don't tend to forget that, so it helps you to cope even when you are very tired, or at times when you might feel resentful . . .'

Acceptance by the broader community – publicity and controversy

In addition to the high expectation ART parents may have of themselves, they may also feel, in common with adoptive parents, that they must frequently justify why they have chosen to become parents in this way. This process may not only provoke parental anxiety and resentment, but also accentuate their 'differentness' for them (Brodzinsky and Huffman, 1988), and have an isolating effect (Mushin, Spensley and Barreda-Hansen, 1985). However, there is very little empirical evidence to support the view that publicity and controversy impact adversely on IVF families. Although Munro, Ironside and Smith (1992) reported deficient social relationships among IVF parents of preschool twins and suggested that these may, in part, be due to a desire to avoid criticism and feelings of unusualness and difference to the community at large, a recent study by Halasz, Munro, Saunders et al. (1993) did not replicate these findings. They reported that IVF parents felt social support was more available and perceived their attachments to be more adequate than those of the control parents. The authors interpreted this finding as an encouraging sign of adaptive modes of social interaction in response to these new family environments.

Nonetheless, for some parents, particularly those who deal with concerns about public scrutiny with secretiveness about ART origins to protect the child or themselves, poorer family and social relationships may ensue. One IVF mother in our study expressed her concerns as follows, 'We haven't told him he's IVF. We don't want him to feel he's different. A lot of people still don't know, like my sister and his godparents. People are still negative about it. It's controversial and where he was conceived isn't significant. Why should we have to tell him? After all, children are not told if they were conceived in the back of a car. We had special treatment to get him, but everything else is normal. Nothing else is different.'

The secrecy issue may be particularly salient for parents whose child is the result of donor sperm, donor eggs or a donated gamete (Durna, Bebe, Leader et al., 1995; Golombok, Cook, Bish et al., 1995). Golombok (1995) notes that although there was no evidence in their study of any parenting difficulties for donor families, not one of the parents whose child had been conceived by donor insemination had told their child about their genetic origins. She concludes that while keeping the method of conception secret from a child aged between four and eight does not appear to have a negative impact upon family relationships or the psychological development of the child, it remains to be seen whether secrecy leads to difficulties when the children are older. It is very difficult to assess this effect, however, because those families who are concerned about secrecy and sensitive about controversy are the ones most likely to decline to participate in research, leading to an overall sampling bias.

As has been noted in the discussion of marital ratings in ART families, sensitivity to scrutiny of their parenting competence may also contribute to a tendency to positive self-reporting in ART families. Halasz, Munro, Saunders et al. (1993) observed that 'Indeed it may seem churlish not to be overwhelmingly positive after achieving, thanks to IVF technology, the "miracle baby" that transforms an infertile couple into a family' (p. 169).

The parent–child relationship

Unrealistic expectations of the child

Despite speculation about parenting difficulties in ART families, most of the research on outcomes has focused on the cognitive development of the children and the presence or absence of behaviour problems. Direct empirical studies of the parent–child relationship are few. Clinical writings have suggested that performance anxiety in the parenting role may be compounded by expectations about the long awaited and highly sought after child. All babies are special to their parents, but the perceived value of something tends to rise according to the difficulty with which it was attained (Lind, Pruitt and Greenfeld, 1989). Dettman and Saunders (1987) suggest that 'After trying so hard for so long, it must be the best behaved, most aware, and cutest baby ever . . . there is a risk of overprotection of a baby whose arrival was so longed for and so delayed' (p. 157).

Miracle babies

Some mothers during long periods of infertility may develop unrealistic fantasies about the perfect child they long for. One IVF mother's eloquent description serves to illustrate just how intense such fantasies can be. 'In the days before IVF and long before I knew Toby [her husband], I knew and began to love my first child Stephen. Stephen slowly formed and developed as part of my expected fertility. Stephen grew and kicked inside me; he kicked for life to begin. Outside him I planned his life. I made the clothes that he would wear, chose the toys that would be a vital part of his development, read books on how to be a good mother and talked about him with my friends . . . Stephen is the child I have been attempting to conceive for the past seventeen years. Stephen is why Toby and I are involved in the IVF program. Stephen is waiting inside my mind. His spirit lives inside me and waits for nature or my doctors to form his body – the body which will set him free to live . . .' (Bainbridge, 1982).

Concern has been expressed about the impact of such an idealized fantasy baby on any real children that may be conceived after infertility. Indeed, Fisher (1989) uses the term 'messianic' with regard to the expectations surrounding the birth of these children. Warnock (1987) is also concerned about the possible consequences for the child of these parental expectations. She writes, 'I am not persuaded by those people who say "the children are bound to be alright; they will be much loved – think how much their parents wanted them". It seems to me that this being wanted, hoped for may put extreme pressure on the child, especially a child without siblings' (Warnock, 1987, p. 155).

Precious (vulnerable) babies

To compound these high parental expectations, the 'miracle' child may also be seen as physically and psychologically vulnerable. The parents may for some time regard the child as not completely theirs, but only on a tenuous loan. Parents may bargain to keep such a child, vowing to 'forgo all aggression and never do anything to upset them' (Green and Solnit, 1964, p. 62). One IVF mother in our sample expressed concern during pregnancy that she would have difficulty relating to her baby after it was born. She said, 'I'll be so afraid of doing something wrong – of hurting it in some way. I want to do everything perfectly . . . I know I won't want to leave the baby – even to go out of the room – I'll want to be with it at all times.'

Of course for those parents whose babies are born prematurely or have illnesses in the perinatal period, anxiety about their child's survival may be particularly intense. Lind, Pruitt and Greenfeld (1989) reported the common occurrence of a proprietorial struggle with staff and quote a mother's comments, 'If anyone is going to harm my baby I would rather it be me. I would want to kill them if they hurt my baby' (p. 129).

It may take some time even after the birth of a healthy child for parents to relinquish their perception of the child as vulnerable and likely to be taken away from them. One mother in our study expressed it like this: 'Through the IVF treatment, you get conditioned to something going wrong at every stage of the process – I kept waiting for God to take him away from me . . .' For many, the fear of cot death in the first twelve weeks is very strong. Another said 'At twelve weeks, I think then I really relaxed because that really high risk of cot death had passed – that was at the back of my mind all the time – and then I thought well that's another big hurdle – we've got a daughter here, its time I started to enjoy her . . .' Another mother reported that she went in every 30 minutes with a torch during the night for the first four months of her baby's life to check that he was still breathing.

'Beggars can't be choosers'
While some parents may approach parenthood with unrealistically high expectations about their babies, this tendency may not generalize to all ART parents. Interestingly, research with non-ART parents has questioned the widely held view that expectant parents romanticize the way in which having a child will affect them and suggests that at least for middle class samples, adaptive, realistic attitudes are common and may be attributable to high levels of education and preparation for becoming parents through reading and classes (Belsky, Ward and Rovine, 1986; Kach and McGhee, 1982).

Many well-informed ART parents, particularly those who have experienced repeated anticipation followed by anxiety and despair while trying to conceive, are well aware of the pitfalls of rigid and unrealistic expectations and may make a particular effort to avoid this. Indeed, Lind, Pruitt and Greenfeld (1989) have suggested that these mothers, being fully acquainted with their 'risk status', may in fact be realistic and even more open than other parents to the possibility of accepting and parenting a child who is less than perfect. As one pregnant IVF mother in our study expressed when asked about her expectations of her child, 'Beggars can't be choosers'.

Post-natally too, some ART mothers feel free to acknowledge a less than perfect infant. One mother, who had twice been admitted to residential care in a community support centre to help her to manage her baby, expressed it as follows, 'I met one IVF mother the other day who kept saying she's a miracle and absolutely perfect. I'd be the first to admit that my daughter is very special – but she's also very difficult! The fact that she's IVF doesn't take away from the problems. It's her saving grace probably, the fact that she was IVF. I would never have put up with her otherwise. The fact is she's been a rotten child some days. I just couldn't take it any more and the fact that she was IVF was irrelevant . . .'

Overprotective parenting

The most common theme emerging from clinical observations and speculations about the parent–child relationship after ART is the suggestion that these parents, as a consequence of their high expectations of themselves and perceptions of their child as both special and vulnerable, are likely to feel excessively anxious about their child's well-being. They are believed to be at risk of becoming overprotective in their parenting.

How useful are theoretical writings on overprotective parenting for exploring the parent–child relationship and parenting styles in the ART context? There are many parallels with the clinical phenomenon of maternal overprotection described by Levy (1966) and Parker (1983), and the complementary 'vulnerable child syndrome' (Green and Solnit, 1964). These authors describe how a history of infertility in the mother and risk factors in the perinatal period for the child may create particularly salient anxiety in the mother. This may lead to an overprotective parenting style which has the potential to interfere with the development of healthy attachment relationships between parents and children.

Parker (1983) suggests that overprotective mothers may excessively and inappropriately stimulate their infants, leading to infants with exaggerated attachment behaviours and failure to progress to independence and separation from their mother. Mahler, Pine and Bergman (1975) describe problems in the child's ability to differentiate self and other if the mother is too intrusive or smothering, and Bentovim (1972) describes a phenomenon of 'too good mothering' in which the mother fails to appreciate that some degree of frustration is essential for a child's healthy development of a sense of self.

While the overprotective parenting paradigm seems at face value to 'fit' the ART context, certain limitations need to be acknowledged. Perhaps most importantly, Parker (1983) has emphasized the importance of distinguishing between highly caring overprotective parenting (which he refers to as 'affectionate restraint') and overprotective parenting characterized by excessive control and inadequate care ('affectionless control') which is more pathogenic. This distinction may be very important in the case of ART parents. A longitudinal follow-up of adopted children (Hoopes, 1982) has noted a tendency to overprotective parenting styles and subsequent timidity in the children. However, Hoopes noted that this parenting was highly caring, and no adverse consequences for the children up to preschool age were observed.

While it is important for health professionals to avoid labelling the group as a whole, for some ART parents overprotectiveness can be a problem, particularly in the early months. Separation, which may be necessary if the mother has to return to work, may be a source of great anxiety and stress, and ART mothers may need additional support at such times. One mother in our study expressed this as follows: 'I don't want to leave her at all with anyone. I go to Tech one day studying and she comes with me . . . but I can't do that much longer. My sister has offered to take her, but I really don't want to leave her. I've contemplated giving up the course. I'm finding it really difficult and I'm feeling a lot of judgement from people around me that I should leave her . . .'

Events such as weaning may be particularly complicated for these mothers. Another mother in our study reported becoming quite depressed after failing with breastfeeding: 'I was so paranoid about the removal of antibodies and the risk of cot death . . . I felt I couldn't let him be exposed to other children as I was so worried about infectious diseases – I became a bit of a prisoner at home.' Those IVF parents who are inclined to feel overprotective toward their child may need more reassurance from health professionals that their child is healthy, well and progressing normally. Additional support may be needed for stressful transitions like separation and weaning.

Empirical research on the parent–child relationship in ART families
The above discussion is based largely on case reports of experiences of individual parents. Empirical data on the quality of parenting in ART groups is limited and, with the exception of Colpin, Demyttenaere and Vandemeulebroecke (1995) and our own research which included videotaped observations of parent–child interaction (McMahon, Ungerer, Tennant et al., 1997), studies have not included independent observations of the quality of parenting or the parent–child relationship. Three recent studies of ART families with two-year-old children (Colpin, Demyttenaere and Vandemeulebroecke, 1995; Halasz, Munro, Saunders et al., 1993) and four to eight year olds (Golombok, Cook, Bish et al., 1995) have failed to find any support for hypotheses of parenting difficulties in the group overall. Indeed, Golombok, Cook, Bish et al. (1995) reported that the quality of parenting was superior and perceived stress was less in families of children conceived by assisted reproduction (including both IVF children and children conceived by donor insemination) compared to families with a naturally conceived child. Whether the child was genetically unrelated to one parent or both parents (as in the case of the adopted group), the quality of parenting in families where the mother and father had gone to great lengths to become parents was superior to that shown by mothers and fathers who had achieved parenthood in the usual way.

Specifically, parents who had conceived by assisted reproduction expressed greater warmth toward their child, showed greater emotional involvement and higher quality of interaction with their children than did parents of naturally conceived children. Furthermore, parents of naturally conceived children reported significantly more parental distress than did parents of IVF children.

A recent study by Durna, Bebe, Leader et al. (1995) also reported that over 90 per cent of parents of donor children felt very close to these children, and in those cases where the men had other children not conceived by donor insemination, the men were significantly closer to their children by donor insemination than to their other children. Other factors, such as the fact that the other children were often from a previous relationship and not living with the father and the failure to include a comparison group, limit the conclusions that can be drawn from these findings.

Despite frequent references to a tendency to 'overprotective parenting' in the clinical literature on ART parents, the research so far has not systematically explored the phenomenon of overprotective parenting in ART families. One study by Halasz, Munro, Saunders et al. (1993) which examined parents' concerns about their two-year-old children by questionnaire, reported no more concerns in the IVF group than in the control group, suggesting that IVF parents are not unduly overprotective and anxious about their children's development. Colpin, Demyttenaere and Vandemeulebroecke (1995) report similar findings. They included a measure of parental attitudes and emotions of parents towards their young children which included a subscale of anxious overconcern and found no differences between IVF parents and control parents on this measure. Further research is needed to determine first, whether ART parents are, in fact, overprotective, and second, whether their 'style' of overprotectiveness is characterized more by control or care.

A common and plausible explanation for positive parenting outcomes in the ART context is that these parents may be more resilient than others in the face of the stresses inherent in the transition to parenthood, having endured the rigours of infertility and IVF treatment. As one mother in our sample (and veteran of 15 IVF attempts!) described it, 'Through all this IVF stuff, I learned to switch off and Graeme was the same. I really learned how to not let myself get overwhelmed by what I was feeling . . . You learn to just hold on to things and control your emotions . . .'

Those who have persevered to this stage of achievement of a pregnancy may be a self-selected group of 'copers' whose relationship and lifestyle have already been seriously challenged and remained intact (Halasz, Munro, Saunders et al., 1993; Mushin, Spensley and Barreda-Hansen, 1985). These couples may see parenthood as yet another challenge to master. Using the coping skills acquired during their period of infertility, they may be able to respond positively and effectively to their child's needs (Lind, Pruitt and Greenfeld, 1989).

Development of the children

The relatively high incidence of perinatal morbidity in IVF births (Doyle, Beral and Maconochie, 1992; Lancaster, Shafir, Hurst et al., 1997) has raised concerns about possible adverse effects of IVF procedures on the development of the children. In addition, concerns about the psychological adjustment of parents conceiving by IVF become translated into concerns about the quality of the rearing environment these parents are able to provide for their children (Weaver, Clifford, Gordon et al., 1993). In order to address these broad concerns, both cognitive and social/emotional outcomes of the children must be assessed.

Cognitive development

A number of studies have considered the cognitive development of children born after IVF conception. These studies vary considerably in methodological rigour, but are consistent in demonstrating no evidence of impaired cognitive development when those born prematurely and those with perinatal problems are excluded. Studies using developmental tests, such as the Bayley scales of infant development, suggest IVF children have normal physical and mental development across the age range from 12 to 48 months (Brandes, Scher, Itzkovits et al., 1992; Gibson, Ungerer, Leslie et al., in press; Halasz, Munro, Saunders et al., 1993; Morin, Wirth, Johnson et al., 1989).

Furthermore, a study which included multiple births and children with birthweights less than 2.5 kg in both IVF and control groups (Halasz, Munro, Saunders et al., 1993) showed that while birthweight, gestational age and multiple birth were strong indicators of adverse outcomes in both

IVF and control groups, there was no independent IVF effect for these children.

Social/emotional development

Although a number of studies have examined the cognitive and developmental outcomes for ART children, fewer studies have assessed aspects of their social/emotional development. Difficulties would be most likely to arise if the method of conception and associated stresses of infertility could be shown to interfere in some way with the quality of interaction between the parents and the child. Literature discussed earlier has shown that no such adverse effects have been identified on quality of parenting, and the study by Golombok, Cook, Bish et al. (1995) found no differences between children four to eight years of age conceived by assisted reproduction (including IVF and donor insemination), adopted children and normally conceived children on a range of standardized measures of emotional well-being in the child (such as the separation anxiety test, and the pictorial scale of perceived competence and social acceptance).

In addition, the child's psychiatric state was assessed using a standardized interview (Graham and Rutter, 1968). Detailed descriptions were obtained of any behavioural or emotional problems shown by the child and these were rated using the Rutter A scale for mothers and Rutter B scale for teachers. There were no differences between the ART children and control groups, and scores were closely comparable to general population norms. Golombok, Cook, Bish et al. (1995) comment in particular on their failure to find any adverse child outcomes in the donor group and suggest that these findings support the view that genetic ties are less important for parenting than a strong desire for parenthood.

Halasz, Munro, Saunders et al. (1993), using the infant behaviour record of the Bayley scales of infant development to examine behaviour in two-year-old children, concluded that there was no evidence of behaviour problems and furthermore, the communication and social maturity skills of the IVF children in their sample were superior to those of the control group children and seemed advanced for their age. However, the authors acknowledged that this may be a result of the extra attention and resources which may be available to 'only children'. They note from anecdotal evidence that many of the IVF children attended formal and informal playgroups, and classes for learning, singing, dancing and exercise.

In our own research (Gibson, Ungerer, Leslie et al., in press), first-born IVF children aged twelve months were compared with matched first-born controls on a range of measures of child behaviour including the infant behaviour record from the Bayley scales of infant development, and the infant behaviour checklist (a downward adaptation of the preschool behaviour checklist (McQuire and Richman, 1988). We did not replicate the finding of superior communication and social maturity skills in the IVF children. Both IVF and control group infants showed low levels of behavioural difficulty and there were no differences between the groups on either of the above measures.

Overall, there is as yet no evidence of cognitive, emotional or behavioural difficulties in IVF children. Suggestions from some studies of superior parenting outcomes (Golombok, Cook, Bish et al., 1995) and child behaviour outcomes (Halasz, Munro, Saunders et al., 1993) require further investigation, and matching the groups for birth order is necessary to establish whether there is a positive IVF effect independent of the 'first-born child effect'.

Conclusions and future directions

The empirical research discussed in this chapter does not support speculation that parents who conceive by IVF will have any particular difficulties adjusting to parenthood. There is also no convincing evidence to date that there are any problems with the parent–child relationship in ART families or that ART children differ on either cognitive or emotional indices of development. While these results are reassuring, group comparisons do not allow the exploration of individual differences in adjustment to parenthood after infertility and assisted reproduction.

The clinical case material we have discussed suggests that while experiences with infertility and ART may engender resilience and adaptive coping styles in many parents, some are particularly vulnerable during the transition to parenthood. Although it may be only a minority of parents who have difficulties, health professionals need to be aware of unique features of the ART experience which complicate the process of adjustment and potentially the quality of the parent–child relationship for these families.

While psychological and developmental theories have been useful in conceptualizing hypotheses about potential difficulties for ART parents and describing stages in adjustment to infertility, the foregoing discussion has shown that in many instances relationships between risk factors and outcomes which apply in other settings cannot be easily generalized to the ART context.

For example, the relationship between anxiety and attachment to the child in ART parents is a complex one. Where anxieties are reality based, adverse effects of parental anxiety on parent–child relationships which have been described in non-ART contexts may not apply. Similarly, although the construct of overprotective parenting is useful in describing the tendencies of ART parents, in the ART context the overprotectiveness (if present) may tend to be more caring than controlling. Consequently, this parenting style may not be associated with the adverse parent–child outcomes which have been described in clinical groups. More empirical research in this area is needed.

IVF technology remains controversial, particularly in terms of concern about the financial, physical and emotional demands that IVF treatment imposes. 'Costs' must be balanced against 'benefits' and follow-up studies of couples successful with IVF treatment are of the utmost importance. It is vital to document that the expected benefit has occurred and that no hidden costs have gone undetected (Weaver, Clifford, Gordon et al., 1993).

Although a 'cost-benefit' approach is clearly important, it is also necessary to broaden our research questions to focus on the nature of the experience of pregnancy and parenthood after IVF. Research with ART families provides an excellent opportunity for researchers to tease out the interactions between

Applications

1. Avoid making assumptions
The research so far suggests that the majority of ART parents are adjusting well to pregnancy and parenthood and have positive relationships with their children. Moreover, they are sensitive to being 'labelled' and do not wish to be seen as different. It is of interest to note that adjustment to pregnancy and early parenthood may take a different course in ART women. Specifically, high anxiety in ART women may not translate into later mother–infant attachment difficulties, as would be expected in naturally conceiving groups.

2. Be alert to individuals who may be vulnerable
Although the majority of ART parents are adjusting well, for some the process is more complicated. Vulnerability markers specific to the ART context include donor families, multiple births, experiences of extensive treatment failure and/or reproductive loss and premature birth. In addition those parents who are vulnerable anyway because of life history factors and poor marital or social support may be particularly troubled by the additional stresses of ART.

3. Be aware of a tendency to under-report problems
Practitioners need to be aware that despite overall positive adjustment, some ART parents may pretend they are coping and fail to report problems because they feel guilty, ashamed and ungrateful if they admit they are not coping. Research has also demonstrated a tendency to suppress emotions in ART parents which may have assisted them to cope with the demands of ART treatment, but may be maladaptive in coping with early parenthood. Practitioners need to give ART parents permission and opportunities to admit they are having difficulties.

4. Be alert to issues that may pose particular difficulties for ART parents
Although there is no empirical support for the idea that ART parents are overprotective, our case material suggests that some ART parents may need extra support during transitions such as weaning, returning to work or putting their child into childcare. Feelings of anxiety and guilt may be intense at these times.

factors unique to this social context and psychological and developmental theories regarding the transition to parenthood. Such information would enable health professionals to be better informed about the adjustment process and also enable the provision of appropriate interventions for any couples whose experiences are likely to be problematic.

Further reading

Dettman, C. and Saunders, D. (1987). *The Chance of a Lifetime: Infertility and IVF*. Melbourne, Victoria: Penguin.
Patient letters: Personal experiences of IVF (1995). IVF Friends inc. GPO Box 482G, Melbourne, 3001, Australia.
Raphael-Leff, J. (1991). *Psychological Processes of Childbearing*. London: Chapman and Hall.
Rothman, B. (1988). *The Tentative Pregnancy: Prenatal Diagnosis and the Future of Motherhood*. London: Pandora.

References

ART World Report (1995). Presented at 10th World Congress on IVF and Assisted Reproductions, Vancouver, May 24–28, 1997.
Bainbridge, I. (1982). In *Test Tube Babies: A Guide to Moral Questions, Present Techniques and Future Possibilities* (W. A. Walters and P. Singer, eds). Melbourne, Victoria: Oxford University Press.
Beaurepaire, J., Jones, M., Thiering, P., Saunders, D. and Tennant, C. (1994). Psychosocial adjustment to infertility and its treatment: male and female responses at different stages of IVF/ET treatment. *Journal of Psychosomatic Research*, **38**, 229–40.
Belsky, J., Ward, M. J. and Rovine, M. (1986). Prenatal expectations, postnatal experiences, and the transition to parenthood. In *Thinking about the Family* (R. D. Ashmore and D. M. Brodzinsky, eds). Hilldale, New Jersey: Lawrence Erlbaum Associates.
Bentovim, A. (1972). Handicapped preschool children and their families: attitudes to the child. *British Medical Journal*, **3**, 579–81.
Blenner, J. L. (1990). Passage through infertility treatment: a stage theory. *Image: Journal of Nursing Scholarship*, **22**, 153–8.
Blumer, H. (1969). *Symbolic Interactionism: Perspective and Method*. Englewood Cliffs, NJ: Prentice-Hall.
Boivin, J., Takefman, J. E., Tulandi, T. and Brender, W. (1995). Reactions to infertility based on extent of treatment failure. *Fertility and Sterility*, **63**, 801–7.
Brandes, J. M., Scher, A., Itzkovits, J., Thaler, I., Sarid, M. and Gershoni-Baruch, R. (1992). Growth and development of children conceived by in vitro fertilization. *Pediatrics*, **90** (3), 424–9.
Brodzinsky, D. M. and Huffman, L. (1988). Transition to adoptive parenthood. *Marriage and Family Review*, **12**, 267–86.
Brown, L. and Brown, J. with Freeman, S. (1979). *Our Miracle Called Louise: A Parents' Story*. London: Paddington Press.
Colpin, H., Demyttenaere, K. and Vandemeulebroecke, L. (1995). New reproductive technology and the family: the parent–child relationship following in vitro fertilization. *Journal of Child Psychology and Psychiatry*, **36** (8), 1429–41.
Condon, J. T. (1993). The assessment of antenatal emotional attachment: development of a questionnaire instrument. *British Journal of Medical Psychology*, **66**, 167–83.
Condon, J. T. and Dunn, D. J. (1988). The nature and determinants of parent-to-infant attachment in the early post-natal period. *Journal of the Academy of Child and Adolescent Psychiatry*, **27**, 293–9.

Cook, R., Parsons, J., Mason, B. and Golombok, S. (1989). Emotional, marital and sexual functioning in patients embarking on IVF and AID treatment for infertility. *Journal of Reproductive and Infant Psychology*, **7**, 87–93.

Cox, M. J., Owen, M. T., Lewis, J. M. and Henderson, V. K. (1989). Marriage, adult adjustment and early parenting. *Child Development*, **60**, 1015–24.

Cranley, M. S. (1981). Development of a tool for the measurement of maternal attachment in pregnancy. *Nursing Research*, **30**, 281–4.

Dettman, C. and Saunders, D. (1987). *The Chance of a Lifetime: Infertility and IVF*. Melbourne, Victoria: Penguin.

Doyle, P., Beral, V. and Maconochie, N. (1992). Preterm delivery, low birthweight and small-for-gestational-age liveborn singleton babies resulting from in-vitro fertilization. *Human Reproduction*, **7** (3), 425–8.

Dunnington, R. M. and Glazer, G. (1991). Maternal identity and early mothering behaviour in previously infertile and never infertile women. *Journal of Obstetric, Gynecologic, and Neonatal Nursing*, **20**, 309–17.

Durna, E. M., Bebe, J., Leader, L., Steigrad, S. J. and Garrett, D. G. (1995). Donor insemination: effects on parents. *Medical Journal of Australia*, **163**, 248–51.

Fisher, A. (1989). *I.V.F.: The Critical Issues*. Blackburn, Victoria: Collins Dove.

Freeman, E. W., Boxer, A. S., Rickels, K., Mastroianni, L. and Tureck, R. W. (1985). Psychological evaluation and support in a program of in vitro fertilization and embryo transfer. *Fertility and Sterility*, **43**, 48–53.

Garner, C. H. (1985). Pregnancy after infertility. *Journal of Obstetric, Gynecologic, and Neonatal Nursing*, **14** (Suppl.), 58s–62s.

Gibson, F., Ungerer, J., Leslie, G., Saunders, D., and Tennant, C. (in press). Development, behaviour and temperament. A prospective study of infants conceived through in vitro fertilisation. *Human Reproduction*.

Golombok, S. (1995). What about the children? *Organon's Magazine on Women and Health*, **3**, 14–16.

Golombok, S., Cook, R., Bish, A. and Murray, C. (1995). Families created by the new reproductive technologies: quality of parenting and social and emotional development of the children. *Child Development*, **66**, 285–98.

Graham, P. and Rutter, M. (1968). The reliability and validity of the psychiatric assessment of the child: II. Interview with the parent. *British Journal of Psychiatry*, **114**, 581–92.

Green, M. and Solnit, A. J. (1964). Reactions to the threatened loss of a child: a vulnerable child syndrome. *Pediatrics*, **34**, 58–66.

Greenfeld, D. A., Diamond, M. P. and DeCherney, A. H. (1988). Grief reactions following in-vitro fertilization treatment. *Journal of Psychosomatic Obstetrics and Gynaecology*, **8**, 169–74.

Halasz, G., Munro, J., Saunders, K., Astbury, J. and Spensley, J. (1993). The growth and development of children conceived by IVF. Melbourne: Monash University Press.

Hoopes, J. L. (1982). Prediction in child development: a longitudinal study of adoptive and non-adoptive families. *The Delaware Family Study*. New York: Child Welfare League of America Inc.

Kach, J. and McGhee, P. (1982). Adjustment to early parenthood: the role of accuracy of preparenthood expectations. *Journal of Family Issues*, **3**, 361–72.

Klein, R. (ed.) (1989). *Infertility: Women Speak Out*. London: Pandora.

Kubler-Ross, E. (1975). *Death, The Final Stage of Growth*. New Jersey: Prentice-Hall.

Lancaster, P., Shafir, E., Hurst, T. and Huang, J. (1997). Assisted Conception, Australia and New Zealand 1994 and 1995. Sydney: AIHW National Perinatal Statistics Unit (Assisted Conception Series, No. 2).

Leiblum, S. R., Kemmanen, E. and Lane, M. K. (1987). The psychological concomitants of in vitro fertilization. *Journal of Psychosomatic Obstetrics and Gynaecology*, **6**, 165–78.

Levy, D. M. (1966). *Maternal Overprotection*. New York: W.W. Norton.

Lind, R., Pruitt, R. L. and Greenfeld, D. (1989). Previously infertile couples and the newborn intensive care unit. *Health and Social Work*, **14**, 127–33.

Litt, M. D., Tennen, H., Affleck, G. and Klock, S. (1992). Coping and cognitive factors in adaptation to *in vitro* fertilization failure. *Journal of Behavioral Medicine*, **15**, 171–87.

Mahler, M., Pine, F. and Bergman, A. (1975). The psychological birth of the human infant. New York: Basic Books.

McQuire, J. and Richman, N. (1988). *The Preschool Behaviour Checklist*. Windsor: NFER, Nelson.

McMahon, C. A., Ungerer, J. A., Beaurepaire, J., Tennant, C. and Saunders, D. (1997). Anxiety during pregnancy and fetal attachment after IVF conception. *Human Reproduction*. **12** (1), 176–182.

McMahon, C. A., Ungerer, J., Tennant, C. and Saunders, D. (1997). Psychosocial adjustment and the quality of the mother–child relationship at four months post-partum after conception by in vitro fertilization. *Fertility and Sterility*, **68** (3), 492–500.

Morin, N. C., Wirth, F. H., Johnson, D. H., Frank, L. M., Presburg, H. J., Van de Water, V. L., Chee, E. M. and Mills, J. L. (1989). Congenital malformations and psychosocial development in children conceived by in vitro fertilization. *Journal of Pediatrics*, **115**, 222–7.

Munro, J. M., Ironside, W. and Smith, G. C. (1992). Successful parents of in vitro fertilization (IVF): the social repercussions. *Journal of Assisted Reproduction and Genetics*, **9**, 170–76.

Mushin, D., Spensley, J. and Barreda-Hansen, M. (1985). Children of IVF. *Clinics in Obstetrics and Gynaecology*, **12**, 865–76.

Mushin, D. N., Barreda-Hansen, M. C. and Spensley, J. C. (1986). In vitro fertilization children: early psychosocial development. *Journal of in Vitro Fertilization and Embryo Transfer*, **3**, 247–52.

Newton, C. R., Hearn, M. T. and Yuzpe, A. A. (1990). Psychological assessment and follow-up after in vitro fertilisation: assessing the impact of failure. *Fertility and Sterility*, **54**, 879–86.

Olshansky, E. (1987). Identity of self as infertile: an example of theory-generating research. *Advances in Nursing Science*, **9**, 54–63.

Parker, G. (1983). *Parental Overprotection: A Risk Factor in Psychosocial Development*. New York: Grune and Stratton.

Raoul-Duval, A., Bertrand-Savais, M., Letur-Konirsch, H. and Frydman, R. (1994). Psychological follow-up of children born after in-vitro fertilization. *Human Reproduction*, **9**, 1097–101.

Raphael-Leff, J. (1991). *Psychological Processes of Childbearing*. London: Chapman and Hall.

Reading, A. E., Chang, L. C. and Kerin, J. F. (1989). Attitudes and anxiety levels in women conceiving through in vitro fertilization and gamete intrafallopian transfer. *Fertility and Sterility*, **52**, 95–9.

Sandelowski, M. (1987). The color gray: ambiguity and infertility. *Image: Journal of Nursing Scholarship*, **19**, 70–74.

Stanton, F. and Golombok, S. (1993). Maternal-fetal attachment during pregnancy following in vitro fertilization. *Journal of Psychosomatic Obstetrics and Gynaecology*, **14**, 153–8.

Thiering, P., Beaurepaire, J., Jones, M., Saunders, D. and Tennant, C. (1993). Mood state as a predictor of treatment outcome after *in vitro* fertilization/embryo transfer (IVF/ET). *Journal of Psychosomatic Research*, **37**, 481–91.

Walters, W. A. and Singer, P. (eds) (1982). *Test Tube Babies: A Guide to Moral Questions, Present Techniques and Future Possibilities*. Melbourne, Victoria: Oxford University Press.

Warnock, M. (1987). The good of the child. *Bioethics*, **1**, 141–55.

Weaver, S. M., Clifford, E., Gordon, A. G., Hay, D. M. and Robinson, J. (1993). A follow-up study of 'successful' IVF/GIFT couples: social-emotional well-being and adjustment to parenthood. *Journal of Psychosomatic Obstetrics and Gynaecology*, **14**, 5–16.

World Collaborative Report Bilan Mondial (1991). *7th World Congress on In Vitro Fertilization and Assisted Procreations*. Paris, June 30–July 3, 1991.

3

Variations in family circumstances: implications for children and their parents

David White

In the previous chapter, the implications of changing technology for parents and children were considered. In this chapter, David White is concerned with the implications of different family structures on children and parents. He asks about the consequences of divorce or family break-up; about experiences such as adoption, being in a step-family, or having gay or lesbian parents; and about the effect of illness, disability (in children or parents), lifestyle and economic circumstances. The social construction of parenthood described in Chapter 1 suggests that all of these variations from the supposedly 'traditional' family will have negative consequences. This chapter challenges this idea and suggests that children can develop healthily in a wide range of different social circumstances, and that some experience of uncertainty as well as consistency can enhance the development of adaptive life skills.

In this chapter consideration is given to the variability of families and family life and how this may be experienced by parents, young children and the wider family. Many families are headed by a heterosexual couple and contain one or two healthy children who have genetic, biological and social links with both of their parents and where fathers are breadwinners and mothers are full-time caretakers. These traditional families, however, vary enormously in all sorts of ways. Many will include caring, committed parents with good parenting skills. Other parents, however, will be less committed or less caring or less skilled. Some of those families will include an alcoholic or illicit drug using parent, others an abusing parent, others still a parent with physical or mental health difficulties.

The children in families are not all the same; they vary in characteristics such as gender, age and temperament. Consequently, even within traditional families the experiences, adjustments and development of family members varies greatly. However, families are not all of this traditional form. They differ in the number and timing of children; in the age of parents; in employment/unemployment patterns.

Not all families are headed by two parents. Some women have children on their own. Especially when they are young, single mothers are supported frequently by their own families (Phoenix, 1991; see Chapter 4 for further discussion). Other parents become single parents following family break-up; these single parents are usually the mother, although fathers may bring up children, especially boys and older children. Other children live in effective one parent families because parents (usually fathers) are in prison, work away from home or have jobs which involve considerable travel. Families with adopted children, step-children or children who are born as a result of using reproductive technologies (discussed in Chapter 2) add further to the variability in family life, as do extended families living together in one household unit. In considering variety in family life, brief consideration will be given to some of the more common family forms before identifying some issues about families that are raised. Finally consideration will be given to parents' experiences, adjustments and coping, to children's experiences, adjustment and development and to qualities of good parenting.

Family circumstances

Working mothers, role reversal families and dual earning families

In the UK, 71 per cent of children live in a family with a working head of household and one in five mothers are in paid employment (Central Statistics Office, 1994). These figures point to the variation in patterns of employment in families. Either, both or neither of the parents may be in paid employment. Mothers' and fathers' experiences as parents are, to some extent, influenced by their working roles outside the home (Bronfenbrenner, 1986). Dual earner families and role reversal families both involve the mother in working outside the home.

In dual earner families both mother and father are in paid employment combining the roles of wage earner, home maker and parent. Concern about dual earner families focuses on the ability of working parents to provide adequate and sensitive care for their children. The balance of who provides care for children is influenced by which parent is available to take part in childcare. The more hours mothers work outside of the home the more likely it is that fathers will become involved in childcare. This relationship is moderated by fathers' views about women's role in the home and their attitudes towards working women (Deutsch, Lussier and Servis, 1993). However, in practice children from dual earner families are treated similarly to other children. Working and non-working parents are equally likely to supervise their children closely, be aware of what their child is doing throughout the day and to make maturity demands of their young children (Crouter, MacDermid, McHale et al., 1990). How parents view work can be important. Working parents who enjoy their work are likely to treat their young children more sensitively and warmly (Grossman, Pollack and Golding, 1988; Silverberg and Steinberg, 1990). Parents' working status need not detract from their commitment to parenting and may enhance it. Children from dual earner families have a different balance of contact with parents including more experience of play with mothers but less with fathers compared with children in conventional families (Lamb, Hwang, Broberg et al., 1988). However, there is no evidence that parents' working experiences make them poorer parents and indeed if their work experience enhances their self-esteem they may become more confident and effective as parents (Barnett and Marshall, 1993; Crouter and McHale, 1993; Greenberger, O'Neil and Nagel, 1994).

So-called role reversal families where fathers remain at home and act as the principal caretaker and mothers work outside the home have also been studied. There are costs and benefits to parents who choose this form of parenting (Russell, 1983). For mothers the principal benefit is the satisfaction that they may derive from their jobs and they also may enjoy increased assertiveness and social influence, but there can be physical and psychological costs (Grbich, 1994). The increased workload and tiredness resulting from their commitment to parenting and to work can be physically draining. Secondary caretaking mothers frequently feel guilty about relinquishing primary responsibility for the care of their children and experience stress at being separated from their young children and regret missing their early developmental years (Grbich, 1994). They may regret the reduced contact with their children and for some their guilt may be fuelled by the belief that the father is not terribly good as a homemaker. The quality of parents' relationship can be adversely affected with more conflicts, often centring around housework and child rearing practices.

For their part, primary caretaking fathers can benefit by forming closer relationships with their children and so feel more positively about them. Their self-confidence can be enhanced by their perception of having taken on a new role successfully. However, there can be considerable costs in that they may spend much of the time feeling bored and they can feel starved of adult company. Also because they spend more time at home they may experience an increase in conflicts with their children. In their turn the children who are looked after principally by their fathers show greater internal locus of control and higher verbal intelligence scores. In contrast children who are brought up by a primary caretaking mother explore less and show more emotional dependence upon the mother. Growing up in a role reversal family does not appear to adversely affect children.

Families created or extended through adoption

At one time adoption involved the adoption of babies soon after birth by childless couples, but now adoption is increasingly of older children and children with disabilities. Nevertheless there are still about 3000 young children of four years and younger adopted each year, of whom 800 are babies. Increasingly people who have children already are becoming adoptive parents. There is more emphasis now on finding good homes for children than on finding babies for childless couples. Nevertheless, many adopting parents are still childless at the time of the adoption.

Adoptions are largely successful leading to cohesive, supportive families in which children develop in a satisfactory way. This is especially true during the preschool years when children adopted when under the age of two years show good intellectual and social development (Tizard, 1991). Adoptees as a whole are equal to or even superior to non-adopted children in their self-image, sense of security, sense of control over their lives and they present positive personality traits (Wegar, 1995). Although in general adopted children are well adjusted, they are over-represented in clinical populations. In middle childhood and adolescence some adopted children begin to show signs of emotional disturbance. More boys have emotional problems than girls (Hersov, 1990).

Emotional disturbances in adopted children are likely to arise from a variety of causes; it is unlikely that there is a common profile. Contributory factors can include adverse pre-adoption experiences of children and their exposure to stigmatization, especially from peers, if their adopted status is known. Some adoptive parents form unattainable aspirations for their adopted children so placing too much pressure on their children to succeed. Becoming an adoptive parent can be stressful for parents, especially their experience of the adoption process. Parents typically find the adoption process intrusive and stressful and this can undermine their parenting skills (Wegar, 1995). Many adoptive parents will have undergone infertility investigations and treatments prior to the adoption, and part of the pre-adoption process focuses upon the success of parents' resolution of their infertility and relationship problems that may have arisen in the process (Daly, 1990). When the adoption takes place the family may have no option but to disclose how the family has been formed. Disclosure exposes parents to possibly stigmatized views about themselves and their adopted children and indeed Miall (1987) found that two-thirds of adoptive mothers in her study were disturbed by the dominant societal belief of the inferiority of adoptive motherhood. Raising adoptive children can be stressful for parents and being an adopted child can be stressful for children. These various experiences can place a strain on the relationship between adoptive parents and their adopted children.

It is not surprising that many adopted children see themselves as different from their peers because their biological parents are not known by them. As they get older they identify a gap in their histories, they do not know the full details of why they were placed for adoption and they may perceive themselves as having a marginal status (March, 1995). This encourages them to trace their parents in an attempt to help define themselves.

Family break-up

At any one time about 19 per cent of children in Britain are living with a lone parent, most usually following family break-up (Central Statistics Office, 1994). Approximately 30 per cent of dependent children (under 16 years of age) will experience family break-up (Wicks and Kiernan, 1990). Families do not usually break up without any warning. For some time before they separate most couples are aware of a deterioration in their relationship that is frequently expressed in terms of arguments and conflict in the home. Conflict and tension in the family is distressing for all family members. Because of deteriorating family relationships prior to the break-up it is likely that children already suffer adverse consequences, and that these accelerate with the break-up. However, even when relationships are unsatisfactory their termination calls for adjustments on the part of all family members which draw on parents' and children's emotional resources. Consequently, the year following family break-up is a period when family members are unlikely to function well. At some point during this time most men and women, regardless of whether they were the initiator of the separation or the non-initiator, feel depressed, incompetent, angry and rejected (Pettit and Bloom, 1984).

For the majority of custodial parents (usually the mother) the first year of bringing up children on their own is demanding; most report having too much to do and too little time and energy available. They report also being socially isolated (Weinraub and Wolf, 1983). Custodial parents tend to be poor at maintaining consistent routines for themselves and their children and established routines may be disrupted by the break-up. Thus the average custodial parent is less likely to read to children or to play with them and are more erratic in getting their children to bed (Hetherington, 1993). Further, custodial parents make fewer maturity demands, communicate less, show less affection and are inconsistent in enforcing rules. These changes lead to poor child behaviour which in turn leads to a further deterioration in parenting (Fauber, Forehand, Thomas et al., 1990; Hetherington, 1993; Stoneman, Brody and Burke, 1989). The difficulties experienced by custodial parents decrease as they and their children adapt to their new situation, but establishing new routines can take a number of years. Bringing up children as a lone parent is demanding and this is reflected in the health of parents. The health of lone parents is significantly worse than the health of parents in two parent families (Popay and Jones, 1990). When parents' health is poor this may impact on their parenting skills and on their relationships with their children. This is discussed further in a later section. Following family break-up there is reduced contact with the non-custodial parent (usually the father) and a reduction in the non-custodial parent's influence upon their child's development (Hetherington, 1993; Kline, Tschann, Johnston et al., 1989).

Following family break-up children show a short-term reaction of distress with increased aggression, poorer attention spans, more disobedience and other behavioural problems (Amato and Keith, 1991; Barber and Eccles, 1992; Brown, 1994; Hetherington, 1993), although this reaction is expressed somewhat differently by children, dependent upon their age at the time (Kurdek, 1986). Infants and toddlers up to two years show their distress by failing to form secure attachments. Preschool children tend to be the most frightened and confused, they are most likely to worry about their own contribution to their parent's departure, to believe that the separation is temporary, and to be confused by a parent assuring the child of his or her love yet moving away. Older children with greater understanding of relationships can understand that their parents might be incompatible and incapable of living together. They usually want to see their parents reconciled but realize that this is unlikely. In the longer term (e.g. ten years after the separation), young children can remember little of their pre-divorce lives and are the most contented. They perceive themselves as having a close relationship with their mothers and they are optimistic about their own futures, including their expectations of their own future marriages, which they expect to last (Wallerstein, Corbin and Lewis, 1988).

In general girls adjust better to family break-up than boys (Zaslow, 1989). In part this is because in the majority of cases the custodial parent is the mother. Mothers' relationships with boys can continue to be troublesome even six or more years after the break-up (Hetherington, 1988). In the longer term following family break-up, children show minor impairment in their academic performance and less conventional sex-role typing and preferences (Stevenson and Black, 1988). However, there are very large differences in adjustments with some children being very severely affected while others show no impairment (Furstenberg and Seltzer, 1986). In adolescence girls who have hitherto seemed well adjusted frequently develop behaviour problems. It is reported that about a third of girls from divorced homes experience difficulty with intimate relationships in adulthood (Long, 1987; Wallerstein, Corbin and Lewis, 1988).

The findings from studies of family break-up are not always consistent. For instance British studies are more likely to reveal more adverse consequences for children reared in single parent homes than do studies conducted in the USA. An example is Cockett and Tripp (1994) who, following an examination of children who had experienced family break-up, concluded that family break-up had consequences that were more severe than the adverse effects of experiencing conflict within the home. This finding runs counter to the evidence from the USA which shows that family break-up unaccompanied by conflict has little impact on children's longer term adjustments (e.g. Davies and Cummings, 1995). This inconsistency may reflect genuine cultural differences in the reactions to family break-up and single parenting, including different levels of support to parents and to children in the two countries. However, they may instead reflect methodological differences. For instance many British studies are longitudinal studies following children of divorce/family break-up over many years (e.g. Wadsworth, 1985). These have reported on outcomes for the offspring of family break-up occurring up to 30 years previously, in many cases predating liberalization of the divorce laws introduced during the 1970s. In these cases family break-up occurred many years ago when the climate in which divorce occurred was very different from the prevailing climate now. In contrast studies from the USA examine divorce and family break-up over a shorter period, but a period when prevailing attitudes and support for families experiencing break-up may be more similar to the situation today. Furthermore, many of these British studies rely on one source of information about children's adjustment to divorce/family break-up, the children themselves. Again in contrast, studies from USA are more likely to collect data from a number of sources, e.g. the children themselves including psychometric data, both parents and school teachers.

Amato and Keith (1991) undertook a meta-analysis of divorce studies. This confirmed that children of divorce were less well adjusted than children from intact families with an average effect size of 0.14 of a standard deviation (a sizeable, but not massive effect). However, they concluded that studies conducted more recently were less likely to show strong adverse effects. Moreover, methodologically stronger studies, relying less on retrospective and clinical data showed smaller effects. This analysis of studies also emphasized the importance of parental conflict in leading to adverse consequences for children. While their analysis is not conclusive it seems more probable that differences in the findings of studies from USA and Britain reflect methodological differences rather than differences in the experience of divorce/family break-up in the two countries, but definite confirmation of this requires the execution of some more complex and methodologically sophisticated studies in Britain.

A difficulty in assessing the impact of family break-up on children is that family break-up is not a single event, but a long sequence of events, some of which will impact on children more than others. Family break-up will have been preceded by a deterioration in relationships, with possibly an increase in verbal or physical conflicts, and conflicts may have been resolved in increasingly inadequate ways. Some children, but not others, will have been prepared for the break-up of the family by one or both parents, although any preparation is harder for younger children with their less sophisticated understandings of family dynamics. The break-up and the period following the break-up will be associated with an increase in family tensions in some cases but with a decrease in others. Following the break-up family circumstances may change dramatically and involve a change in housing, in area of residence, in family income and presence of family possessions; it may also result in reduced contact with familiar people. Because family break-up is associated with so many changes it is difficult to tease out the impact of any one of the events. Longitudinal studies covering the period before, during and after the break-up can contribute to knowledge in this area, but they are expensive in time and money to mount and so few have been conducted.

Reconstituted families

Many family break-ups are followed by entry into a reconstituted family. In Britain one in twelve children live in a step-parent family (Central Statistics Office, 1994). Being part of a reconstituted family, especially if it is a blended family involving other children, calls for many adjustments (Santrock, Warshak and Elliott, 1982). It is often difficult to disentangle the impact for children of living in step-parent families from their experiences arising from family break-up. If there are unresolved issues for the child remaining from the break-up at the time they join a reconstituted family, these will colour the child's perceptions of their new family and their reactions to it (Gorell-Barnes, 1991). Furthermore, each family transition introduces additional interpersonal problems to be solved and can tax children's coping resources (Furstenberg and Seltzer, 1986). Some children in step-parent families are very demanding and step-parents and their partners may have insufficient time together away from the children to develop their intimate relationship and consequently reconstituted families frequently break-up.

Becoming part of a step-parent family may result in improvements in children's experiences. Frequently their relationship with their custodial parent improves and strong relationships can form with the step-parent and the step-parent's own family. However, children's experiences may not improve and their exposure to family conflict may increase. Children in step-parent families can be exposed to two sources of family conflict, (i) conflict in their current homes which may involve their biological parent, step-parent, step-siblings or themselves and (ii) conflict between biological parents who live apart. On average, children living in step-parent families experience more conflict than children in single parent families or in original two parent families because of the double exposure to inter-parental conflict (Hanson, McLanahan and Thomson, 1996).

In general step-fathers are absorbed into reconstituted families more easily than are step-mothers. The arrival of a step-father is often associated with warmer, firmer treatment of the children by their mothers and by an improvement in family finances (Hetherington, 1993). Step-mothers have a more difficult time than step-fathers. They experience more interpersonal conflict, more anxiety, more anger and depression than any other group of women, and children perceive them as unaffectionate and unfair (Ganong and Coleman, 1987). Step-mothers usually take over the day-to-day care for someone else's children, thus exposing themselves to more areas of conflict with their step-children than do step-fathers who usually are more peripheral in their children's lives. Furthermore, if a step-mother is introduced into a family where the father was awarded custody it is likely that the biological mother was deemed to be unsuitable. Some of the difficulties step-mothers experience in establishing good relationships with step-children may reflect the unresolved tensions between those children and their biological mother (Gorell-Barnes, 1991).

There are some small but consistent differences between children from step-parent and intact families (Zill, 1988). Compared to children from intact homes, children from both single parent homes and step-parent homes show more problem behaviours including: antisocial destructive behaviours; verbal and physical aggression; poor attention span; high levels of anxiety; social withdrawal and depressed mood; when older they perform less well at school and they miss more school because of illness. There are somewhat more problems amongst children in step-mother families and girls show more adverse reactions to being in a step-parent family than do boys (Zill, 1988). As with family break-up there are variations in the adjustments of children in step-parent families; some form good relationships with the new parent and are well adjusted, others have greater difficulties.

Gay and lesbian parents

The opportunities for family building are more limited for would-be parents who are gay or lesbian. Adoption and medicalized reproduction are not normally available to homosexual men and women. Lesbian women who want assisted reproduction usually have to resort to self administered AID using unscreened donated semen with its attendant risk of exposure to sexually transmitted diseases (Macaulay, Kitzinger, Green et al., 1995). But some young children are brought up by a gay or lesbian parent, either living in a single parent family or in a family with two same sexed 'parents'. Children most frequently live with a gay or lesbian parent following family break-up and so children in these families have to face the adjustments to family break-up in addition to any further adjustments their particular living arrangements may impose. Even this route to parenthood may pose problems as gay fathers and lesbian mothers are commonly denied custody if custody is disputed (Rivera, 1991).

Interest in gay and lesbian parents focuses upon their parenting effectiveness, the stigma children may experience and the gender development of children in these households. Consequently, there are studies which examine the development of children raised by gay or lesbian parents. Because of their experience of family break-up it is most appropriate when evaluating the outcomes for children raised by gay or lesbian parents to compare their adjustments to children who have also experienced family break-up, but been raised by a heterosexual mother. Such comparisons are few in number; nevertheless their findings are consistent. These studies in general collect their information from more than one source, usually mothers and teachers, and children's performance is assessed on standardized psychometric tests. Comparisons of children reared in lesbian and single heterosexual mother headed households find no differences during childhood in gender role, emotional adjustment, self-esteem or quality of friendships. They find no differences in mothers' availability to their children nor in their nurturance and warmth in interacting with their children. In adulthood they find no differences in the sexual orientations of the two sets of children (e.g. Tasker and Golombok, 1995). The available evidence points to the similarities in the experiences of these and conventional families. However, as with all research into the family, studies rely on willing participants and willing participants may be non-representative. As with heterosexual headed families, there is diversity within gay and lesbian headed families and some parents create a better climate for their children's development than others.

Children with chronic illness or disabilities and their families

Approximately 14 per cent of children experience a chronic illness; included in this figure are 3–4 per cent of children with physical disabilities (Cadman, 1987). If children suffer from a chronic illness or are disabled, this may have implications for the experiences and adjustments of each family member, including the children themselves. The most commonly studied group of children with disabilities are those with Down's syndrome (e.g. Carr, 1988) but there is a growing literature looking at other conditions, including cancers, sickle cell disease and diabetes (Midence, Fuggle and Davies, 1993; Midence, 1994). Different diseases and disabilities may make somewhat different demands on the family, but there is a core of common experience. Ill or disabled children require more intensive care over a longer period than do healthy children. In order to give this care mothers usually become the principal carer for the ill or disabled child and fathers take greater responsibility for other children, in their turn older brothers and sisters are expected to take more responsibility for household chores. Families with a chronically ill or disabled child report more financial hardship, experience a more restricted lifestyle, more social isolation and more stigmatization than other families (Holroyd and Guthrie, 1986).

Parents of chronically ill or disabled children may experience considerable stress. This can result in an increase in the incidence of minor illness and increased anxiety and depression (Faust, Rosenfeld, Wilson et al., 1995). Fathers seem more at risk from psychological problems than mothers, especially when they withdraw from the care of the ill or disabled child (Longo and Bond, 1984). There are reports of more marital conflict in families with a sick or disabled child and of increased rates of family break-up; however, the evidence is contradictory (Faust, Rosenfeld, Wilson et al., 1995). It may be that different childhood conditions make different demands on parents and that the contradictory results arise when looking across conditions. Despite the negative consequences outlined above, many families cope well and enjoy life. Overcoming the challenges presented by sick or disabled young children can provide a growth point for family members and in retrospect this is reported by the majority of siblings of such children, most of whom claim that the experience made them more mature, more tolerant and more responsible (Carr, 1988). Sick or disabled young children, like healthy children, pass developmental milestones, develop their own personalities and can present the family with satisfying experiences.

Children who are chronically ill or disabled may experience more emotional problems and a lowering of self-esteem, but this may be condition specific (Garralda, 1994). However, the large body of evidence on chronically ill and disabled children suggests resilience, that they are able to draw strength from their experiences, make good adjustments, integrate successfully into society and enjoy a good quality of life (Hauser, DiPlacido, Jacobson et al., 1993; Zani, Di Palma and Vullo, 1995). Nevertheless, features of the condition such as symptom unpredictability, uncertain prognosis, associated sensory problems and visibility of condition all increase the likelihood of emotional problems occurring (Ireys, Werthamer-Larsson, Kolodner et al., 1994; Thompson, 1992).

Health and lifestyle of parents

Parents may become depressed, develop a severe illness or exhibit a chaotic lifestyle. Each of these events will affect family functioning and parenting skills and so might impact on the family and on developing children in the family. Because of mothers' more central role in childrearing within most families, more attention is given to maternal than to paternal depression and ill health. Maternal depression may interfere with mothers' relationships with their children, but this is not always the case. When it does, mothers tend to be more irritable, punitive and angry with their children, they tend to be less responsive and interact with their children less. When parents are under strain themselves they attend to their children less, noting what their children are doing only when their children's behaviour demands attention. Consequently, at such times parents see their children as behaving badly when they really are behaving normally; this encourages mothers to restrict their children's freedoms more, creating resentment and a worsening of mother–child relationships (Stoneman, Brody and Burke, 1989). Mothers' depression can have an impact on childrens' development, leading to poorer language development and more emotional and behavioural problems (Puckering, 1989).

Parental physical ill health may also impact on children's development. Many parents experience severe and debilitating medical conditions and even more experience conditions such as migraine which are not life threatening but are likely to affect parental behaviour. There is very little literature addressing the impact of parental illness on child functioning, but what there is suggests that children in these families function less well than children with healthier parents (Armistead, Klein and Forehand, 1995; Armistead and Forehand, 1995) and that this may be mediated by reduced parental support of the child, uncertain family routines, few efforts to discipline children, more neglect of the child and inter-parental conflict. If the mother is in poor health with too little energy to care for her children, the relationship of children with their fathers becomes particularly important. Good father–child relationships can help to buffer the child from the adverse effects of weakened mother–child relationships and the adverse consequences to the child of worrying about their mother's future and well-being.

Parents do not all have well ordered lives. For instance some parents abuse alcohol and other substances. In USA it is estimated that 27 per cent of pregnant 18–25-year-old women have used illicit drugs during the previous year and that 10–17 per cent use cocaine during pregnancy (Peterson, Burns and Widmayer, 1995). Maternal alcohol and drug use can affect the developing child through the direct impact of pre-natal exposure to drugs on personality and behaviour and also through the impact of alcohol and drug use on parenting skills. Child abuse and child neglect is higher among infants exposed to drugs pre-natally (Jaudes, Ekwo and Vanvoorhis, 1995).

One aspect of parenting that may be affected by parental substance use is parental monitoring. Chassin, Pillow, Curran et al. (1993) looked at mediating mechanisms between parental alcoholism and child adjustments. Parental alcoholism increased the child's exposure to stressful events and increased their unhappiness, alcoholic parents monitored their children's activities less and in older children these things increased children's association with peers supportive of drug using behaviours, encouraging their own substance use. Parents who use substances are not all negligent or inept as parents; improved parenting skills among drug using parents are associated with low impulsivity, low sensation seeking and high educational expectations (Brook, Whiteman, Balka et al., 1995). Reinforcing findings in earlier sections about the adverse effects of experiencing family conflict, it is reported that having a parent with a drinking problem does not have long term adverse consequences for children provided that the child does not also experience family disharmony (Orford and Velleman, 1995).

Issues raised by differing family circumstances

Personal, social, economic and cultural context of parenting

In the preceding section consideration was given to some of the ways in which family circumstances vary, but families in apparently similar situations are characterized by their diversity; they are not all alike. Family dynamics are influenced by the total context in which the family operates. Some of these contextual features such as the health of family members, family conflict and the relationship between the family and paid employment have been touched on already, some additional features are considered next.

An important determinant of parenting behaviour and satisfaction with parenting is the characteristics displayed by children. The term temperament is used to describe young children's characteristic ways of responding. Some children are happy, adaptable, inquisitive and sociable; these are referred to as temperamentally easy children. Other children are moody, react poorly to changes in their environment and experiences, are overactive and unsociable; these are referred to as temperamentally difficult children. Parents experiencing all sorts of family circumstances invest effort and emotion to promote their children's well-being. If their child develops as a happy, easy child parents can see that their effort has been worthwhile, their confidence in their parenting skills is boosted and the family atmosphere is enhanced. In contrast if the same effort results in a moody, difficult child it is harder for parents to view their efforts as worthwhile, it is harder to view themselves as successful parents and the family atmosphere may suffer. The impact of child temperament is discussed further in a later section.

Another feature influencing parenting behaviour is the depth of parents' knowledge of their children. In conventional families where the mother remains with the children as the principal caretaker she knows in great detail what her child has experienced. Employed fathers in such families will have less detailed knowledge of their child's experiences, but will know about these in broad terms. This knowledge of a child's history may be lacking with other family forms. Step-parents and adoptive parents may treat their children inappropriately because of a lack of knowledge of a critical event in their child's life. Additionally, lacking knowledge of the child's life events means that there may be important aspects of the children's lives that are not shared with the parents and cannot readily be discussed with them. With other family forms such as dual earning parents where alternative day care is used there may be small, but important events that are not shared, e.g. it may be the childminder and not a parent who experiences important milestones such as seeing the first steps taken by an infant.

Guilt is an emotion that is often experienced by parents – for instance when they respond inappropriately to their child with anger – but usually this sense of guilt is transitory. However, for some parents a sense of guilt is a more enduring experience and this will affect parenting. Substance using parents may experience guilt about their chaotic lifestyle and their deviation from conceptions of what constitutes a 'good' parent (Abdulrahim, White, Phillips et al., 1994). Guilt reactions may be felt by parents following family break-up as parents regret being unable to offer their children regular contact with both parents (Kline, Tschann, Johnston et al., 1989). In some families high levels of parental guilt are experienced following the birth of a child with a congenital defect such as Down's syndrome. In these circumstances parents frequently search for explanations of their child's condition in their own behaviour, blaming themselves for imagined transgressions (Gath, 1978). It has been suggested that parents who experience such guilt also believe that they can optimize their children's life experiences and development and so work harder towards this end (Beresford, 1994).

In many families there are insufficient resources, including financial resources, time, energy, space, love, affection and attention. When resources are scarce there are likely to be conflicts as, for example, fathers and children struggle for mothers' attention or mothers and fathers try to find time for themselves (Moss, Bolland, Foxman et al., 1986). Children are a financial drain on the family budget, they have to be housed and fed, they wear through clothes, damage the home and 'need' lots of toys and other equipment. For unemployed parents and families on low income financial hardship and worries about money can interfere with their enjoyment of parenting and with their ability to respond sensitively to their children. Conversely becoming a dual earning family or a step-parent family results in improved finances and a reduction in worry about money. Parents in such families should become more available to their children and this is reported by and of mothers in step-father families (Hetherington, 1993). A group of families who experience more financial burden than others are families with a chronically ill or disabled child. These children cost more because of visits to clinics and the need for special equipment. The earning power of these families may be reduced since mothers of ill or disabled children are less likely to be employed outside of the home, and family commitments may mean that fathers are less likely to seek promotion or to work overtime.

The experience of families is influenced by the reactions of society in general to their circumstances. The wider community has expectations of what it is to be a mother or a father. The role of men in parenting is much less clearly defined than is that of women and this adds to the tensions around fatherhood. This societal reaction may be supportive, but it may be hostile. Single parent families, lesbian headed families, families with an adopted or disabled child may all suffer from the adverse reaction of broader society. For instance children with highly visible disabilities experience stigmatization. One result of this is that some fathers of such children are less willing to be seen in public with their children, so curtailing their activities with them (Cooke and Lawton, 1984).

When children are conceived, born and brought up in conventional families, parenting is seen largely as a private matter. However, alternative forms of family building bring private behaviour into the public arena and make it clear that parenting and having children is not just an issue for individuals but for the wider society as well. The opportunity to become a parent through adoption, AID or IVF is tightly controlled and is available only to those who fit society's ideas of what constitutes good parents (Haimes, 1989). This means heterosexual couples, married or in stable long term relationships, who are not too old (sometimes this is defined as 35 or 40 for women, but often older for men). This scrutiny is justified in terms of what society thinks is an appropriate context for the creation of families and the upbringing of children (Phoenix, Woollett and Lloyd, 1991 and Chapter 1). As with adoption there is increased scrutiny of would-be parents before access to medical intervention is allowed. Similarly when a parent has a psychological or physical illness there is more scrutiny of the family.

Secrets in the family

An issue for families is maintenance of secrets within the family and keeping secrets from some family members. The stigma of infertility and adoption have meant that parents whose families were built through adoption or the use of reproductive technology often remained silent about their children's origins. Parents often fear the reactions and the curiosity of others and so prefer to remain silent about how their families have been formed (Pfeffer and Woollett, 1983). The differences between some families and conventional families are obvious and cannot be hidden, such as when parents adopt an older child or a child from a different ethnic community. But in other cases the differences are less obvious. With AID and IVF, for instance, children are born to their mothers and information about their conception is not generally public knowledge and attempts at secrecy can be made (Haimes, 1989). Similarly, gay or lesbian headed families may wish to protect their children from possible stigma and societal reactions to their sexuality and protect themselves from gossip about their suitability as parents.

Maintaining secrets can be costly in psychological terms and keeping secrets is not easy. Secrecy is an active process which requires deliberate behavioural and mental work. Working at maintaining secrets increases their accessibility in memory, and persevering in concealing a secret can increase the likelihood of that secret being unwittingly revealed (Lane and Wegner, 1995). Disclosure of secrets is psychologically therapeutic as it reduces the person's level of emotional inhibition and so releases the person from a constant demand.

If secrets are maintained, energy goes into hiding rather than dealing with issues and avoiding situations where the truth might be revealed. When secrecy is maintained people never have the opportunity to talk to other people and obtain support. The advantages of secrecy have to be balanced against children's rights to know about their origins and the costs of their discovering such information under distressing circumstances. With the reproductive technologies the advice given to parents is not to disclose such information and often parents have little information to give (Haimes, 1989; Rowland, 1985). Secrets are not, of course, just an issue for families built in unconventional ways. There are secrets in many families who work hard to keep them hidden. These can include children being conceived before marriage or extra-maritally, domestic violence or child abuse. With step-parenting, secrets may centre around the discord in the family prior to divorce, or relations with the non-custodial parent. Sexual abuse when it occurs in families points to the ability of many families to contain its secrets. Often family members are blind to the abuse that is occurring.

Family coping

Parenting is often seen as adding to the meaning of life and ensuring personal development and continuity. At the same time parenting is costly and becoming a parent involves making sacrifices. Whatever the circumstances of the family there will be occasions when parents experience difficulties, are uncertain about childcare, how to deal with their temperamentally difficult child, etc., requiring adjustments to be made. When asked what they find most helpful in allowing them to cope, parents most frequently report 'talking to their spouse' (Brown and Hepple, 1989). Other frequently reported strategies are 'reminding themselves how much worse it could be', restructuring their situation using humour and using the extended family for emotional and practical support. Amongst parents bringing up disabled children, there have been attempts to relate parents' coping strategies with their measured well-being. Findings are not all consistent. For example the use of emotional release strategies (getting angry, crying, etc.) is reported as beneficial in some studies but as maladaptive in others. Nevertheless, there are some consistent findings. Wishful thinking (wishing that one's circumstances were different) and self-blame are associated with poorer outcomes for parents whereas seeking social support, positive restructuring (changing the way the difficulty is viewed so that it does not cause distress) and active coping (planning, direct problem solving and information seeking) are associated with adaptive outcomes (Beresford, 1994).

There are few comparisons of mothers' and fathers' coping, but it is suggested mothers find it easier to adjust to a demanding or ill child than do fathers. This is partly because the average mother does more for her children than do fathers and has more opportunity to get to know the child including their strengths and accomplishments. Additionally, mothers are better than fathers at eliciting and utilizing social support (e.g. Tunali and Power, 1993).

In all families siblings and the extended family can be an important coping resource, offering support, practical and financial help and serving as advisors and confidants. Siblings and the extended family may be particularly important for single mothers, for families following family break-up, reconstituted families and families with a sick or disabled child. Single mothers are frequently supported by their own mothers and following family break-up families often spend some time living with or close to grandparents (Wilson and Tolson, 1988). For children living in families that are under stress due to family break-up, family illness, parental substance use, etc., siblings may provide support for one another. However, this support is most frequently offered by sisters (Hetherington, 1988). In families where there is an ill or disabled child or where a parent is ill, older children, and especially older sisters, get called on to do more household chores and more caretaking than in other families (Carr, 1988: Gath, 1978). At the time they may resent this and see themselves as robbed of their childhood, but when they are adult and are asked to look back on their experiences most claim that the experience made them more mature, more tolerant and more responsible (Carr, 1988).

An important coping resource for parents is the support they provide for one another. When parents have a good relationship not only do they offer mutual support, they also provide a harmonious atmosphere in which to raise children. The quality of the relationship between mothers and fathers also has a strong bearing on the involvement of both parents and especially the warmth and involvement of fathers with children (Floyd and Zmich, 1991; Kerig, Cowan and Cowan, 1993; Levy-Shiff, 1994). If they are preoccupied with problems with their partner they are less attentive and responsive to the child. The demands of a child may be experienced as emotional overload, as competition for a partner's attention or as a shared activity and commitment. The extent to which each partner respects and acknowledges the parenting skills of the other influences men's and women's satisfaction with parenting (Belsky, Robins and Gamble, 1984; Bronfenbrenner, 1986).

The characteristics of children can moderate parents' experience of stressful or demanding situations. Most parents can cope effectively with challenges when they are presented singly, but when too many challenges occur simultaneously this can tax parents' coping resources (Rutter, 1985). A child who is temperamentally difficult presents a challenge that most parents can meet when other aspects of their lives are undemanding. However, when they are having to deal with additional challenges such as relationship or financial problems, their ability to cope sensitively with a temperamentally difficult child declines rapidly (Levy-Shiff, Goldsmidt and Har-Even, 1991). Furthermore, looking after a temperamentally difficult child can put relationships between parents under strain too.

The temperament of the child is also an important factor influencing how well young children themselves cope with adversity such as family conflict. In one study temperamentally difficult children living in low conflict families showed very similar levels of anxiety, depression and social withdrawal as temperamentally easy children living in similar low conflict families. However, temperamentally difficult children in high conflict families showed very high levels of anxiety, depression and social withdrawal, unlike temperamentally easy children in such families. Similarly temperamentally difficult children in high conflict families showed high levels of aggression and destructive behaviour (Tschann, Kaiser, Chesney et al., 1996). It may be that the distress shown by young temperamentally difficult children exposed to conflict is mediated by parent–child relationships. Parents who themselves are distressed by conflict in the family may be less accessible to their temperamentally difficult children, but not their temperamentally easy children, increasing the distress of difficult children.

Children's experiences and adjustments

Because they are cognitively immature and have limited life experiences, pre-school children may have a poor understanding of their experience in families. For adoptive children, children in step-parent families, children who experience chronic illness or disability and children of assisted concep-tions there are complex issues to understand. Young children following family break-up and children who have a chronic illness often share the reaction of believing that their experiences result from something that they have done wrong. Brewster (1982) examined chronically ill children's under-standing of the cause of their illness and the purpose of specific medical procedures. Children's understanding of illness correlated with their cogni-tive development as measured on Piagetian tasks. Children of five years and younger viewed illness as the result of direct human transgressions (their own or others) and medical procedures were seen as punishments for wrongdoing. In a similar way pain is seen as punishment by young children (McGrath, 1995).

Children who have experienced family break-up, entry into a reconstituted family, a chaotic parent, etc., have to master the same skills and face the same challenges as do other children, but in addition they have to cope with disruptions in routines and the reactions of others to them and their family status. For children with a chronic illness or disability they have to cope as well with the physical and physiological aspects of the disease, medication and other treatments, frequent hospitalization and visits to clinics and assess-ment centres, disruptions in daily activities and the reactions of others to their disability. These features have the potential to restrict the normal devel-opment of children. Despite this, most children cope well, but there are individual differences, inviting the question of what allows children to cope effectively. Unfortunately there is little work on the coping of children of preschool age. When distressed children as young as two years old show different reactions in different circumstances, this suggests an adaptiveness in their response. For instance in one study it was observed that children who had undergone painful surgery used self-distraction when undergoing medical examinations, but anger and other emotional responses in other situations (Woodgate and Kristjanson, 1995). Similarly, pre-school children undergoing routine examination by doctors were observed to use comfort seeking from caregivers and information seeking as strategies to help them cope (Hyson, 1983). With slightly older children aged six years and above it is possible to question them about what they find helpful when they are dis-tressed. In a study of children of battered mothers and children who had themselves been abused, the most helpful strategy was seeking support from a caregiver, or from a friend. Use of self-distraction, self-calming and anger were also reported as strategies adopted (Rossman and Rosenberg, 1992). Band and Weisz (1988) presented children with a number of hypothetical stressful situations and asked them what they would do to cope. For most situations they favoured problem-solving strategies aimed at changing the condition. However, for medical situations they recognized that the condition may be unalterable and instead adopted strategies intended to maximize the goodness of fit between themselves and the condition.

What makes a good parent?

This is not a simple question to answer. For instance what are desirable outcomes for children? It might be thought that it would be desirable for children to be sociable, compliant to authority, and be successful educationally, whereas aggressiveness and insensitivity to others would be undesirable. Consequently parenting styles which result in compliant, sociable and intellectually curious children would be seen as the ideal. 'Good' parents would not punish their children physically, instead they would explain why rules are set and why they need to be followed. This may be good preparation for those children who experience consistency in their lives but may be inadequate preparation for children who face a world in which rules are poorly defined or ignored by the adults around them. For a child growing up in a poor inner city area or preparing for life in the enterprise culture, aggressiveness, deviousness and unconcern for the welfare of others may be signs of successful adaptation rather than signs of psychopathology.

Some of the child development literature describes parenting behaviours in terms of a few parenting styles and assumes that a style that is effective in one situation will be equally successful in others. But in reality parents and children have different needs at specific life stages. Parents adopt their own individual styles for caring for their children. Parenting style is influenced by a wide range of factors including: their own experiences of being a child; their personality and that of their children; constraints of time and money; the number, age and gender of the children; individual beliefs about child-rearing. The range of different styles is vast and it is impossible to say for each individual family experiencing their own unique life circumstances which particular parenting styles are most likely to produce intended results. Nor should it be assumed that a style that is effective in one circumstance at one point in time would be equally effective when adopted at a different time or in different circumstances.

Despite the words of caution above, some patterns about effective parenting emerge from an examination of the variety of family circumstances. Hetherington (1988) when talking about the effects of divorce upon children uses the pejorative term 'inept parenting' to describe a raft of parenting features that appear to be associated with distress in their children. This includes lack of daily routines, inconsistent enforcement of rules, introduction of new arbitrary rules, lack of monitoring of child activities in and out of the home and giving children insufficient attention. This list points to features of parenting that might be distressing and implies that the reverse features may be associated with adaptive development. Consistency is a feature that is stressed. However, there is also evidence that the experience of inconsistency is important for developing children. For many children an experience of inconsistency comes from playing with fathers, which is non-repetitive and variable. It is therefore hard to predict what fathers will do next and to fit into their activities. Father play therefore presents children with problems to try and solve and to do this they have to be alert to any cue that fathers may present. They also have to learn quickly to communicate effectively with the father to ensure that the play continues to be enjoyable and does not become boring because it is not in synchrony or is confusing and frightening because it is too unpredictable. This means that they have to communicate efficiently their emotional reactions of enjoyment, fear or boredom. It is suggested the striving for understanding that is involved in father play helps to develop children's problem solving skills and their ability to take the perspective of others (Parke, MacDonald, Burks et al., 1989). Such problem solving skills lay the foundation for successful interaction with peers and siblings and others. Such skills may also help protect the child in times of adversity, since children who have not experienced challenges in their lives and who have been overprotected are unprepared for adversity when they do experience it.

Can parenting skills be improved?

A variety of different family forms have been discussed in this chapter and they point to the similarity of experience in different families despite differing circumstances. However, they also point to diversity of experience within each family structure. Families are not identical and some provide better environments for their children's developments than others. This invites the question of how readily parents can be trained to provide improved environments for their children. There have been a number of attempts recently to develop programmes to improve parenting skills and these have been targeted at different populations of parents, including parents suspected of child abuse and families perceived to be at high risk of substance misuse. The goals of the interventions include a reduction in family conflict and improved conflict resolution skills, increasing parents' awareness of child development thereby enabling parents to recognize what are reasonable and unreasonable expectations of young children, improved attentiveness and responsiveness to children (e.g. O'Donnell, Hawkins, Catalano et al., 1995; Szapocznik, Santisteban, Rio et al., 1989). The results of family intervention studies are promising but not conclusive (Campbell and Patterson, 1995). This is partly because the effectiveness of interventions has not yet been followed up for long enough periods to evaluate whether gains are maintained.

Methodological considerations

There are a number of methodological issues that recur when exploring families with differing life circumstances. In general there is a need for more longitudinal research to allow some of the relationships within families to be explored more effectively and to inform the actions of professionals who may need to be involved with families or offer families advice. When longitudinal studies are conducted they are frequently of relatively short duration. Erroneous conclusions about the determinants of successful adaptation may be made if too short a time frame is considered. Successful later adaptation may be seen in children who at an earlier time point did not show this characteristic, but if studies do not extend into later life these connections will be missed. Our understanding of families is limited by the paucity of data on most family members. Too little is known of fathers and their range of influence, but equally data are too limited regarding the range of influence of the extended family and of siblings. A difficulty in understanding family processes is that the influences are complex as are the theoretical concepts to be explored. Usually, however, the measures of these complex issues are crude and approximate poorly to the construct of interest. In these circumstances it is difficult to explore theoretical ideas with confidence. Unfortunately, there is inconsistency in the adoption of these (inadequate) measures by investigators, hampering the attempt to make meaningful comparisons across studies and so limiting the extent to which the available evidence can be integrated. Finally, there is great diversity amongst families, even those in apparently similar circumstances. Our informants about family life (the families studied) may not be fully representative of this diversity, again limiting our knowledge of some of the range of experiences and outcomes within families.

Conclusion

Psychologically healthy personalities can develop in many different social groupings and departures from the conventional norm of family structure are not necessarily harmful to children. All family forms have strengths and weaknesses and no one form has the monopoly on how to best meet children's needs at all times (Schaffer, 1986). Regardless of the family circumstances, children can develop as resilient capable individuals. The material reviewed in this chapter points to some similar themes whatever the precise circumstance of the family. Regardless of the family circumstances, children who are exposed to conflict, and especially conflict that is not resolved, are placed at a disadvantage. In two parent households a good relationship with one parent can offer support to developing children even if their relationship with the other parent is impaired (e.g. through substance misuse, illness, conflict). In all families it is important that children experience both consistency and uncertainty so that they can learn adaptive life skills and have the resources to overcome life's challenges. Most children are resilient and cope with the inconsistent behaviour that most parents, siblings and peers demonstrate.

Applications

1. High conflict in families threatens children's well-being

Professionals working with high conflict families should work towards a reduction in conflict and assist families to deal with their emotional reactions. In cases where decisions about post-separation access are being made, attention needs to be paid to the potential harm of applying joint custody or frequent access when this increases the risk of experiencing family conflict.

2. Parenting skills can be improved

Professionals involved in the development of programmes to enhance parenting skills need to recognize that there are a wide range of acceptable strategies for bringing up children. One approach will not suit all parents.

3. Families are embedded in a personal, social, economic and cultural context

There are limits to what professionals can achieve when working with families, unless the context in which parenting occurs is addressed. Mothers or fathers with low self-esteem, perhaps resulting from the neglect they experienced as children, or anxieties about debts will not readily be taught to persevere patiently with explaining family rules to a difficult and demanding child unless their own sense of inadequacy or their economic problems are addressed first.

4. Disclosing secrets

Parents need to consider the desirability of disclosing secrets. In the short term a disclosed secret may increase the distress of those concerned, but in the longer term disclosure is usually therapeutic.

Further reading

Armistead, L., Klein, K. and Forehand, R. (1995). Parental physical illness and child functioning. *Clinical Psychology Review*, **15** (5), 409–22.

Beresford, B. A. (1994). Resources and strategies: How parents cope with the care of a disabled child. *Journal of Child Psychology and Psychiatry*, **35**, 171–209.

Eiser, C. (1990). Psychological effects of chronic disease. *Journal of Child Psychology and Psychiatry*, **31**, 85–98.

Fincham, F. D. (1994). Understanding the association between marital conflict and child adjustment: Overview. Special Section: Contexts of interparental conflict and child behavior. *Journal of Family Psychology*, **8**, 123–7.

Golombok, S., Cook, R., Bish, A. and Murray, C. (1995). Families created by the new reproductive technologies: Quality of parenting and social and emotional development of the
children. *Child Development*, **66**, 285–98.
Hersov, L. (1990). The seventh Jack Tizard Memorial Lecture. Aspects of adoption. *Journal of
Child Psychology and Psychiatry*, **31**, 493–510.
Levy-Shiff, R., Goldsmidt, I. and Har-Even, D. (1991). Transition to parenthood in adoptive
families. *Developmental Psychology*, **27**, 131–40.

References

Abdulrahim, D., White, D., Phillips, K. et al. (1994). *Ethnicity and Substance Use: Towards the
Design of Community Interventions*. North East Thames Regional Health Authority.
Amato, P. R. and Keith, B. (1991). Parental divorce and the well-being of children: a meta-
analysis. *Psychological Bulletin*, **110**, 26–46.
Armistead, L. and Forehand, R. (1995). For whom the bell tolls: parenting decisions and
challenges faced by mothers who are HIV seropositive. *Clinical Psychology – Science and
Practice*, **2**(3), 239–50.
Armistead, L., Klein, L. and Forehand, R. (1995). Parental physical illness and child function-
ing. *Clinical Psychology Review*, **15** (5), 409–22.
Band, E. B. and Weisz, J. R. (1988). How to feel better when it feels bad: children's perspectives
on coping with everyday stress. *Developmental Psychology*, **24**, 247–53.
Barber, B. L. and Eccles, J. S. (1992). Long-term influence of divorce and single parenting on
adolescent family – and work-related values, behaviors and aspirations. *Psychological Bulletin*,
111, 108–26.
Barnett, R. C. and Marshall, N. L. (1993). Men, family-role quality, job-role quality, and
physical health. *Health Psychology*, **12**, 48–55.
Belsky, J., Robins, E. and Gamble, W. (1984). The determinants of parental competence. In
Beyond the Dyad (M. Lewis, ed.). New York: Plenum Press.
Beresford, B. A. (1994). Resources and strategies: how parents cope with the care of a disabled
child. *Journal of Child Psychology and Psychiatry*, **35**, 171–209.
Brewster, A. B. (1982). Chronically ill hospitalised children's concept of their illness. *Pediatrics*,
69, 355–62.
Bronfenbrenner, U. (1986). Ecology of the family as a context for human development: research
perspectives. *Developmental Psychology*, **22**, 723–42.
Brook, J. S., Whiteman, M., Balka, E. B. and Cohen, P. (1995). Parent drug use, parent person-
ality, and parenting. *Journal of Genetic Psychology*, **156** (2), 137–51.
Brown, C. (1994). The impact of divorce on families: the Australian experience. *Family and
Conciliation Courts Review*, **32**, 149–67.
Brown, A. and Hepple, S. (1989). *How Parents Cope*. Hertford: Barnardo's.
Busfield, J. (1987). Parenting and parenthood. In *Social Change and the Life Course* (G. Cohen,
ed.). London: Tavistock.
Cadman, D. (1987). Chronic illness, disability and mental and social well-being: findings of the
Ontario Child Health Study. *Pediatrics*, **79**, 805–12.
Campbell, T. L. and Patterson, J. M. (1995). The effectiveness of family interventions in the
treatment of physical illness. *Journal of Marital and Family Therapy*, **21** (4), 545–83.
Carr, J. (1988). Six weeks to twenty one years old: a longitudinal study of children with
Down's syndrome and their families. *Journal of Child Psychology and Psychiatry*, **29**,
407–31.
Central Statistics Office (1994). *Social Focus on Children*. HMSO.
Chassin, L., Pillow, D. R., Curran, P. J., Molina, B. S. G. and Barrera, M. (1993). Relation of
parental alcoholism to early adolescent substance use – a test of 3 mediating mechanisms.
Journal of Abnormal Psychology, **102** (1), 3–19.
Cockett, M. and Tripp, J. (1994). Children living in re-ordered families. *Social Policy Research
Findings*, No. 45.

Cooke, K. and Lawton, D. (1984). Informal support for carers of disabled children. *Child: Care, Health and Development*, **55**, 782.

Crouter, A. C., MacDermid, S. M., McHale, S. M. and Perry Jenkins, M. (1990). Parental monitoring and perceptions of school performance and conduct in dual- and single-earner families. *Developmental Psychology*, **26**, 649–57.

Crouter, A. C. and McHale, S. M. (1993). Temporal rhythms in family life: seasonal variations in the relation between parental work and family processes. *Developmental Psychology*, **29**, 198–205.

Daly, K. (1990). Infertility resolution and adoption readiness. *Families in Society*, **71**, 483–92.

Davies, P. T. and Cummings, E. M. (1995). Children's emotions and organizers of their reactions to interadult anger – a functionalist perspective. *Developmental Psychology*, **31** (4), 677–84.

Deutsch, F. M., Lussier, J. B. and Servis, L. J. (1993). Husbands at home: predictors of paternal participation in childcare and housework. *Journal of Personality and Social Psychology*, **65**, 1154–66.

Fauber, R., Forehand, R., Thomas, A. M. and Wierson, M. (1990). A mediational model of the impact of marital conflict on adolescent adjustment in intact and divorced families: the role of disrupted parenting. *Child Development*, **61**, 1112–23.

Faust, J., Rosenfeld, R. G., Wilson, D., Durham, L. and Vardopoulos, C. C. (1995). Prediction of depression in parents of Turner Syndrome adolescents as a function of growth hormones, family conflict, and coping style. *Journal of Developmental and Physical Disabilities*, **7** (3), 221–33.

Floyd, F. T. and Zmich, D. E. (1991). Marriage and the parenting partnership: perceptions and interactions of parents with mentally retarded and typically developing children. *Child Development*, **62**, 1434–48.

Furstenberg, F. F. and Seltzer, J. A. (1986). Divorce and child development. In *Sociological Studies of Child Development, Vol. 1* (P. A. Adler and P. Adler, eds). London: J.A.I. Press.

Ganong, L. H. and Coleman, M. M. (1987). Step children's perceptions of their parents. *Journal of Genetic Psychology*, **148**, 5–17.

Garralda, M. E. (1994). Chronic physical illness and emotional disorder in childhood. *British Journal of Psychiatry*, **164**, 8–10.

Gath, A. (1978). *Down's Syndrome and the Family*. London: Academic Press.

Gorell-Barnes, G. (1991). Step families in context: the post divorce process. *Association for Child Psychology and Psychiatry Newsletter*, **14**, No. 5, 3–11.

Grbich, C. (1994). Women as primary breadwinners in families where men are primary caregivers. *Australian and New Zealand Journal of Sociology*, **30**, 105–18.

Greenberger, E., O'Neil, R. and Nagel, S. K. (1994). Linking workplace and homeplace: relations between the nature of adults' work and their parenting behaviours. *Developmental Psychology*, **30**, 990–1002.

Grossman, F. K., Pollack, W. S. and Golding, E. (1988). Fathers and children: predicting the quality and quantity of fathering. *Developmental Psychology*, **24**, 82–91.

Hackel, L. S. and Ruble, D. N. (1992). Changes in the marital relationship after the first baby is born: predicting the impact of expectancy disconfirmation. *Journal of Personality and Social Psychology*, **62**, 944–57.

Haimes, E. (1989). Recreating the family: policy considerations relating to the 'new' reproductive technologies. In *The New Reproductive Technologies* (M. McNeil, I. Varcoe and S. Yearley, eds). London: Macmillan.

Hanson, T. L., McLanahan, S. S. and Thomson, E. (1996). Double jeopardy: parental conflict and stepfamily outcomes for children. *Journal of Marriage and the Family*, **58**, 141–54.

Hauser, S. T., DiPlacido, J., Jacobson, A. M. and Willetts, J. (1993). Family coping with an adolescent's chronic illness: an approach and three studies. *Journal of Adolescence*, **16**, 305–29.

Hersov, L. (1990). The seventh Jack Tizard Memorial Lecture. Aspects of adoption. *Journal of Child Psychology and Psychiatry*, **31**, 493–510.

Hetherington, E. M. (1988). Parents, children and siblings: six years after divorce. In *Relationships within Families: Mutual Influences* (R. A. Hinde and J. Stevenson-Hinde, eds). Oxford: Clarendon Press.

Hetherington, E. M. (1993). An overview of the Virginia Longitudinal Study of Divorce and Remarriage with a focus on early adolescence. Special Section: families in transition. *Journal of Family Psychology*, **7**, 39–56.

Holroyd, J. and Guthrie, D. (1986). Family stress with chronic childhood illness: cystic fibrosis, neuromuscular disease and renal disease. *Journal of Clinical Psychology*, **42**, 552–61.

Hyson, M. C. (1983). Going to the doctor: a developmental study of stress and coping. *Journal of Child Psychology and Psychiatry*, **24**, 247–59.

Ireys, H. T., Werthamer-Larsson, L. A., Kolodner, K. B. and Gross, S. S. (1994). Mental health of young adults with chronic illness: the mediating effect of perceived impact. *Journal of Pediatric Psychology*, **19**, 205–22.

Jaudes, P. K., Ekwo, E. and Vanvoorhis, J. (1995). Association of drug abuse and child abuse. *Child Abuse and Neglect*, **19** (9), 1065–75.

Kerig, P. K., Cowan, P. A. and Cowan, C. P. (1993). Marital quality and gender differences in parent–child interaction. *Developmental Psychology*, **29**, 931–9.

Kline, M., Tschann, J. M., Johnston, J. R. and Wallerstein, J. (1989). Children's adjustments in joint and sole physical custody families. *Developmental Psychology*, **25**, 430–38.

Kurdek, L. A. (1986). Children's reasoning about parental divorce. In *Thinking about the Family: Views of Parents and Children* (R. D. Ashmore and D. M. Brodzinsky, eds). Hillsdale, NJ: Lawrence Erlbaum Associates.

Lamb, M. E., Hwang, C.-P., Broberg, A., Bookstein, F. L., Hult, G. and Frodi, M. (1988). The determinants of paternal involvement in primiparous Swedish families. *International Journal of Behavioural Development*, **11**, 433–49.

Lane, J. D. and Wegner, D. M. (1995). The cognitive consequences of secrecy. *Journal of Personality and Social Psychology*, **69**, 237–53.

Levy-Shiff, R. (1994). Individual and contextual correlates of marital change across the transition to parenthood. *Developmental Psychology*, **30**, 591–601.

Levy-Shiff, R., Goldsmidt, I. and Har-Even, D. (1991). Transition to parenthood in adoptive families. *Developmental Psychology*, **27**, 131–40.

Long, B. H. (1987). Perceptions of parental discord and parental separation in the United States: effects on daughters' attitudes toward marriage and courtship progress. *Journal of Social Issues*, **127**, 573–82.

Longo, D. and Bond, L. (1984). Families of the handicapped child: research and practice. *Family Relations Journal of Applied Family and Child Studies*, **33**, 57–65.

Macaulay, L., Kitzinger, J., Green, G. et al. (1995). Unconventional conceptions and HIV. *AIDS Care*, **7**, 261–76.

McConachie, H. (1982). Fathers of mentally handicapped children. In *Fathers: Psychological Perspectives* (N. Beail and J. McGuire, eds). London: Junction Books.

McGrath, P. J. (1995). Annotation: aspects of pain in children and adolescents. *Journal of Child Psychology and Psychiatry*, **36**, 717–30.

March, K. (1995). Perception of adoption as social stigma: motivation for search and reunion. *Journal of Marriage and the Family*, **57** (3), 653–60.

Miall, C. (1987). The stigma of adoptive parent status: perceptions of community attitudes toward adoption and the experience of informal sanctioning. *Family Relations*, **36**, 34–9.

Midence, K. (1994). The effects of chronic illness on children and their families: an overview. *Genetic, Social and General Psychology Monographs*, **120**, 309–26.

Midence, K., Fuggle, P. and Davies, S. C. (1993). Psychosocial aspects of sickle cell disease in childhood and adolescence: a review. *British Journal of Clinical Psychology*, **32**, 271–80.

Moss, P., Bolland, G., Foxman, R. and Owen, C. (1986). Marital relations during transition to parenthood. *Journal of Reproductive and Infant Psychology*, **4**, 57–67.

O'Donnell, J., Hawkins, D., Catalano, R. F., Abbott, R. D. and Day, L. E. (1995). Preventing school failure, drug use, and delinquency among low-income children: long-term intervention in elementary schools. *American Journal of Orthopsychiatry*, **65** (1), 87–100.

Orford, J. and Velleman, R. (1995). Childhood and adulthood influences on the adjustment of young adults with and without parents with drinking problems. *Addiction Research*, **3** (1), 1–15.

Parke, R. D., MacDonald, K. B., Burks, V. M. et al. (1989). Family and peer systems: in search of the linkages. In *Family Systems and Lifespan Development* (K. Kreppner and R. M. Lerner, eds). Hillsdale, NJ: Lawrence Erlbaum Associates.

Peterson, L. M., Burns, W. J. and Widmayer, S. M. (1995). Developmental risk for infants of maternal cocaine abusers: evaluation and critique. *Clinical Psychology Review*, **15**, 739–76.

Pettit, A. J. and Bloom, B. L. (1984). 'Who's decision was it?' The effects of initiator status on adjustments to marital disruption. *Journal of Marriage and the Family*, **46**, 587.

Pfeffer, N. and Woollett, A. (1983). *The Experience of Infertility*. London: Virago.

Phoenix, A. (1991). *Young Mothers?* Cambridge: Polity Press.

Phoenix, A., Woollett, A. and Lloyd, E. (eds) (1991). *Motherhood: Meanings, Practices and Ideologies*. London: Sage.

Popay, J. and Jones, G. (1990). Patterns of health and illness amongst lone parents. *Journal of Social Policy*, **19**, 499–534.

Puckering, C. (1989). Maternal depression. *Journal of Child Psychology and Psychiatry*, **30**, 807–18.

Rivera, R. R. (1991). Sexual orientation and the law. In *Homosexuality: Research Implications for Public Policy* (J. C. Gonsiorek and L. D. Weinrich, eds). Newbury Park, CA: Sage Publications.

Rossman, B. B. R. and Rosenberg, M. S. (1992). Family stress and functioning in children: the moderating effects of children's beliefs about their control over parental conflict. *Journal of Child Psychology and Psychiatry*, **33**, 699–715.

Rowland, R. (1985). The social and psychological consequences of secrecy in artificial insemination by donor (AID) programmes. *Social Science and Medicine*, **21**, 391–6.

Russell, G. (1983). *The Changing Role of Fathers*. Milton Keynes: Open University Press.

Rutter, M. (1985). Resilience in the face of adversity: protective factors and resistance to psychiatric disorder. *British Journal of Psychiatry*, **147**, 598–611.

Santrock, J. W., Warshak, R. A. and Elliott, G. L. (1982). Social development and parent–child interaction in father custody and stepmother families. In *Non-traditional Families: Parenting and Child Development* (M. E. Lamb, ed.). Hillsdale, NJ: Lawrence Erlbaum Associates.

Schaffer, H. R. (1986). Child psychology: the future. *Journal of Child Psychology and Psychiatry*, **27**, 761–79.

Silverberg, S. B. and Steinberg, L. (1990). Psychological well-being of parents with early adolescent children. *Developmental Psychology*, **26**, 658–66.

Steinberg, L. (1987). Single parents, stepparents and the susceptibility of adolescents to antisocial peer pressure. *Child Development*, **58**, 269–75.

Stevenson, M. R. and Black, K. N. (1988). Paternal absence and sex-role development: a meta-analysis. *Child Development*, **59**, 793–814.

Stoneman, Z., Brody, G. H. and Burke, M. (1989). Marital quality, depression and inconsistent parenting: relationship with mother–child conflict. *American Journal of Orthopsychiatry*, **59**, 105–17.

Szapocznik, J., Santisteban, D., Rio, A., Perez-Vidal, A., Santisteban, D. and Kurtines, W. M. (1989). Family effectiveness training: an intervention to prevent drug abuse and problem behaviours in hispanic adolescents. *Hispanic Journal of Behavioral Sciences*, **11** (1), 4–27.

Tasker, F. and Golombok, S. (1995). Adults raised as children in lesbian families. *American Journal of Orthopsychiatry*, **65** (2), 203–15.

Thompson, R. J. (1992). Stress, coping and psychological adjustment of adults with sickle cell disease. *Journal of Consulting and Clinical Psychology*, **60**, 433–40.

Tizard, B. (1991). Inter country adoption: a review of the evidence. *Journal of Child Psychology and Psychiatry*, **32**, 743–56.

Tschann, J. M., Kaiser, P., Chesney, M. A., Alkon, A. and Boyce, W. T. (1996). Resilience and vulnerability among preschool children: family functioning, temperament, and behavior problems. *Journal of the American Academy of Child and Adolescent Psychiatry*, **35** (2), 184–92.

Tunali, B. and Power, T. G. (1993). Creating satisfaction: a psychological perspective on stress and coping in families of handicapped children. *Journal of Child Psychology and Psychiatry*, **34**, 945–57.

Wadsworth, M. E. (1985). Parenting skills and their transmission through the generations. *Adoption and Fostering*, **9**, 28–32.

Wallerstein, J. S., Corbin, S. B. and Lewis, J. M. (1988). Children of divorce: a ten year study. In *The Impact of Divorce, Single Parenting and Step-parenting on Children* (E. M. Hetherington and J. Arasteh, eds). Hillsdale, NJ: Lawrence Erlbaum Associates.

Wegar, K. (1995). Adoption and mental health: a theoretical critique of the psychopathological model. *American Journal of Orthopsychiatry*, **65** (4), 540–48.

Weinraub, M. and Wolf, B. M. (1983). Effects of stress and social supports on mother–child interactions in single- and two-parent families. *Child Development*, **54**, 1297–311.

Wicks, M. and Kiernan, K. (1990). *Family Change and Future Policy*, Joseph Rowntree Memorial Trust.

Wilson, M. N. and Tolson, T. F. J. (1988). Single parenting in the context of three generational black families. In *The Impact of Divorce, Single Parenting and Step-parenting on Children* (E. M. Hetherington and J. Arasteh, eds). Hillsdale, NJ: Lawrence Erlbaum Associates.

Woodgate, R. and Kristjanson, L. J. (1995). Young children's behavioural responses to acute pain: strategies for getting better. *Journal of Advanced Nursing*, **22**, 243–9.

Zani, B., Di Palma, A. and Vullo, C. (1995). Psychosocial aspects of chronic illness in adolescents with thalassaemia major. *Journal of Adolescence*, **18**, 387–402.

Zaslow, M. J. (1989). Sex differences in children's responses to parental divorce: 2. Samples, variables, ages and sources. *American Journal of Orthopsychiatry*, **59**, 118–41.

Zill, N. (1988). Behavior, achievement, and health problems among children in stepfamilies: findings from a national survey of child health. In *The Impact of Divorce, Single Parenting and Step-parenting on Children* (E. M. Hetherington and J. Arasteh, eds). Hillsdale, NJ: Lawrence Erlbaum Associates.

4

Age and parenting

Julia C. Berryman and Kate C. Windridge

Is there a 'right time' to have a baby? Much of the current media and political discussion about parenting suggests that there is – at least for mothers. We are concerned about both 'teenage' mothers and older women who have children, especially post-menopausal women. In this chapter, Julia Berryman and Kate Windridge investigate the experience of pregnancy, birth and parenting for mothers who have their first babies at the 'wrong time' and the outcomes for their children. Are the children of younger mothers neglected and abused, while those of older mothers are pampered and spoilt? Are older women more likely to experience pregnancy complications and post-natal depression? Is age itself important, or are the social and economic circumstances of women having children 'out of time' of greater significance? For example, is it the youth of teenage mothers which causes problems, or their poverty? Is age the only difference between 'older' and 'on-time' mothers, or are they also different in terms of education, social class and wealth?

Introduction

Patterns of childbearing vary in different cultures and at different historical times (for example, see Coale, 1992), yet for each culture at any given point in history there is a notion of the 'right time' to have a baby, and this view tends to be more tightly constrained for women than for men. Although the biological capacity of a woman to bear children spans almost 40 years (from 11–12 to 50–51 years on average), and that of men a rather longer period, there tends to be a consensus that it is desirable to restrict childbearing to a relatively short period in life. Those who become parents outside this time period – 'off-time' parents – are viewed rather negatively. These views on the timing of parenthood are reflected in some theories of the life-cycle, such as those of Erikson (1965) and Bühler (1968) where childbearing is generally seen as a task of the earlier part of adult life. With the greater availability of effective forms of contraception, it is generally assumed (in the developed world at least) that families are planned, and those who appear not to plan are often seen as lacking the qualities desirable in parents.

This chapter explores a range of issues surrounding parental age and the problems of carrying out research on this topic. It includes some discussion of current statistics on childbearing by parental age and the popular perceptions of parents of different ages. The chapter also includes discussion of the events before conception, i.e. decision making and family planning; the chances of conception at different ages; the age-related risks and problems for women becoming pregnant and giving birth at various ages; and finally the effects of parental age on child outcomes. The emphasis is on maternal rather than parental age, because researchers have so far focused on the former rather than the latter, although there are signs that this imbalance is slowly being rectified.

The chapter presents up-to-date information from a wide range of disciplines, which has central relevance to understanding whether, and if so why, a person's age might affect parenthood and parenting. We shall present the issue of parental age in the context of many other complex relationships of variables, all of which can have an impact on parenting. Parental age provides an interesting focus for research because it is an easily measured, 'visible' variable: however, as we hope to make clear, there are many issues that are much less quantifiable but probably much more important in predicting outcomes for parents and their children. These include well known ones such as socio-economic status, marital status and level of education (Hart and Risley, 1992; Arntzen, Moum, Magnus et al., 1995; Byrd and Weitzman, 1994; Chandola, Robling, Peters et al., 1992; Bradley, 1993) as well as exciting new evidence from the US that genes may influence a wider range of life-long processes than has been realized formerly (Reiss, 1995).

Problems of research on ageing

Psychologists are familiar with the problems of interpreting the findings of longitudinal and cross-sectional studies but, despite this, comparisons between older and younger parents have often failed to control adequately the many confounding variables already mentioned (e.g. socio-economic status). Cohort effects must also be considered: for example in comparing women who became mothers in the 1940s with those who had children in the 1960s any differences observed would be just as likely to result from variation between cohorts as from the age at which they became mothers (in addition to the factors already considered). Stereotypically, being an 'older' or 'younger' mother is associated with particular life features, although in reality these features are not intrinsic to a given age. For example, very young mothers are more likely to be unmarried (are bound to be if they are below the legal age for marriage), unemployed, and hence are also likely to be poor – these characteristics play a part in their capacity to be 'good' parents. Research comparing different age groups must compare groups of women whose background characteristics are equivalent, so that age effects are not confounded with other characteristics. Alternatively, regression analyses can identify the effects of variables such as age, education and so on, on outcomes for children and parents. Geronimus, Korenman and Hillemeier (1994) discuss the problems of age research in detail and they themselves use sister and cousin comparisons (i.e. women who experienced first births at different ages) to control for family background. This, of course, can provide an excellent match for family characteristics but has the disadvantage of tending to over-represent women from larger families in the sample. Berryman and Windridge, in their longitudinal study of older and average age mothers (1993, 1995) adopted a technique of pairing each older first-time mother ('target' mother) with a younger woman sharing her background characteristics (marital/partnership status, education, etc.). However, as they and other researchers have found (e.g. Constantine, Haynes, Spiker et al., 1993), recruitment of participants and/or drop out rates can also vary as a function of the ages of participants.

Reports of research that uses age as the explanation for differences between individuals of different ages must thus be interpreted with caution

– and due attention should be paid to how samples were recruited and the data analysed.

Age and fertility

Current fertility statistics

Over the last few decades, there has been a trend towards later parenthood. Currently the average age for all births, in England and Wales, is 28.1 years (data for 1993, Birth Statistics, 1995). This is the highest mean age for almost forty years. The percentage of all births by maternal age in England and Wales indicates that whilst 64.3 per cent of births are still to women under 30 years of age, over 10.3 per cent are to women aged 35 and over, whilst only 6.7 per cent are to women under the age of 20. Indeed, over the last ten years, the number of births to women over the age of 30 is increasing more rapidly than in any younger age group. Fertility fell in all other younger age groups (Birth Statistics, 1995).

The trend towards delayed parenthood is not unique to England and Wales. It is apparent throughout the developed world, as birth statistics from many countries show. For example, in Europe, Australasia and the Middle East, births to women aged 35 and over increased from between 5 and 6 per cent of all births in 1983 to between 8 and 14 per cent in 1989–91 (Demographic Yearbook, 1994) and similarly births in the younger age groups were decreasing during this time. Early parenthood is particularly prevalent in the United States, which has the highest rates of adolescent pregnancy and childbirth amongst western industrialized nations. Statistics show that 40 per cent of North American adolescent women become pregnant (at least once) before the age of 20, and 20 per cent of adolescent women bear a child (Rhode and Lawson, 1993).

The pattern of paternal age at birth is different from that of mothers. On average, fathers tend to be older than mothers, and the span of years during which they become parents is greater. Statistics for live births within and outside marriage show that men continue to become fathers well into old age (Birth Statistics, 1995). The number of live births within and outside marriage in 1993 to men aged 40 and over was 8.7 per cent, compared with just 1.6 per cent of live births to women in this age group. The bulk of live births are attributed to men under the age of 30, with a mere 1.7 per cent recorded to fathers under twenty. However, this last figure, which is much lower than the equivalent figure for women of this age (6.7 per cent) is more likely to reflect the fact that the father's name was not registered, than a true representation of paternities (over 50,000 births in 1993 in England and Wales were solely registered by women, across all age groups of mother, and one quarter of sole registrations are by mothers under the age of 20 (Birth Statistics, 1995)). Data on mothers under twenty tend to indicate, where age of the child's father is given, that the majority of these fathers are in their early 20s (Adams, Pitman and O'Brien, 1993).

Birth statistics alone do not give a complete picture of all maternities and it is not possible to gather a wholly complete picture of the outcome of all conceptions because some pregnancies end in miscarriage or stillbirth; and many of the former are unrecorded. However, one major category of pregnancy outcome which is recorded is legal abortion, and statistics for these reveal a very different picture of maternities by age. There were 157,846 abortions across all age groups in England and Wales in 1993 (Abortion Statistics, 1995). Of these 18.3 per cent were to women under the age of 20 and 12.2 per cent were to women aged 35 and over. Almost two-thirds of abortions were to single women and, as with births, the majority were to women in their 20s.

The proportion of abortions relative to live births tends to be greater in both younger and older mothers. In examining statistics on the outcome of maternities the proportion of abortions to live births by age group shows that in teenage girls and women abortions comprise nearly 40 per cent of the sum of these two categories of pregnancy outcome. It is of interest to note that until 1982 in England and Wales the number of abortions to women aged 40 and over exceeded the number of births and the only other age group that is equally high or higher than this in recent years has been girls under the age of 16 (Birth Statistics, 1989; 1995), thus suggesting that having a baby at either the top or the bottom of the age range is not perceived as right or desirable.

These figures reveal much about attitudes towards the age at which child-bearing is considered appropriate and indicate that being single, 'young' or 'old' are characteristics that increase the likelihood of abortion.

The popular perception of older and younger mothers

It has already been noted that the age when most women give birth is neither consistent over time nor across cultures. From the medical perspective there has been a tendency to stress that the 20s are the best time to have a baby; being very young or very old has been viewed as problematic. The psychological perspective on individuals as parents provides a slightly different view, but here too there is a tendency to justify the status quo. Price, in 1977, argued that there is a 'prejudice against the older parent' and Phoenix (1993) has described the social construction of teenage motherhood as 'overwhelmingly negative'.

At both ends of the natural age range for potential childbearing women are seen in terms of problems: social problems, medical problems for them and their babies, and in some cases psychological problems too – such as increased rates of depression and child abuse.

Phoenix (1993) summarizes the problem for the '*teenage, adolescent,* and *young mother* (especially in combination)' as follows: such mothers have been reported to have a 'high rate of unplanned pregnancies, to suffer from complications during pregnancy, to be depressed after birth, to gain few educational qualifications, and to be reliant on state provision of housing and money. Their children have similarly been found to achieve less than children born to older mothers and to be more likely to suffer accidental and non-accidental injuries' (Phoenix, 1993; Simms and Smith, 1986, p. 79).

The popular perception of the older mother is surprisingly similar. Pregnancy and birth complications are widely commented on in connection with older motherhood and Mansfield (1988) lists eight pregnancy outcomes commonly linked to the mother's increased age. In addition to these the age of the mother is associated with a variety of chromosomal abnormalities, in particular the increased risk of Down's syndrome (Nortman,

1974). Older mothers are perceived as not up to the task, physically, and Kern (1982) also stresses the fatigue aspects of later motherhood. Other researchers highlight the long term physical problems following childbirth that older mothers are more likely to experience (MacArthur, Lewis and Knox, 1991).

Wilkie (1981) has observed that older first-time motherhood is 'a recent strategy adopted by women interested in careers, especially those with higher education'. Such women are viewed as fitting motherhood into their lives, in a rather calculating way, around their paid work commitments and aspirations. However, in the past delayed marriage was a strategy which was used as a form of family planning at times when women were not expected to be sexually active outside marriage. Older women adding to their families are characterized as being women in second marriages or partnerships (see Berryman, Thorpe and Windridge, 1995). Younger and older fathers have, in general, received rather less attention than mothers in these age groups. Research on young fathers tends to highlight the ambivalence surrounding their position (Kiselica and Sturmer, 1993) and the relative lack of services available for teenage fathers compared to teenage mothers (see Cervera, 1991). Older fathers are rarely perceived as a problem or form the subject of research (see Berryman, Thorpe and Windridge, 1995).

Fecundity and fertility

Most young women assume that they are fecund – that they will become pregnant if they try to do so – but what is the risk of pregnancy after one act of intercourse? Establishing the likelihood of becoming pregnant for all women of a given age is a task that takes different forms at different ages. Fertility statistics merely tell us the number of babies born; they indicate nothing of the extent to which abstinence, contraceptive practices, abortion and so on influence the figures.

One factor that has, until recently, defined the outer limits of the ages for childbearing has been the age at menarche (first menstruation) and menopause (last menstruation). Today, the latter is not necessarily the upper limit because egg donation to a post-menopausal woman (or indeed the use of her own fertilized eggs stored at an earlier time in her life) extends the potential for childbearing.

Space does not permit a detailed discussion of menarche and the menopause but suffice it to say that, in the western world, there has been a dramatic decline in the age of the former of around four years since the 1800s, with current estimates indicating an average age of menarche of around 12.4 to 13.5 years (Tanner, cited in May, 1978). In England the menopause occurs around age 50, and at around 51 in North America (Gray, 1976; Khaw, 1992). Some authorities believe that the latter may also have changed in an upward direction but it is hard to establish the truth of this (Gray, 1976).

Menarche marks the first menstruation but not necessarily the first ovulation. Döring (1969, cited in Short, 1976) estimated, in a study of German girls, that 60 per cent of cycles are anovulatory in girls aged 12–14, 45 per cent in those aged 15–17 and 25 per cent in the 18–20 age group in this study. The maximum percentage of ovulatory cycles (95 per cent) did not occur until 26 to 30 years old. Ovulation was assessed using basal body temperature records and whilst this is not a perfect method of assessment Short (1976) argues that 'there are good reasons for believing that ovulatory failure is common in the post-menarchal years' (Short, 1976, p. 10). Thus fecundability (the probability of conception per menstrual cycle) is likely to be lower in sexually active post-menarcheal girls than in women in their late teens or 20s. Whilst this finding may lend support to an often quoted view by young girls that you cannot get pregnant at first-time intercourse, the latter has been shown to be a far from reliable belief.

Fertility statistics for natural populations with few or no restrictions on fertility come from historical data, and from a few selected groups of contemporary women. In a large study in France, of 15,000 women who were contestants in a large family competition after World War I, Vincent (1961, cited in Short, 1976) found that fecundability rose from 15 per cent at the age of 16, to 24 per cent at age 18–19 and reached a peak of 27 per cent at age 25. Similar figures have been found for the North American Hutterites (Eaton and Mayor, 1953). It should be noted that the fertile period per cycle usually lasts less than 48 hours and coital frequency to achieve the maximum probability of conception is 12 times per cycle (Short, 1976). Despite this the human conception rate compares very unfavourably with that in cattle where 75 per cent of animals conceive after a single artificial insemination at ovulation (Short, 1976).

Fecundability statistics are probably most reliable when taken from statistics of the success of artificial insemination as a function of age. These data are preferable to those for natural populations because they are not confounded by male infertility, and changes in the frequency of intercourse associated with increasing age and length of marriage or partnership, but of course they are not available for very young women.

Data from Schwartz and Mayaux (1982) are widely quoted in this area and these authors report a cumulative percentage success rate (achieving a pregnancy) of 73, 74.1, 61.5 and 53.6 for under 25, 26–30, 31–35 and over 35 years respectively. These results may appear relatively low – as Gosden (1985) has pointed out, partly due to factors such as stress associated with the secrecy generally surrounding AID and the use of frozen rather than fresh sperm. However, in a recent paper Gosden and Rutherford (1995) suggest that 'women planning to start a family late do well to weigh the biological consequences', because oocytes disappear faster from the ovary after the age of 37 and in their view fertility 'is almost gone by 40'. Estimates of sterility by age produce a much more optimistic picture: Henry's data puts this at 3 per cent in married women at 20 years, 10 per cent at 30 years and 31 per cent at 40 years (Henry, 1961).

Family planning and age

In what way does age influence the extent to which women and men plan their families? There is a widely held assumption that the pregnancies of very young mothers are unplanned, whilst those of older women are more calculated – what is the evidence to support this contention?

In a paper on unintended pregnancies Fleissig (1991) showed that about one-third of pregnancies are unintended (in England and Wales); this study was concerned with pregnancies that lead to babies and excludes those that are terminated. If abortion statistics are added to this figure we find that approximately half of all pregnancies are unintended and/or terminated. Such a high figure tends to suggest that use of reliable contraception is much less widespread than is commonly assumed. Planning of pregnancies is probably the highest in women in their 30s; Fleissig's (1991) survey found that approximately one quarter of babies born to women over 30 are unintended (25.4 per cent), compared to 26.6 per cent in the 25–29 age group, 44.4 per cent in the 20–24 age group and 56.9 per cent in the under 20s. Frankel and Wise (1982) who compared older mothers (women aged 33 and over) with younger mothers (those in their 20s) found that all the older ones had postponed childbearing voluntarily whereas the younger women had made less conscious choices about when to bear a child. Welles-Nystrom and de Chateau (1987) found a similar pattern. Research on mothers over 40 however produced a rather different picture. Berryman and Windridge (1991) reported that less than half the babies in a study of mothers of 40 and over were planned, and amongst first-time mothers 40 per cent were linked to fertility problems – making the 'planning' aspects hard to gauge (one participant in this study had planned her baby 21 years before its eventual arrival).

Amongst much younger mothers the reasons behind teenage pregnancies are widely discussed. In the United States around 80 per cent of pregnancies to girls and women of this age are unintended: this is often described as the problem of 'children having children' (Rhode and Lawson, 1993) and there is much moral panic surrounding this issue (Phoenix, 1993). However, it must be stressed that this pattern is common in some communities and ethnic groups. Pearce (1993) points out that teenage motherhood 'is both normative and traditional' for some groups, such as black women in the US, among whom 40 per cent have become mothers before the age of 20 throughout the twentieth century.

Most would view pregnancies to teenagers of 18 or 19 as entirely different from those of much younger teenagers; the latter are viewed as problematic for a variety of reasons. Boxer (1992) argues that many people are distinctly uncomfortable about adolescent girls expressing their sexuality whereas this generally does not apply to boys who are perceived as focused on obtaining sexual pleasure at this stage. Such young women may be perceived as lacking sexual desire and as being passive victims. This leads to an ambivalent attitude towards contraception. Rhode and Lawson (1993) suggest that 'by letting intercourse "just happen" female adolescents seek to avoid being stigmatised as either prudish or promiscuous' (p. 8). Other research indicates that many teenage sexual experiences may be due to coercion, rather than choice. Moore, Nord and Peterson (1989) indicate that 5.8 per cent of white women and 2.0 per cent of black women between the ages of 18 and 22 report having non-voluntary sexual intercourse when they were less than 14 years old.

In contrast to this highly negative view, Phoenix (1993) points out that the problem aspects of many teenage pregnancies are overstated. In a national study of British teenage mothers and their partners, Simms and Smith (1984) found that only 11 per cent of those interviewed one year after their child was born reported that they were sorry they had become mothers when they did. In her own study, Phoenix (1991a) also found positive attitudes towards becoming a mother at this age in her sample of 16–19 year olds. Twenty two per cent of her sample wanted to conceive, and a further 25 per cent did not mind whether or not they conceived, 28 per cent had not thought about it and 35 per cent considered it important not to conceive. Almost all her sample knew about and had used contraception, so that lack of knowledge of contraception could not be used as an explanation for these pregnancies.

Miscarriage

Once conception has occurred, what is the effect of the age of the mother on the viability of the pregnancy? One of the most obvious possibilities is the likelihood of miscarriage and here the higher the age of mother the greater the risk of miscarriage. Estimates of the incidence of miscarriage vary from study to study (see Warburton and Fraser, 1964; Hansen, 1986; Virro and Shewchuk, 1984). In one study the rate was reported to be 12.2 per cent for women under the age of 20, 18.7 per cent at ages 35–39 and 25.5 per cent at age 40 (Warburton and Fraser, 1964). Hansen (1986) estimates the incidence to be from 7.2–15 per cent for women in their 20s, with a rate of increase of about 50 per cent from the 20s to the 30s and a two- to four-fold increase in women above 40 when compared with those in their 20s. From the point of view of staying pregnant, the younger the mother the better. However, one factor which militates against this is the likelihood of inadequate health care in pregnancy found in very young pregnant girls and women (to be discussed later).

Assisted conception

For those women who cannot achieve a pregnancy there is the possibility of becoming pregnant by one of the many forms of treatment now available. Infertility can be a problem at any age but as a woman gets older her fertility declines and thus the older would-be mother is very likely to seek help to conceive and/or maintain a pregnancy (see Berryman, Thorpe and Windridge, 1995). Today it is theoretically possible for a woman of almost any age, both before and after the menopause, to achieve a pregnancy if she has a uterus and is in good health. The technique that is now used (see Sauer, Paulson and Lobo, 1992) involves the use of an egg from a younger woman that is fertilized and inserted into the uterus of the older woman who has been stimulated hormonally so that she can receive it (see Berryman, Thorpe and Windridge, 1995, for fuller discussion). The 'younger' fertilized egg has a good chance of implanting in the wall of the uterus because most of the problems of the older mother (prior to the menopause) are with the quality of her eggs, rather than her uterus (Abdalla, Burton, Kirkland et al., 1993) and thus, with hormone treatment, a woman approaching the menopause or a post-menopausal woman can achieve conception and maintain a pregnancy.

The issue of motherhood after the natural age for menopause (around 50) is a very controversial one. Mary Warnock (who chaired the Committee of Inquiry into Human Fertilization in 1982–84) believes it is 'inherently wrong and offensive' but her view is opposed by others (Warnock, 1993). Natural motherhood still occurs in a small proportion of women after the age of 50 (in Britain the oldest natural mother of recent years was aged 59 – see Narayan, Buckett, McDougall et al., 1992) and worldwide there are many other cases (see Berryman, Thorpe and Windridge, 1995). For example, figures for Europe alone show that in one year (1989) there were 716 live births to women of 50 and over, and this does not include 10 European nations for which data were not available (Demographic Yearbook, 1994). Sauer (1993) in the US feels strongly that we are prejudiced against the older woman in a way that we are not against older men who wish to become parents. He argues for the use of donor eggs to enable an older woman to conceive 'if it's OK for a man . . . if it's fine to use donor sperm for his young wife, why isn't it OK for the 55 year-old woman if she wants to have a 25 year-old husband?' In her paper 'Something old, something new, something borrowed, and something taboo?' van den Akker (1994) argues forcefully the case that the right to reproduce should not be withheld from older women. It should be borne in mind that many older women care for younger children very successfully as foster mothers or grandparents, and in the authors' view, assisting older women to become mothers should neither be encouraged nor discouraged – it should be a personal matter for the woman, her partner and the doctor from whom treatment is sought (see Berryman, Thorpe and Windridge, 1995, for fuller discussion of the issue). There is no doubt that the issue of post-menopausal motherhood will continue to be discussed and, in future, the options for women delaying motherhood will be the storage of eggs collected when she is young for later use. Potentially a woman could store her eggs in her 20s and not use them for several decades. Such a possibility puts the notion of 'family planning' into a whole new perspective.

Age and pregnancy

Having discussed the effects of age on fertility and conception, we shall now look at how parental age affects the well-being of parents and child once pregnancy is achieved. One of the most obvious issues in this context is the question of ability to maintain a healthy developing fetus. There are several important factors to take into account when interpreting research which examines possible links between maternal age and complications of pregnancy, such as how long ago the research was carried out (for instance, women of 35 and over in the 1990s tend to be healthier than women of that age even 20 years ago), the number of women who were studied, how they were selected, what sort of women they were, and whether the study took into account variables such as socio-economic status, income, occupation, health behaviours and so on which may vary *with* age but are not necessarily *caused* by age. Age is something which cannot be changed. Risk factors that vary with age (such as smoking, or lack of education) can be changed.

It has been argued that pregnant women over 35 are at increased risk of a range of medical problems when compared to women of 'average age'. Mansfield (1988) argues that the majority of the studies she reviewed in this area suffered from methodological flaws. This conclusion was also reached by Harker and Thorpe four years later (1992). More recently, our review with Thorpe examined the current evidence on increased maternal age

and risks to mother and child of miscarriage, hypertension, placental complications, prolonged labour, pre-term delivery, maternal mortality, infant
perinatal mortality, abnormal birthweight, poor health at delivery and
abnormality in the infant (Berryman, Thorpe and Windridge, 1995). The
evidence cited in this review suggests that women over 35 may be at a slightly
increased risk of some pregnancy complications but that parity, educational
status and occupation need to be taken into account. Research published
since that review tends to support that conclusion. For instance, although
older mothers are slightly more likely to be overweight or to have high blood
pressure *before* pregnancy (Bobrowski and Bottoms, 1995), it is important to
bear in mind that these and some other risks are lower in first-time older
mothers than in women who have already had children. The overwhelming
consensus from many countries in the midwifery literature is that raised
maternal age, as a risk factor during pregnancy and birth, is becoming less
important because the 'risks' are becoming more manageable as antenatal,
obstetric, and perinatal care improve (Prysak, Lorenz and Kisly, 1995;
Roberts, Algert and March, 1994; Fujimoto, Makinoda and Hoshi, 1994).
There is an established link between increased maternal age and risk of some
chromosomal abnormalities, such as Down's syndrome, although a recent
study (Baird, Sadovnick and Yee, 1991) found that so far as non-chromo-
somal abnormalities are concerned (e.g. dislocatable hip) babies of older
mothers are *less* likely to be affected than those of younger or average-age
mothers.

Adolescence is an interesting time because as Hamburg and Dixon (1993)
point out it is the age-range within which there are most likely to be marked
discrepancies between three different ways of looking at age: chronological,
biological, and social. A 12 year old can be biologically older, but chrono-
logically younger, than a 14 year old if the former has reached menarche and
the latter has not; and whether or not the two ages are perceived as having
reached maturity by the rest of society (social construction of age) will
depend on their particular culture. Western, developed societies tend to use
chronological age as a marker, but this does not necessarily match biological
age. Hamburg and Dixon point out that from the social view of age, adolescence now starts earlier and finishes later than formerly because of the downward trend in age at menarche (biological age), and a corresponding upward
trend in the age at which people complete their education and move on to
earning an income. Pregnant teenagers of 18 or 19 have passed biological,
chronological and social markers: they are physically mature, are legally
allowed to marry, and are closer to the normative age for childbearing
than are those of school age. The issues faced by pregnant women of 17
and under are thus rather different from those faced by those aged 18 and 19.

As was pointed out earlier, female humans are reaching puberty earlier
than in former centuries. Therefore, their biological readiness for childbearing is less of a problem than is sometimes portrayed. However, there is
evidence to suggest that sexual maturity is not necessarily accompanied
by cognitive and emotional maturity – as Petersen and Crockett note
(1993) 'Increased menarcheal age was related to only a few cognitive and
achievement measures' (p. 38). Hamburg and Dixon (1993) argue that
psychological immaturity may have an impact on the health of mothers and
children in that it may lead teenage mothers of school age to postpone

pre-natal care. US figures suggest that in recent years nearly two-thirds of pregnant mothers under 15 did not start pre-natal care in the first trimester of pregnancy, and at least one-fifth either failed to obtain pre-natal care or waited until the last trimester to do so. This is worrying not because of these expectant mothers' young age per se but because mothers and infants, regardless of maternal age, are at higher risk of health complications (e.g. delivering a low birthweight baby) if they do not receive attention from health professionals early in pregnancy.

Why do some teenagers delay seeking antenatal care? They may wish to conceal the pregnancy, as may pregnant women of any age. It has also been suggested that young teenagers are prone to believe in a 'personal fable' of invulnerability (see Hamburg and Dixon, 1993), which could lead them to believe that pregnancy will not happen to them and even if it does, no problems will arise: although this argument makes the assumption that all teenage pregnancies are unintended which is not necessarily the case as we noted earlier.

Overall, then, the experience of pregnancy for adolescent mothers may differ (but does not necessarily do so) from that of older women. When it does, it is because of factors other than chronological age per se which are experienced by women of any age, but are more 'noticeable' when pregnancy occurs outside the age-range within which it is seen as normal. In this respect women of 35 and over may share some of the experiences of adolescent mothers. However, they are dramatically different from adolescent women, at least if they are first-time mothers, in their experiences and attitudes to the involvement of health care professionals. Older *multiparous* women may have a 'relaxed' view of seeking help during pregnancy, and after birth there is evidence that this is so (Kaplan and Mascie-Taylor, 1992). However, women of 35 or more, pregnant for the first time, may find their contacts with health professionals play an important role in their pregnancy.

Antenatal screening

Because of the link between raised maternal age and increased incidence of chromosomal abnormalities such as Down's syndrome, women who are pregnant in their late 30s or 40s are likely to take antenatal screening very seriously, although serum screening for Down's syndrome is now offered to increasing numbers of younger women as well. Most women welcome the reassurance of the *results* of antenatal screening and diagnosis; however, the process leading up to the results can be extremely stressful because women and their families are asked to make decisions based on statistical probabilities, which is something that human information processing is not well equipped to do. The statistical information offered after serum screening tends to be framed negatively rather than positively and this has an impact on whether or not prospective parents will opt for amniocentesis (Marteau, 1989). There is also evidence that women of 35 and more compared with those in their 20s, may 'put off' expressing their attachment to the fetus until after mid-pregnancy, although there is little evidence that this has long term effects (Berryman and Windridge, 1993; 1995, 1996). Although prospective parents do find it difficult to use probabilistic information (such as that contained in serum screening results) as a basis for deciding whether

or not to undergo amniocentesis, serum screening can identify many pregnancies where the chances of having a Down's syndrome baby are lower than
would be expected on the basis of maternal age alone (Haddow, Palokami,
Knight et al., 1994). These researchers argue that because of this, more than
half of amniocenteses could be avoided by using serum screening, thus reducing the risk of miscarriage (associated with the procedure of amniocentesis)
for these pregnancies. Interestingly, the tendency to prefer not to have
amniocentesis increases with increased maternal age (Beekhuis, De Wolf,
Mantingh et al., 1994). These issues are covered in depth elsewhere
(Berryman, Thorpe and Windridge, 1995) but are mentioned here to explain
why antenatal screening may differ for older and younger mothers.

In summary, so far as physiological fitness is concerned, there is much
evidence to support the idea that the outlook has never been better, especially
for older women who are pregnant. As one physician put it: 'From an obstetrician's point of view a healthy woman of 38 is less of a risk than an
unhealthy woman of 28' (Collee, 1991, p. 66).

Pregnancy and psychosocial issues

Depression (or its absence) during pregnancy is an important predictor of
depression (or its absence) after birth, which in turn is associated with various problems later on (e.g. Radke-Yarrow, Nottelman, Martinez et al., 1993
and Chapter 6). On the whole, evidence suggests that older women, particularly those expecting their first baby, are not at increased risk of depression,
and may be at less risk of depression than average-aged mothers (see
Berryman, Thorpe and Windridge, 1995). This may be partly explained by
the tendency for such women to be advantaged in terms of health, income,
education and occupational status (De Wit and Rajulton, 1992; Grindstaff,
Balakrishnan and De Wit, 1991).

Pregnant teenagers have often been found to be a distressed group
(Haskett, Johnson and Miller, 1994) although researchers emphasize again
and again that it is not their age per se that places them at a disadvantage in
this or in other respects. Neither is it true that very young mothers are
doomed to social isolation and loneliness: one study showed that in
Britain, women having babies at 16 are 'likely to be living with or near
(their) family, gaining social support and practical services from them. The
loneliest women, and those least well integrated into helpful networks, are
often the geographically mobile middle-class women who do not have their
first babies until their late 20s' (MacIntyre and Cunningham-Burley, 1993,
p. 66).

In the media, teenage motherhood is often perceived as 'a problem', and is
equated with unpartnered or unmarried status. There is a corresponding
tendency for single status to be viewed as problematic. Does the nature (or
existence) of the relationship between prospective parents actually have a big
impact on the outcome of pregnancy, and does this vary with age? The
message to be gleaned from research is that even if very young unpartnered
mothers have sometimes been found to be at a disadvantage, it is not clear
whether this is due to being young, being without a partner, or to a complex
combination of factors. Certainly the few studies on single older mothers
(e.g. Linn, 1991) do not suggest that single status per se is a problem. Where

partners do cohabit or are married, the quality of their relationship (whether they are satisfied with each other's level of understanding and so on) is a good predictor not only of how well they will relate to each other as a couple after birth but also of how smoothly the new baby is incorporated into the family (see, for example, Broom (1994) and discussion in Berryman, Thorpe and Windridge (1995)). There is some evidence that couples of different ages differ in the ways they cope with the everyday problems that arise in any relationship. One researcher reports that coping by showing physical affection and initiating shared activities was common among older couples (those above 40) whereas more negative responses to problems (e.g. worry, difficulty sleeping, conflict, criticism, sarcasm) were at their most frequent in the 20–29-year-old group and then fell to lowest levels with increasing age (Bowman, 1990).

Birth

Does a woman's age make a difference to what happens to her and her baby during labour and delivery? There are two main factors at work here: the first is the issue of whether an older, or younger, than average body can cope with the physiological side of labour and delivery. The second is the psychological side of the equation, which is very hard to separate from the physiological processes. Problems faced by teenagers giving birth tend to be related to factors other than their youth on its own, such as lack of antenatal care. Very young teenage mothers are likely to be having their first baby. However, just because a mother is under 20 does not mean that she will *not* be multiparous. At the opposite end of the age spectrum, most mothers of 35 and over have already given birth before. This means that age and parity tend to be confounded in some older studies. Recent research is more likely to distinguish between nulliparous and multiparous mothers, for instance, taking the case of caesarean section rate, one study found that among multiparous teenagers giving birth to medium-weight infants, caesarean rates were only 3 per cent, compared with 59 per cent for primiparous women of 40 or more with very heavy infants (Parrish, Holt, Easterling et al., 1994). In another recent study (Albers, Lydon-Rochelle and Krulewitch, 1995) 7792 low-risk, first-time mothers with a wide range of ages (teenage to over 30s) were studied. The *only* labour complication that varied significantly across these groups was caesarean section: teenagers were the least likely, and the oldest mothers were the most likely, to have a caesarean delivery (rates were 11.6 per cent and 28.3 per cent respectively). The interesting thing about this age difference was that caesarean delivery rates could not be explained by medical indications alone: caesarean delivery was also associated with being socially advantaged, and as we have already pointed out, older first-time mothers are likely to be advantaged.

A further recent comparison of 25–29 and 35+ women found slightly higher complication rates among the older groups, although despite this maternal and perinatal outcomes were good (Prysak, Lorenz and Kisly, 1995). There is some evidence that women of different ages may use different methods of pain relief (Prysak, Lorenz and Kisly, 1995; Roberts, Algert and March, 1994; Berryman and Windridge, 1995) and may differ in terms of the chances of pre-term delivery or breech presentation (Roberts, Algert and March, 1994).

One Scandinavian study found a steady rise with maternal age in the length of the second (but not the first) stages of labour. This held true for both 'first-time' and multiparous mothers (Rasmussen, Bungum and Hoie, 1994). Berryman and Windridge (1995) also found that multiparous mothers of 35 and over had a longer second stage than multiparae in their 20s, although in this study no such relationship emerged for primiparae. The overall message here is that, when considering a very wide range of ages, there are many factors more important than maternal age alone in determining the incidence of complications during birth.

Physical recovery from pregnancy and birth

Women sometimes express concern about recovering their physical fitness and body image after birth. Older women, in particular, may be concerned about whether their older body will 'let them down' during the rigours of coping with a new baby. There is evidence to suggest that the number of health problems experienced by women of all ages in the months and years following childbirth has been underestimated: MacArthur, Lewis and Knox (1991) followed up more than 11,000 women and said that the study '. . . revealed an enormous and previously unrecognised problem: a level of post-partum morbidity and impaired health far beyond anything which might have been suspected' (p. 57). They point out that not all new post-partum health problems were related directly to obstetric factors. What is of concern here is that many women sought no help with their problems, many of which had become chronic and long term. Does a woman's age affect her chances of suffering from health problems after birth? Research suggests that this may depend on the symptoms being investigated. Taking the most frequently experienced symptoms first, MacArthur et al. found that 23.3 per cent of women experienced post-delivery, longer term backaches. Age did not affect this, although women under 25 were more likely than those over 25 to say that they were suffering from backache for the *first* time. So far as headaches were concerned, long term, frequent headaches and/or migraine, newly occurring after delivery, were reported by 1 in 20 women. The researchers suggest that some headaches were part of a syndrome including backache, associated with epidural anaesthesia – no age effects were present. A second syndrome of post-partum headache consisted of headache unaccompanied by backache – this was not postural nor associated with epidurals, and occurred most frequently among younger (under 25) multiparous women.

Other musculo-skeletal problems (excluding backache and headache) were reported by approximately 1 in 12 women, but maternal age was not a factor associated with frequency of occurrence. Over 20 per cent of women reported stress incontinence within 3 months of delivery: although for one quarter of these the problem was not new, the majority of these had already had a baby. In the case of this symptom, increasing maternal age was associated with an increased likelihood of suffering stress incontinence in both primiparae and multiparae, and following both caesarean section and vaginal delivery, despite the fact that caesarean section was found to be slightly 'protective' against stress incontinence. Stress incontinence was more likely to become chronic with increasing maternal age. Haemorrhoids occurring for the first time after childbirth were reported by 1 in 12 women, but age did not affect their frequency.

Research in the area of fatigue suggests that older women are more likely than younger women to suffer from extreme tiredness after birth (MacArthur, Lewis and Knox, 1991; Berryman and Windridge, 1995). In line with this, older women may be particularly likely to express a need for extra 'practical help' (housework, etc.) after birth (Berryman and Windridge, 1995); but overall the evidence is that the number, and age, of a woman's other children are more important here than maternal age alone. There are many more similarities than differences between different age groups and where there *are* differences older mothers are not necessarily at a disadvantage.

Emotional well-being after birth

Does a woman's age have any bearing on emotional adjustment to parenthood, and does this in turn have any impact on the baby? There is no clear-cut relationship between maternal age and the likelihood of suffering from depression after childbirth, although depression during pregnancy and lack of emotional support do tend to be associated with suffering from depression after birth. At the positive end of the emotional spectrum, Dillon and Totten (1989) reported that older mothers 'used humour significantly more as a coping device, had higher hardiness scores, higher IgA levels in their saliva, and lower rates of upper respiratory tract infections in themselves and their infants' (p. 161) than did younger mothers. Ages in this study ranged from 16 to 41. Although this was a very small study, the interesting point about the findings is that they highlight the relationship between physical and emotional well-being: IgA levels are one measure of the body's immune response, which has been shown to be related to various psychological factors, such as stress and loneliness, according to research cited by Dillon and Totten. Psychological hardiness, as measured in this research, was defined as a combination of feeling a sense of internal control and meaningfulness, and having an attitude of vigorousness towards the environment; it would therefore seem unlikely to be compatible with depression. In one study of mothers of pre-term babies, women of 28 and over were found to be more optimistic about their infant's future and were also more likely to claim that they thought about their infant 'all the time' than mothers in the under 28 age group. Unfortunately, as the researchers point out, age and socioeconomic status were confounded in this study, so although the findings may be of interest it would not be wise to conclude that the difference was entirely due to maternal age (Chatwin and MacArthur, 1993). Brooten, Gennaro, Brown et al. (1988) found no relationship between maternal age and anxiety, depression or hostility. Kelley, Power and Wimbush (1992) suggest that being a younger mother tends to go with higher levels of stress, and that this in turn may lead to a more 'parent-centred' attitude to discipline. However it is unlikely that it is youth per se that causes higher stress.

Feeding, sleeping and caretaking

Breastfeeding is of great interest in the context of this chapter because it is a phenomenon which *does* vary considerably with maternal age. Teenagers are less likely to breastfeed than are older mothers (Peterson and DaVanzo, 1992) and there are a variety of reasons for this including low levels of income and education but also, possibly, developmental aspects of adolescence such as concern about body image. With increasing maternal age the incidence of breastfeeding increases, and this has been reported in more than one country. It is also apparent that older mothers who breastfeed tend to do so for longer than do younger mothers, and that there is a correlation between being older, breastfeeding for longer, and having raised educational and occupational status (Ever-Hadani, Seidman, Manor et al., 1994, in Israel; Vestermark, Hogdall, Plenov et al., 1991, in Denmark; Kern, 1982, in the US; Berryman and Windridge, 1995, in the UK). This gives rise to interesting speculations because some researchers have linked duration of breastfeeding with other parenting practices. For instance, DeMan (1989) argued that extended breastfeeders tended to be less hostile, controlling and rejecting in the way they treated their children later.

Sleeping and lack of sleep are likely to feature prominently in the thoughts of new parents. Does age matter here? Lack of sleep is a problem for parents of any age, although as we have seen older parents may feel the effects of this lack more. In 1991 Becker, Chang, Kameshima and Bloch looked at the relationship between sleep and stress in single mothers and found that adolescent mothers' babies, when compared with adult mothers' babies, did less of their sleeping during the night and that this occurred particularly in association with high levels of stress in a mother. Infants whose mothers had more emotional support had more predictable patterns of sleep than did infants of less well-supported mothers. There is some evidence that parents in different age groups may have different ideas about how to approach sleeping – for instance women of 35 and over are more likely than those in their 20s to have their infants sleeping for all or part of the night in bed with them (Berryman and Windridge, 1995). This may be related to the higher breastfeeding duration in this group. Practices vary historically: Crawford (1994) found that in one particular group (Basque women), elderly women, referring to their own children born half a century earlier, often said that they had had their child sleeping with them in bed until the age of four or five whereas contemporary mothers were less likely to say this. Various reasons have been suggested for historical changes in co-sleeping (see Morelli, Oppenheim, Rogoff et al., 1992); one with relevance to parental age is that the necessity for physical proximity to keep a baby warm has decreased: these days death from hypothermia is very rare among infants. However, medical professionals are beginning to identify a link between low socio-economic status, being a younger mother, and over-heating in babies, and there are some suggestions that there could be links between these factors and Sudden Infant Death Syndrome (Bacon, Bell, Clulow et al., 1991; Arntzen, Moum,

Magnus et al., 1995). It must be stressed that the links between over-heating and SIDS are extremely tentative, but the issues need clarification. The dangers of hypothermia were very real for babies in the 1960s, but now that those babies are becoming parents themselves the prevalence of central heating in the developed world has meant that there is less need for them to use large quantities of insulating bedclothes, compared with their parents.

Will any age-related differences in feeding and sleeping 'show up' in a child's later life? It is difficult to say, because maternal age is not usually the only distinguishing factor in the groups of mothers who are compared. However, looking ahead, Pollock (1994) found that night-waking at age five was linked to some symptoms of emotional distress, and to certain medical conditions, five years later when the children were ten. However, mothers of under 17 were significantly less likely than mothers of 25 and over to report high levels of night-waking. Pollock suggests a tentative link with other factors including the use of forceps or vacuum extraction during delivery.

All the studies cited here are likely to reflect the social and cultural norms not only of the place and group within which they are carried out but also its time: norms change over time even within one group and this is as true of breastfeeding and sleeping practices as it is of other aspects of childrearing.

Outcomes for children of parents of different ages

What are the long term consequences for children of having relatively young or old parents? Although not a widely researched area, it is one that has grown in recent years. We shall outline the effects of parental age, at both the top and bottom of the age-range, and once again there will be greater emphasis on mothers' age effects than fathers' (see Rosenheim and Testa, 1992; Lawson and Rhode, 1993; Berryman, Thorpe and Windridge, 1995).

It is widely believed in the western world that teenage motherhood may produce children who have a range of problems and difficulties later on; evidently Hitler (see Stone cited in Phoenix, 1991b) had this view, and in general children of such mothers are often seen as being subject to child abuse, dependence on welfare benefits and having poor educational outcomes (Phoenix, 1991a and b) to name only a few of their difficulties.

As has already been mentioned, it is vital to disentangle the factors other than age that have confounded many of the studies of teenage motherhood before it is fair to draw conclusions about the effects of age per se. Geronimus, Korenman and Hillemeier (1994) question whether teenagers are 'best understood as teenagers or as socioeconomically disadvantaged women' (p. 585), since there is an over-representation of the latter amongst teenage mothers. When socio-economic differences are controlled the findings have not always been consistent. Some research (e.g. Finkelstein and Ramey, 1980; Brooks-Gunn and Furstenberg, 1986) favours children of older or average-age mothers whereas other research finds very little evidence that teenage motherhood per se has adverse effects on measures of child development once other variables are controlled (e.g. Byrd and Weitzman, 1994; Ketterlinus, Henderson and Lamb, 1991; Chambers and Grantham-McGregor, 1986; Bradley, 1993). Phoenix (1991a) in her studies of mothers aged 16–19 years old, found a number of positive advantages in her sample. Eighty per cent of her sample of women had previous experience of caring for young children, and in general they were aware of ideas about childrearing, thus a charge of ignorance about these matters could hardly be aimed at them – something that other research has not always found in older more economically advantaged women (e.g. Boulton, 1983). Phoenix also found that few of her young mothers had paid work whilst their baby was small and while this is consistent with society's view of the 'good mother' it is often perceived as a problem in women who are both young and single because they are perceived as a drain on the state. Phoenix (1991a) did not find evidence that her sample of teenage mothers were 'bad' mothers, but they were undoubtedly poor and single.

The claim that adolescent parenthood is linked to increased rates of child maltreatment (see Phoenix, 1993 for discussion) has been questioned by Massat (1995). In an analysis of demographic data in Illinois she found no evidence that adolescent parents were over represented amongst maltreating parents. Massat also stresses that age itself is not a very reliable predictor of child outcomes because it is correlated with a large number of other variables that may be of greater significance in determining such outcomes. Connelly and Straus (1992) studied nearly 2000 families and suggested that low income and low educational levels at time of birth could explain the association they found between maternal youth and greater rate of child abuse.

Research on the outcomes for children of older mothers is patchy and incomplete – and much of it lacks adequate controls for background characteristics identified at the start of this chapter. Children's intellectual development has been linked to age of the mother (see Ragozin, Basham, Crnic et al., 1982; Zybert, Stein and Belmont, 1978; Wadsworth, Taylor, Osborn et al., 1984). Ragozin and colleagues (1982) reported that children of older mothers do better: 'consistent results have been obtained from studies of different countries, race, social classes, and child ages' (p. 627). This was evident when variables such as education and social class were controlled. The reason for this difference is not clear but may be related to maternal attitudes and behaviour – for example older mothers are said to encourage verbalization in children more than younger mothers and to foster greater independence in their children (Seth and Khanna, 1978). More recent studies do not necessarily reveal this association of intellectual development with maternal age in a clear-cut way (e.g. Byrd and Weitzman, 1994; Fergusson and Lynskey, 1993).

Styles of interacting with children may differ as a function of parental age. Australian research (Thorpe and Cinnamon, 1992) found that older mothers were more responsive to their infants when they cried; infants were also taken out to more organized activities. Analogous findings are reported by Lojkasek, Goldberg, Marcovitch and MacGregor (1990) and Broom (1994). Other research (MacDonald and Parke, 1986) indicates that older parents engage in less physical play with their children, and that as fathers engage in physical play more than mothers, this negative correlation with parental age may have an impact on sex-role appropriate behaviour in the opinion of the authors of the study. Sons of older fathers might be viewed as relatively disadvantaged compared with those of younger fathers, or alternatively older adults may be viewed as providing less stereotypical sex-role training for their children: the authors cite evidence that older adults are more androgynous than younger ones. Yarrow (1991) has commented that the large generation gap between children and older parents can have an impact on the family climate. He argues that older parents are often perceived as more 'emotionally distant, serious, and formal' (p. 89) but some children of older parents report feeling the freedom of not having to compete with parental ambitions and desires sometimes felt between children and more youthful parents. Yarrow's study was based on anecdotal accounts and thus must be viewed with some caution.

Family life

There are many different types of 'family' so we shall restrict our discussion to aspects of 'being part of a family' that may vary with parental age. Although young mothers are often single, many live with their families of origin and their own mother often helps out with childcare (see Dellmann-Jenkins, Sattler and Richardson, 1993). Such support can be seen as enabling the mother to adequately meet her child's needs whilst also completing her education and preparing for future employment. In their study of adolescent parents, Dellmann-Jenkins, Sattler and Richardson (1993) found that over three-quarters of the mothers of the adolescent mothers believed that their child was likely to turn to them for any kind of support (emotional, financial and so on). Mothers reported feeling fully confident in their children's parenting abilities, but many believed that they needed additional support for their child to be a better and more self-confident parent.

One of the dilemmas for some adolescent mothers is the relationship between them, their baby's father, and their own parents. Cervera (1991) in a small study of unwed teenage pregnancy, found that it was common for the teenage mother's parents to be very distant with the baby's father even when he tried to remain involved. Cervera concluded that some teenage mothers have to choose between their parents', or the baby's father's, support and that this may have consequences for a child's social and cognitive development. Other studies (e.g. Oyserman, Radin and Benn, 1993) suggest that the grandfather's role may become important, and have direct beneficial effects on child outcomes, where the father is not involved. Kelly (1995) was interested in adolescent mothers' preventative health care and found that those 14–17 year olds who maintained a relationship with their child's father were more likely to practise better preventative health care than those who did not.

Some studies have suggested a link between delaying parenthood and being likely to hold non-traditional gender roles, to attempt to pass on egalitarian values to children, or to have been involved in political activism as a younger person (Robinson, Olmsted, Garner et al., 1988; Weisner and Wilson-Mitchell, 1990; Dunham and Bengston, 1994). These findings may have implications for how parents of different ages deal with issues as their children get older as it is found that for women who do paid work their gender role ideology tends to predict their marital stability: women who have a non-traditional view of gender roles tend to have more stable marriages when they do more hours of paid work, whereas no such relationship exists for 'traditional' women (Greenstein, 1995). In the area of family interactions, age (because it is easy to measure) has as usual been the focus of attention in studies which link adolescent motherhood to lower levels of expressiveness, less delight and less positive mother–infant interaction generally (e.g. Culp, Culp, Osofsky and Osofsky, 1991; Baranowski, Schilmoeller and Higgins, 1990) and to lower levels of knowledge about child development at least at some stages (Gullo, 1988). However, researchers looking at parental age increasingly recognize the need to take into account a parent's socio-economic status, because this is linked to child-rearing practices and family roles. For instance, Hart and Risley (1992) suggest that the amount of 'parenting' per hour, and quality of the verbal content of parenting are strongly related to socio-economic status (and the subsequent IQ of the child).

Where a child has two parents, there is evidence that the nature of the parents' relationship with each other is important – for instance Australian researchers have found that even if children are subjected to several changes of parent (through separation, remarriage, etc.) this does not have an impact on measurable aspects of their behaviour such as juvenile offending whereas exposure to discord between parents during early and middle childhood does lead to increased risks of offending. In this case it appears that family changes such as separations and reconciliations between parents, in the absence of discord, were less damaging than discord without separation or other changes (Fergusson, Horwood and Lynskey, 1992). Some researchers (Umberson, 1989; Belsky and Rovine, 1990) suggest that delayed parenthood may be linked with greater marital happiness not only in the 1980s and 1990s, but seventy years ago (Heuvel, 1988). However, not all studies confirm this (Berryman and Windridge, 1995; Windridge and Berryman, in press).

Paid work and age of mother

In recent years, research is blossoming in the area of multiple roles (mother, partner, employed person, etc.) in women's lives, particularly in the US. The economic climate is shifting so that in many respects it 'makes sense', for instance, for women in seriously disadvantaged families in urban North America to start and finish childbearing very early (i.e. in their teens) so that they are still under their own parental roof, and by the time their children are old enough to go to school they themselves are still in their early 20s and can still compete effectively in the job market, such as it is. Such women do not necessarily miss out and may be at an advantage in terms of education or occupational progress when compared with their contemporaries who do not have children while still in their teens.

At the upper end of the spectrum, it makes sense if a woman is living in advantaged circumstances (middle-class, well-educated, etc.) for her and her partner to delay childbearing until their earnings are sufficient to support a family – and this is happening later than it used to, historically, as the nature of paid work shifts with the technological changes of our time.

Parents who undertake paid work, particularly mothers, may be concerned about whether their absence from home will affect their children. The type of work undertaken and the childcare arrangements used may depend on how old a mother is: mothers who start their families early are most likely to live near their own family and may thus use them for childcare, and are quite likely to do this without paying them. Older women are most likely to be in well-paid jobs and may be more likely to pay for childcare (nursery, nanny, rather than childminder, for instance) (Berryman, Thorpe and Windridge, 1995; Berryman and Windridge, 1995).

Conclusions

In this chapter, we have outlined research that has examined 'off-time' parenthood, and in particular motherhood. Our focus has been young (teenage) mothers and older mothers (chiefly those of 35 and over). Research findings show that age per se is responsible for relatively few major differences in pregnancy, birth and child outcomes. More recent research has found that earlier studies often confounded age with other variables such as social class and once these are controlled age effects are relatively minimal. There is no doubt that the experience of pregnancy and motherhood may be different at different ages, but it is vital to remember that the stereotyping of mothers by virtue of age, as we saw in the popular perceptions of older and younger mothers, does little to assist them through a pregnancy and into parenthood. For older women the experience of pregnancy is undoubtedly changed by the ever present worry of the increased risk of chromosomal abnormalities and antenatal screening (see Berryman and Windridge, 1993, 1996; and Berryman, Thorpe and Windridge, 1995). But there is no doubt that as Maroulis (1991) has pointed out in today's developed societies 'women in their early 40s are young . . .' (p. 116) and their chances of a successful pregnancy are probably better than a woman of any age in Third World countries, or younger women in past times in developed countries. True there are slightly increased risks to her and her baby relative to a healthy woman in her 20s, but these should not be over stressed. From the psychological perspective there are a number of real advantages to later motherhood for both mothers and children, and set against some of the slightly increased medical risks and differences in parenting styles shown in parents of different ages the conclusion can only be that each age of parent has something to offer as well as some disadvantages. Becoming a parent is a very personal matter for the two individuals concerned, in itself age should not be viewed as of overriding importance. In general as Geronimus, Korenman and Hillemeier (1994) observed, are teenage mothers 'best understood as teenagers or as socioeconomically disadvantaged women?' (p. 585). Economic and marital status are just two of many factors that have an enormous impact on parenthood and parenting. Our understandable tendency to focus on easily measurable variables such as age should not blind us to the importance of acknowledging that researchers need to broaden their view of what is 'normal' in parenting; as Ambert (1994) points out, research to date has been biased because it arises largely from a western paternalistic definition of mothering (to the exclusion of carers other than the mother). We need to be fully aware, through research, of the conditions that promote successful parenthood/parenting and ensure that appropriate conditions are available to parents at what ever age they opt, by choice or otherwise, to become parents.

(Manuscript received January 1996)

Applications

1. Be cautious in interpreting observed age differences

Do not assume that any differences observed that are linked to a particular age group are always caused by age per se. Just because age is easily identified and recorded, it does not mean that it explains why two age groups differ. Many things correlate with age that are not caused by age (e.g. income) and even when researchers have controlled for these variables, cohort effects may confound the findings.

2. Don't make assumptions about the best time for becoming a parent

There has been a tendency to assume that the 'normal' or right time to have a baby is the average age for births. Yet the average age has varied in different cultures and periods of history. Currently, with the trend to delay childbearing, the average age is increasing. Professionals working with mothers and babies should avoid classifying mothers as too old or young for motherhood. Research evidence finds differences between age groups in parenting styles but value judgements about the age for becoming a parent should be avoided. Parents at any age have much to offer and should be supported.

Further reading

Berryman, J. C., Thorpe, K. C. and Windridge, K. (1995). *Older Mothers: Conception, Pregnancy and Birth After 35*. London: Pandora.

Rosenheim, M. K. and Testa, M. F. (eds) (1992). *Early Parenthood and Coming of Age in the 1990s*. New Brunswick, New Jersey: Rutgers University Press.

Lawson, A. and Rhode, D. L. (eds) (1993). *The Politics of Pregnancy: Adolescent Sexuality and Public Policy*. New Haven: Yale University Press.

References

Abdalla, H. I., Burton, G., Kirkland, A., Johnson, M. R., Leonard, T., Brooks, A. A. and Studd, J. W. W. (1993). Age, pregnancy and miscarriage: uterine versus ovarian factors. *Human Reproduction*, **8** (9), 1512–17.

Abortion Statistics (1995). *Legal Abortions Carried Out Under the 1967 Abortion Act in England and Wales, 1993*. Series AB, No. 20. London: HMSO.

Adams, G., Pitman, K. and O'Brien, R. (1993). In *The Politics of Pregnancy: Adolescent Sexuality and Public Policy* (A. Lawson and D. L. Rhode, eds). New Haven: Yale University Press.

Albers, L. L., Lydon-Rochelle, M. T. and Krulewitch, C. J. (1995). Maternal age and labor complications in healthy primigravidas at term. *Journal of Nurse-Midwifery*, **40** (1), 4–12.

Ambert, A. M. (1994). An international perspective on parenting: social change and social constructs. *Journal of Marriage and the Family*, **56**, 529–43.

Arntzen, A., Moum, T., Magnus, P. and Bakketeig, L. S. (1995). Is the higher postneonatal mortality in lower social status groups due to SIDS? *Acta Pediatrica Scandinavica*, **84** (2), 188–92.

Bacon, C. J., Bell, S. A., Clulow, E. E. and Beattie, A. B. (1991). How mothers keep their babies warm. *Archives of Disease in Childhood*, **66** (5), 627–32.

Baird, P. A., Sadovnick, A. D. and Yee, I. M. L. (1991). Maternal age and birth defects: a population study. *Lancet*, **337** (8740), 527–30.

Baranowski, M. D., Schilmoeller, G. L. and Higgins, B. S. (1990). Parenting attitudes of adolescent and older mothers. *Adolescence*, **25**, 781–90.

Becker, P. T., Chang, A., Kameshima, S. and Bloch, M. (1991). Correlates of diurnal sleep patterns in infants of adolescent and adult single mothers. *Research in Nursing and Health*, **14** (2), 97–108.

Beekhuis, J. R., de Wolf, B. T. H. M., Mantingh, A. et al. (1994). The influence of serum screening on the amniocentesis rate in women of advanced maternal age. *Prenatal Diagnosis*, **14** (3), 199–202.

Belsky, J. and Rovine, M. (1990). Patterns of marital change across the transition to parenthood: pregnancy to three years postpartum. *Journal of Marriage and the Family*, **52** (1), 5–20.

Berryman, J. C. and Windridge, K. C. (1991). Having a baby after 40. I: a preliminary investigation of women's experience of pregnancy. *Journal of Reproductive and Infant Psychology*, **9**, 3–18.

Berryman, J., Thorpe, K. and Windrigde, K. C. (1995). *Older Mothers: Conception, Pregnancy and Birth After 35*. London: Pandora.

Berryman, J. C. and Windridge, K. (1993). Pregnancy after 35: a preliminary report on maternal attachment to the foetus as a function of parity and maternal age. *Journal of Reproductive and Infant Psychology*, **11**, 169–74.

Berryman, J. C. and Windridge, K. C. (1996). Pregnancy after 35 and attachment to the fetus. *Journal of Reproductive and Infant Psychology*, **14**, 133–43.

Berryman, J. C. and Windridge, K. C. (1995). *Motherhood After 35: A Report on the Leicester Motherhood Project*. Leicester University and Nestlé UK Ltd.

Birth Statistics (1995). *Review of the Registrar General on Births and Patterns of Family Building in England and Wales, 1993*. Series FM1, No. 16. London: HMSO.

Birth Statistics (1995). *Review of the Registrar General on Births and Patterns of Family Building in England and Wales, 1993*. Series FM1, No. 22. London: HMSO.

Bobrowski, R. A. and Bottoms, S. F. (1995). Underappreciated risks of the elderly multiparous. *American Journal of Obstetrics and Gynaecology*, **172** (6), 1764–70.

Bogenschneider, K. and Steinberg, L. (1994). Maternal employment and adolescents' academic achievement: a developmental analysis. *Sociology of Education*, **67** (19), 60–77.

Boulton, M. G. (1983). *On Being a Mother: A Study of Women with Pre-School Children*. London: Tavistock Publications.

Bowman, M. (1990). Coping efforts and marital satisfaction: measuring marital coping and its correlates. *Journal of Marriage and the Family*, **52**, 463–74.

Boxer, A. M. (1992). Adolescent pregnancy and parenthood in the transition to adulthood. In *Early Parenthood and Coming of Age in the 1990s* (M. K. Rosenheim and M. F. Testa, eds). New Brunswick, New Jersey: Rutgers University Press.

Bradley, R. H. (1993). Children's Home Environment, health, behaviour and intervention efforts: a review using the HOME inventory as a marker measure. *Genetic, Social, and General Psychology Monographs*, **119** (4), 437–90.

Brooks-Gunn, J. and Furstenberg, F. F. (1986). The children of adolescent mothers: physical, academic and psychological outcomes. *Developmental Review*, **6** (3), 224–51.

Broom, B. L. (1994). Impact of marital quality and psychological well-being on parental sensitivity. *Nursing Research*, **43** (3), 138–43.

Brooten, D., Gennaro, S., Brown, L. P., Butts, P., Gibbons, A. L., Bakewell-Sachs, S. and Kumar, S. P. (1988). Anxiety, depression and hostility in mothers of pre-term infants. *Nursing Research*, **37** (4), 213–16.

Bühler, C. (1968). The development and structure of goal setting in group and individual studies. In *The Course of Human Life* (C. Bühler and F. Massarik, eds). New York: Springer.

Byrd, R. S. and Weitzman, M. L. (1994). Predictors of early grade retention among children in the United States. *Pediatrics*, **93** (3), 481–7.

Cervera, N. (1991). Unwed teenage pregnancy: family relationships with the father of the baby. *Families in Society*, **71** (1), 29–37.

Chambers, C. M. and Grantham-McGregor, S. M. (1986). Patterns of mental development among young, middle class Jamaican children. *Journal of Child Psychology and Psychiatry and Allied Disciplines*, **27** (1), 117–23.

Chandola, C. A., Robling, M. R., Peters, T. J., Melville-Thomas, G. and McGuffin, P. (1992). Pre- and perinatal factors and the risk of subsequent referral for hyperactivity. *Journal of Child Psychology and Psychiatry and Allied Disciplines*, **33**, 1077–90.

Chatwin, S. L. and MacArthur, B. A. (1993). Maternal perceptions of the preterm infant. *Early Childhood Development and Care*, **87**, 69–82.

Coale, A. J. (1992). Age of entry into marriage and the date of the initiation of voluntary birth control. *Demography*, **29** (3), 333–41.

Collee, J. (1991). A doctor writes. *Observer Magazine*, **87**, 69–82.

Connelly, C. D. and Straus, M. A. (1992). Mother's age and risk for physical abuse. *Child Abuse and Neglect*, **16** (5), 709–18.

Constantine, W. L., Haynes, C. W., Spiker, D., Kendall-Tackett, K. and Constantine, N. A. (1993). Recruitment and retention in a clinical trial for low birth weight, premature infants. *Journal of Developmental and Behavioural Pediatrics*, **14** (1), 1–7.

Crawford, C. J. (1994). Parenting practices in the Basque Country: implications of infant and childhood sleeping location for personality development. *Ethos*, **22** (1), 42–82.

Culp, A. M., Culp, R. E., Osofsky, J. D. and Osofsky, H. J. (1991). Adolescent and older mothers' interaction patterns with their six-month-old infants. *Journal of Adolescence*, **14**, 195–200.

De Wit, M. L. and Rajulton, F. (1992). Education and timing of parenthood among Canadian women: a cohort analysis. *Social Biology*, **39**, 109–22.

Dellmann-Jenkins, M., Sattler, S. H. and Richardson, R. A. (1993). Adolescent parenting: a positive, intergenerational approach. *Families in Society*, **74** (10), 590–601.

DeMan, A. (1989). Early feeding practices and subsequent childrearing attitudes of French Canadian women. *Perceptual and Motor Skills*, **68** (3 Pt 1), 879–82.

Demographic Yearbook (1994). Department for Economic and Social Information and Policy Analysis: New York, United Nations.

Dillon, K. M. and Totten, M. C. (1989). Psychological factors, immunocompetence, and health of breast-feeding mothers and their infants. *Journal of Genetic Psychology*, **150** (2), 155–62.

Döring, G. K. (1969). Cited in Short, R. V. (1976). The evolution of human reproduction. *Proceedings of the Royal Society of London*, B. **195**, 3–24.

Dunham, C. C. and Bengston, V. L. (1994). Married with children: protest and the timing of family life course events. *Journal of Marriage and the Family*, **56**, 224–8.

Eaton, J. W. and Mayor, A. J. (1953). The social biology of very high fertility among the Hutterites: the demography of a unique population. *Human Biology*, **25** (3), 206–64.

Erikson, E. H. (1965). *Childhood and Society*. Harmondsworth: Penguin.

Ever-Hadani, P., Seidman, D. S., Manor, O. and Harlap, S. (1994). Breast-feeding in Israel; Maternal factors associated with choice and duration. *Journal of Epidemiology and Community Health*, **48** (3), 281–5.

Fergusson, D. M. and Lynskey, M. T. (1993). Maternal age and cognitive and behavioural outcomes in middle childhood. *Paediatric and Perinatal Epidemiology*, **7** (1), 77–91.

Fergusson, D. M., Horwood, L. J. and Lynskey, M. T. (1992). Family change, parental discord and early offending. *Journal of Child Psychology and Psychiatry and Allied Disciplines*, **33** (6), 1059–75.

Finkelstein, N. W. and Ramey, C. (1980). Information from birth certificates as a risk index for educational handicap. *American Journal of Mental Deficiency*, **84** (6), 546–52.

Fleissig, A. (1993). Unintended pregnancies and the use of contraception: changes from 1984 to 1989. *British Medical Journal*, **302**, 147.

Frankel, S. A. and Wise, M. J. (1982). A view of delayed parenting: some implications of a new trend. *Psychiatry*, **45** (3), 220–25.

Fujimoto, S., Makinoda, S. and Hoshi, N. (1994). Elderly pregnancy and labor. *Asian Medical Journal*, **37** (3), 117–30.

Geronimus, A. T., Korenman, S. and Hillemeier, M. M. (1994). Does young maternal age adversely affect child development? Evidence from cousin comparisons in the United States. *Population and Development Review*, **20** (3), 585–609.

Gosden, R. G. (1985). *Biology of Menopause: The Causes of Consequences of Ovarian Ageing*. London: Academic Press.

Gosden, R. G. and Rutherford, A. (1995). Delayed childbearing: fertility declines at 30 and is almost gone by 40. *British Medical Journal*, **311**, 1585.

Gray, R. H. (1976). The menopause–epidemiological and demographic considerations. In *The Menopause* (R. J. Bearch, ed.). Lancaster: MTP Press.

Gray, R. H., Campbell, O. M., Ruben, A., Eslami, S. S., Zacur, H., Ramos, R. M., Gehret, J. C. and Labbok, M. H. (1990). Risk of ovulation during lactation. *The Lancet*, **335** (Jan. 6), 25–9.

Greenstein, T. N. (1995). Gender ideology, marital disruption and the employment of married women. *Journal of Marriage and the Family*, **57**, 31–42.

Grindstaff, C. F., Balakrishnan, T. R. and De Wit, D. J. (1991). Educational attainment, age of first birth, and lifetime fertility: an analysis of Canadian fertility survey data. *The Canadian Review of Sociology and Anthropology*, **28**, 324–9.

Gullo, D. F. (1988). A comparative study of adolescent and older mothers' knowledge of infant abilities. *Child Study Journal*, **18** (3), 223–31.

Haddow, J. E., Palomaki, G. E., Knight, G. J. et al. (1994). Reducing the need for amniocentesis in women 35 years of age or older with serum markers for screening. *New England Journal of Medicine*, **330** (16), 1114–18.

Hamburg, B. A. and Dixon, S. L. (1993). Adolescent pregnancy and parenthood. In *Early Parenthood and Coming of Age in the 1990s* (M. K. Rosenheim and M. F. Testa, eds). New Jersey: Rutgers University Press.

Hansen, J. (1986). Older maternal age and pregnancy outcome: a review of the literature. *Obstetrical and Gynecological Survey*, **41** (11), 726–34.

Harker, L. and Thorpe, K. (1992). 'The last egg in the basket?' Elderly primiparity – A review of findings. *Birth*, **19**, 23–30.

Hart, B. and Risley, T. R. (1992). American parenting of language-learning children: persisting differences in family–child interactions observed in natural home environments. *Developmental Psychology*, **28** (6), 1096–105.

Haskett, M. E., Johnson, C. A. and Miller, J. W. (1994). Individual differences in risk of child abuse by adolescent mothers: assessment in the perinatal period. *Journal of Child Psychology and Psychiatry and Allied Disciplines*, **35** (3), 461–76.

Henry, L. (1961). Some data on natural fertility. *Eugenics Quarterly*, **8**, 81–91.

Heuvel, A. V. (1988). The timing of parenthood and intergenerational relations. *Journal of Marriage and the Family*, **50**, 483–91.

Kaplan, B. A. and Mascie-Taylor, C. G. (1992). Mother's age, birth order and health status in a British national sample. *Medical Anthropology*, **13** (4), 353–67.

Kelley, M. L., Power, T. G. and Wimbush, D. D. (1992). Determinants of disciplinary practices in low-income black mothers. *Child Development*, **63**, 573–82.

Kelly, L. E. (1995). Adolescent mothers: what factors relate to level of preventive health care sought for their infants? *Journal of Pediatric Nursing*, **10** (2), 105–13.

Kern, I. (1982). '. . . an endless joy', the culture of motherhood over 35. *Papers in the Social Sciences*, **2**, 43–56.

Ketterlinus, R. D., Henderson, S. and Lamb, M. E. (1991). The effects of maternal age at birth on children's cognitive development. *Journal of Research on Adolescence*, **1** (2), 173–88.

Khaw, K. T. (1992). Epidemiology of the menopause. *British Medical Bulletin*, **48** (2), 249–61.

Kiselica, M. S. and Sturmer, P. (1993). Is society giving teenage fathers a mixed message? *Youth and Society*, **24** (4), 487–501.

Lawson, A. and Rhode, D. L. (1993). *The Politics of Pregnancy: Adolescent Sexuality and Public Policy*. New Haven: Yale University Press.

Linn, R. (1991). Mature unwed mothers in Israel: socio-moral and psychological dilemmas. *Lifestyles: Family and Economic Issues*, **12** (2), 145–70.

Lojkasek, M., Goldberg, S., Marcovitch, S. and MacGregor, D. (1990). Influences on maternal responsiveness to developmentally delayed preschoolers. Special issue: families. *Journal of Early Intervention*, **14** (3), 260–73.

MacArthur, C., Lewis, M. and Knox, E. G. (1991). *Health After Childbirth*. London: HMSO.

MacDonald, K. and Parke, R. D. (1986). Parent–child physical play: the effects of sex and age of children and parents. *Sex Roles*, **15** (7–8), 367–78.

MacIntyre and Cunningham-Burley (1993). Cited in *The Politics of Pregnancy: Adolescent Sexuality and Public Policy*. (A. Lawson and D. L. Rhode, eds). New Haven: Yale University Press.

Mansfield, P. K. (1988). Midlife childbearing: strategies for informed decision making. Special issue: women's health: our minds, our bodies. *Psychology of Women Quarterly*, **12** (4), 445–60.

Maroulis, K. T. (1992). Epidemiology of the menopause. *British Medical Bulletin*, **48** (2), 249–61.

Marteau, T. M. (1989). Framing of information: its influence upon decisions of doctors and patients. *British Journal of Social Psychology*, **28**, 89–94.

Massat, C. R. (1995). Is older better? Adolescent parenthood and maltreatment. *Child Welfare*, **74** (2), 325–36.

May, R. M. (1978). Human reproduction reconsidered. *Nature*, **272**, 491–5.

Moore, K. A., Nord, C. W. and Peterson, J. L. (1989). Nonvoluntary sexuality among adolescents. *Family Planning Perspectives*, **21**, 110–14.

Morelli, G. A., Oppenheim, D., Rogoff, B. and Goldsmith, D. (1992). Cultural variations in infants' sleeping arrangements: questions of independence. *Developmental Psychology*, **28** (4), 604–13.

Narayan, H., Buckett, W., McDougall, W. and Cullimore, J. (1992). Pregnancy after fifty: profile and pregnancy outcome in a series of elderly multigravidae. *European Journal of Obstetrics, Gynaecology and Reproductive Biology*, **47** (1), 47–51.

Nortman, D. (1974). Parental age as a factor in pregnancy outcome and child development. *Reports of Population/Family Planning*. No. 16, New York: Population Council.

Oyserman, D., Radin, N. and Benn, R. (1993). Dynamics in a three-generational family: teens, grandparents and babies. *Developmental Psychology*, **29** (3), 564–72.

Parrish, K. M., Holt, V. L., Easterling, T. R. et al. (1994). Effect of changes in maternal age, parity, and birth weight distribution on primary cesarean delivery rates. *Journal of the American Medical Association*, **271** (6), 443–7.

Pearce, D. M. (1993). Children having children: teenage pregnancy and public policy from the women's perspective. In *The Politics of Pregnancy: Adolescent Sexuality and Public Policy* (A. Lawson and D. L. Rhode, eds). New Haven: Yale University Press.

Petersen, A. C. and Crockett, L. J. (1993). Adolescent sexuality, pregnancy, and child rearing: developmental perspectives. In *Early Parenthood and Coming of Age in the 1990s* (M. K. Rosenheim and M. F. Testa, eds). New Brunswick: Rutgers University Press.

Peterson, C. E. and Da Vanzo, J. (1992). Why are teenagers in the United States less likely to breast-feed than older women? *Demography*, **29**, 431–50.

Phoenix, A. (1991a). *Young Mothers?* Cambridge: Polity Press.

Phoenix, A. (1991b). Mothers under twenty: outsider and insider views. In *Motherhood: Meanings, Practices and Ideologies: Gender and Psychology* (A. Phoenix, A. Woollett and E. Lloyd, eds). London: Sage Publications.

Phoenix, A. (1993). The social construction of teenage motherhood: a black and white issue? In *The Politics of Pregnancy: Adolescent Sexuality and Public Policy* (A. Lawson and D. L. Rhode, eds). New Haven: Yale University Press.

Pollock, J. I. (1994). Night-waking at five years of age: predictors and prognosis. *Journal of Child Psychology and Psychiatry and Allied Disciplines*, **35** (4), 699–708.

Price, J. (1977). *You're Not Too Old To Have a Baby*. New York: Faivar, Straus and Giroux.

Prysak, M., Lorenz, R. P. and Kisly, A. (1995). Pregnancy outcome in nulliparous women 35 years and older. *Obstetrics and Gynaecology*, **85** (1), 65–70.

Radke-Yarrow, M., Nottelman, E., Martinez, P., Fox, M. B. and Belmont, B. (1993). Young children of affectively ill parents: a longitudinal study of psychosocial development. *Annual Progress in Child Psychiatry and Child Development*, 191–212.

Ragozin, A. S., Basham, R. B., Crnic, K. A., Greenberg, M. T. and Robinson, N. M. (1982). Effects of maternal age on parenting role. *Developmental Psychology*, **18** (4), 627–34.

Rasmussen, S., Bungum, L. and Hoie, K. (1994). Maternal age and duration of labor. *Acta Obstetrica et Gynecologia Scandinavica*, **73** (3), 231–4.

Reiss, D. (1995). Genetic influence on family systems: implications for development. *Journal of Marriage and the Family*, **57**, 543–60.

Rhode, D. L. and Lawson, A. (1993) Introduction. In *The Politics of Pregnancy: Adolescent Sexuality and Public Policy* (A. Lawson and D. L. Rhode, eds). New Haven: Yale University Press.

Roberts, C. L., Algert, C. S. and March, L. M. (1994). Delayed childbearing – are there any risks? *Medical Journal of Australia*, **160** (9), 539–44.

Robinson, G. E., Olmstead, M., Garner, D. M. et al. (1988). Transition to parenthood in elderly primapiras. *Journal of Psychosomatic Obstetrics and Gynaecology*, **9**, 89–101.

Rosenheim, M. K. and Testa, M. F. (eds) (1992). *Early Parenthood and Coming of Age in the 1990s*. New Brunswick: Rutgers University Press.

Sauer, M. (1993). In *Cheating Time*. A Horizon programme transmitted on 11 January on BBC2. (Quotation from the published text, page 11.)

Sauer, M. V., Paulson, R. J. and Lobo, R. A. (1992). Reversing the natural decline in human fertility. An extended clinical trial of oocyte donation to women of advanced reproductive age. *Journal of the American Medical Association*, **9:268**, 1275–9.

Schwartz, D. and Mayaux, M. J. (1982). Female fecundity as a function of age. *New England Journal of Medicine*, **306** (7), 404–6.

Seth, M. and Khanna (1978). Childrearing attitudes of the mothers as a function of age. *Child Psychiatry Quarterly*, **11** (1), 6–9.

Short, R. V. (1976). The evolution of human reproduction. *Proceedings of the Royal Society of London*, **195**, 3–24.

Simms, M. and Smith, C. (1986). *Teenage Mothers and Their Partners*. Department of Health and Social Security Research Report. No. 15. London: HMSO.

Stets, J. (1990). Verbal and physical aggression in marriage. *Journal of Marriage and the Family*, **52**, 501–14.

Tanner, J. M. Cited in R. M. May (1978). Human reproduction reconsidered. *Nature*, **272**, 491–5.

Thorpe, K. and Cinnamon, J. (1992). The timing of motherhood. Unpublished Research Report. University of Queensland, Department of Psychology.

Umberson, D. (1989). Relationships with children: explaining parents' psychological well-being. *Journal of Marriage and the Family*, **51**, 999–1012.

van den Akker, O. B. A. (1994). Something old, something new, something borrowed, and something taboo. *Journal of Reproductive and Infant Psychology*, **12**, 179–88.

Vestermark, V., Hogdall, C. K., Plenov, G., Birch, M. and Toftager-Larsen (1991). The duration of breastfeeding. A longitudinal prospective study in Denmark. *Scandinavian Journal of Social Medicine*, **19** (2), 105–9.

Vincent, P. (1961). Cited in Short, R. V. (1976). Evolution of human reproduction. *Proceedings of the Royal Society of London*. B. **195**, 3–24.

Virro, M. R. and Shewchuk, A. B. (1984). Pregnancy outcome in 242 conceptions after artificial insemination with donor sperm and effects of maternal age on the prognosis for successful pregnancy. *American Journal of Obstetrics and Gynaecology*, **148**, 518–24.

Wadsworth, J., Taylor, B., Osborn, A. and Butler, N. (1984). Teenage mothering: child development at five years. *Journal of Child Psychology and Psychiatry and Allied Disciplines*, **25** (2), 305–13.

Warburton, D. and Fraser, F. C. (1964). Spontaneous abortion risks in man. Data from reproductive histories collected in a medical genetics unit. *American Journal of Human Genetics*, **16**, 1–25.

Warnock, M. Cited in A. Neustatter (1993). Pioneer in the laboratory of life. *The Independent*, 3 August.

Weisner, T. S. and Wilson-Mitchell, J. E. (1990). Nonconventional family lifestyles and sex typing in six-year-olds. *Child Development*, **61**, 1915–33.

Welles-Nystrom, B. L. and de Chateau, P. (1987). Maternal age and transition to motherhood: prenatal and perinatal assessments. *Acta Psychiatrica Scandinavia*, **76** (6), 719–25.

Wilkie, J. R. (1981). The trend towards delayed parenthood. *Journal of Marriage and the Family*, **43** (3), 583–91.

Windridge, K. C. and Berryman, J. C. (1996). Maternal adjustment and maternal attitudes during pregnancy and early motherhood in women of 35 and over. *Journal of Reproductive and Infant Psychology*, **14**, 45–55.

Yarrow, A. L. (1991). *Latecomers – Children of Parents Over 35*. The Free Press, Macmillan.

Zybert, P., Stein, Z. and Belmont, L. (1978). Maternal age and children's ability. *Perceptual and Motor Skills*, **47**, 815–18.

5

Post-partum experiences

Anne Woollett and Paula Nicolson

From a medical perspective, most women are 'fit and well' after childbirth, immediately capable of taking on the physical and emotional demands of infant care, as the current trend towards 'drive-thru deliveries' suggests. From a 'bonding theory' perspective, immediate contact with the newborn baby is essential for the development of good relationships. From a woman's perspective, the post-partum days are a time of intense and changeable emotions, from euphoria to the 'baby blues'. Can all these different perspectives be understood and reconciled? Post-partum experiences for both mothers and fathers have largely been neglected in both health care, and research. Although we know a great deal about psychological aspects of childbirth itself (see Chapters 9, 10 and 11 in Volume 2) and the feelings women describe in the weeks and months after childbirth (see Chapter 6), very little attention has been paid to the first days after birth. In this chapter, Anne Woollett and Paula Nicolson begin to remedy this omission by describing the research which does exist and bring together the different perspectives on post partum by considering the tasks and issues which mothers (and fathers) need to address in these early days.

Introduction

The term 'post partum' is used to refer to the days and weeks after childbirth (sometimes also called 'post natal'). Interest in the post partum takes a variety of forms, ranging from the physical recovery of mothers from childbirth, the establishment of infant feeding, attachment and mother–child relations, the well-being and 'adjustment' of mothers (and sometimes fathers) including post-natal depression. The post partum, and especially the experiences and perspectives of women themselves, has generated less interest compared with pregnancy and childbirth from the health professions and social sciences, and from consumer groups such as National Childbirth Trust.

This chapter draws on research and discussion of the post partum from a variety of perspectives, medical/health, psychological and social sciences, to identify a range of issues of relevance and salience to women and their families and to health care providers. We examine some of the differing theoretical approaches, the medical management of the post partum, in the hospital and home environment, and the feelings and experiences of mothers, fathers and the wider family.

Throughout the chapter we draw on research findings (and omissions in research/theorizing) to identify some of the key tasks and issues for women in the post partum and to argue that women's experiences encompass complex bodily changes, feelings and emotions, and changing identities and social relations. We point to the diversity of women's experiences, well-being and adjustment and suggest how these might be associated with differences amongst women and their coping strategies, as well as the social and economic circumstances in which they are having children (see also Chapter 3). In doing this we encourage the reader to examine critically some assumptions about what are 'normal' feelings and adjustment in the post partum, and some implications for practice.

Theoretical approaches to the post partum

In contrast to medical approaches to pregnancy and delivery as potentially problematic and as requiring active management, in the post partum women are viewed as 'fit and well' and requiring little medical care. This approach is challenged by research which details the longer term medical problems of birth interventions (Davis-Floyd, 1994; Glazener, Abdalla, Russell and Templeton, 1993). The medical management of childbirth is also criticized because it can detract from women's emotional and psychological experience and the establishment of mother–child relations in the early post-partum days (Kitzinger, 1978; Oakley, 1979). This is argued in a recent UK Government Report 'Changing Childbirth' (1993) in which good post-partum care is defined as placing women 'at the centre of maternity services which should be planned and provided with their interests and those of their babies in mind' (Changing Childbirth, Department of Health, 1993, p. 3).

Psychological approaches to the post partum have focused on the child rather than the mother and on the impact of early experiences for their later development and social relations. Psychological research points to the range of perceptual abilities which babies demonstrate and their potential for sociability (Fogel, 1993; Stratton, 1982, and see Chapters 8 and 9). Theories of attachment, drawing on psychological and psychodynamic approaches to the early weeks and months of life, consider that early mother–child relations provide the basis for the development of attachment. An extreme version of attachment theory (so-called 'bonding' theory) takes this further to argue that mother–infant contact in the first hours of life is an essential ingredient for later attachment (Klaus and Kennell, 1982). While there is little evidence to support 'bonding' theory (Niven, 1992; White and Woollett, 1992; Svedja, Campos and Emde, 1980), recognition of the early competence of babies and the desire of mothers (and fathers) to have contact with their babies as soon as they are born has brought about changes in the management of delivery. It is now common for mothers (and others) to hold (and even to feed) their babies as soon as they are born, and for babies to stay with mothers on the post-natal wards.

Psychological approaches to the post partum also consider the emotional significance for women (and sometimes fathers) as they become parents and begin to develop a relationship with their baby. For first time parents the post partum marks an important phase in the transition to parenthood as parents take on their new identities and acquire parenting skills. Even when parents are looking forward to their new role, the post partum is not necessarily an easy time and their feelings and experiences do not necessarily match their expectations (Clulow, 1982; Belsky and Kelly, 1994; Parr, 1996; White and Woollett, 1992; Nicolson, 1986). Psychological research and interest is largely concerned with identifying problems and pathology (especially post-natal depression). As a result, there is less consideration given to the range, diversity and complexity of feelings and experiences, and the implication of these for parents, their wider social networks and health professionals (Nicolson, 1986; Nicolson, 1991/2).

In contrast the social sciences place greater emphasis on the social and cultural significance and implications of the post partum. Anthropological approaches, for example, emphasize the cultural significance of the post partum for women and their families. The early post-partum days are viewed as an intermediate state/time between being childless and being a mother, when women are often considered to be 'polluted' and women and babies as vulnerable, not only physically but spiritually and socially (Jones and Doughtery, 1982; Kitzinger, 1978). As a result, women are often excluded from activities such as preparing food, and engaging in social gatherings (Raphael-Leff, 1991; Woollett and Dosanjh-Matwala, 1990a; Davis-Floyd, 1994; Dobson, 1988). Feminist and social science approaches point to the significance of childbirth for women's identities and relationships, as they incorporate the new baby into the network of the family and other relationships, and as they renegotiate a relationship with their partner.

The medical management of the post partum

The post-partum hospital stay

In western societies childbirth usually takes place in hospital and the process of medical management started in pregnancy continues into the post partum (Niven, 1992; Jones and Doughtery, 1982). Women spend time in hospital after delivery, but in the UK and in the USA the length of hospital stay is now much shorter than in the past, often less than 48 hours, prompting the use of the term 'drive thru deliveries' in the USA. The emphasis in this immediate post-partum period is on the physical recovery of the mother and the baby from childbirth and the establishment of infant feeding (Niven, 1992). While medical approaches continue to view pregnancy and childbirth as risky and problematic, ideas about the post partum are changing. In the past newly delivered women were considered to need hospital care to allow them to rest and recover from childbirth. Increasingly they are considered 'fit and well' and hence as capable of taking responsibility for looking after themselves and their babies, and as requiring only a minimum of hospital care (Davis-Floyd, 1994; Niven, 1992). In emphasizing that women are 'fit and well' the impact of delivery and medical intervention for many women is underestimated. Delivery itself is tiring and while some women do feel well and welcome the opportunity to care for their babies, others (especially those who have experienced extensive intervention in childbirth) find it difficult to feed and care for their babies (Moss, Bolland, Foxman and Owen, 1987a; Woollett and Dosanjh-Matwala, 1990b).

The role of health professionals in the early hours/days is consequently seen not so much as caring for babies and providing help for mothers as monitoring 'well' women and babies and as providing advice. However, the shortness of women's stay in hospital means that health professionals have less opportunity to support breastfeeding and advise women about issues such as baby care and contraception.

Women's experiences of their post-partum care are rarely examined. This is in part because this aspect of maternity care has not caught the imagination of consumer groups who have raised awareness of women's perspectives in pregnancy and childbirth. However, when given an opportunity to talk about their post-partum experiences, women do express strong views (e.g. Woollett, Dosanjh, Nicolson et al., 1995; Woollett and Dosanjh-Matwala, 1990b; Moss, Bolland, Foxman and Owen, 1987b). They often experience the hospital environment as unsympathetic to their needs and are concerned about issues such as lack of privacy, quality of food, and hospital rules and routines. Women are unhappy about hospital policy and procedures which require them to look after themselves and their baby when they do not feel well and do not allow them to get sufficient rest, and rules which limit the opportunities for families to visit. Not surprisingly, therefore, many women are pleased to return home as soon as possible after delivery, especially when fathers want to share the care of the baby or mothers can call on help and support from friends and relatives. However, other women find the early post-partum days tiring and difficult, especially those who are ill or are recovering from extensive medical intervention and are unable to care for their babies. Yet other women prefer a longer stay in hospital which allows them to rest before returning to heavy domestic responsibilities at home. While fathers are encouraged to be present and to have a role at delivery, in the post partum fathers (as well as women's wider family and social networks) are marginalized (White and Woollett, 1991).

Medical problems
When there are medical problems the management of the post partum takes a somewhat different form (Niven, 1992). Major interventions in delivery, such as caesarean section, usually mean that mothers take longer to recover from childbirth. They are weak and in pain from stitches for many weeks after delivery (Garel et al., 1987). Women delivered by caesarean section often complain about the lack of support they receive in caring for their babies (Woollett and Dosanjh-Matwala, 1990b; Moss, Bolland, Foxman and Owen, 1987a, and see Chapter 10 in Volume 2). In addition, women who experience major interventions often need to come to terms with their feelings, for example, their disappointment at not being able to give birth 'naturally', and the 'failure' of their body (Raphael-Leff, 1991). When fathers are absent from delivery women may be concerned about whether fathers will get attached to their babies. Women may also be concerned about the impact of a complex delivery on their sexual attractiveness and sexuality (Alder, 1994; Raphael-Leff, 1991).

While most babies are well and able to go home with their mothers, some need to stay in hospital longer because they are of low birthweight, premature or sick. This is more likely to be the case for multiple births who make up a small proportion of births, but are more common as a result of assisted conception procedures (Botting, Macfarlane and Price, 1990). Babies in special care are separated from parents, especially when the mother leaves hospital before the baby. Parents are anxious about their child's health and may have to cope with the death of their baby or the news that they are handicapped or disabled. Even when the baby is doing well parents may be concerned about whether not being able to hold and care for them may affect their ability to love their babies and, given the emphasis on 'bonding', they may also be concerned about the effects on the baby of being separated from his/her mother while they are in special care (Niven, 1992). Women regret being unable to take responsibility for the care of their babies and miss the pleasure of introducing the new baby to family, friends and wider society.

Even once babies are well and have gone home, parents may continue to be concerned about their baby's health and possible longer term effects. McHaffie (1990) argues that it is important to ensure that before mothers take babies home, they feel ready and confident to care for what were tiny or sickly babies. Parents may also need to come to terms with feelings associated with not having produced the 'perfect baby', in spite of following advice and attending antenatal clinics regularly (Davis-Floyd, 1994).

The post partum in the home context

With hospital stay getting shorter, recovery from childbirth and establishment of feeding increasingly takes place in women's homes rather than in hospital. The medical care of women in their own homes differs in a number of respects from care in hospital. One important difference relates to the interpersonal dynamics between health professionals and mothers. Lomax (1995) examined the ways in which the physical examination of the perineum (a key aspect of monitoring the physical recovery of the woman) is managed in the home, that is in the mother's rather than the health professional's space or 'territory'. In hospital women's status is primarily and straightforwardly that of 'patient' and so such examinations are easily managed by health professionals, whereas in the home they raise complex issues about managing privacy and boundaries between acceptable and nonacceptable physical contact (Niven, 1992; Savage, 1987). Lomax (1995) found, for example, that the living room was the usual location for preliminary questions and discussion but that midwives preferred to conduct the physical examination in the woman's bedroom and had, therefore, to negotiate the change of location. Because in their homes women are fully dressed midwives have also to manage the removal of the women's clothes as part of the shift from 'discussion about how things are going' to 'physical examination'.

A benefit of post-partum care in the home setting is that the support and advice health professionals provide can be made appropriate to the woman's situation. In this way health professionals may be able to recognize the limitations of advice which, for example, suggests that a woman without access to a car 'goes out to the shops each day' to alleviate post-natal depression when the nearest shops are a distant out-of-town shopping development inaccessible by public transport. Working in the women's home also enables the recognition that mother and baby are an intermeshing 'system', and that, for example, the crying of the baby and the tiredness of the mother are closely related and cannot usefully be dealt with independently. However the extent to which health professionals can use such contextualized knowledge is often limited by the demands of their own work loads, for example to ensure that they visit a requisite number of women per day.

At home women have to fit the baby into family routines and combine childcare with other household tasks (Tulman and Fawcett, 1991; Niven, 1992). They are more able to manage the post partum in ways which are appropriate to their own ideas and those of their religion and culture. For example, they may not engage in cooking when in their culture women are viewed as 'polluted' in the post partum and they may share care of the baby because their culture views women who have recently given birth as 'vulnerable', or because they and their partners are committed to sharing childcare (Woollett and Dosanjh-Matwala, 1990a; Dobson, 1988; Jones and Doughtery, 1982).

There is little information about women's experiences once they go home, although some studies suggest that women's well-being and adjustment are related to factors such as the health of the mother and the baby, and the extent to which women's expectations of mothering have prepared them for looking after a small baby (Green, Coupland and Kitzinger, 1990). Psychological research on mother–baby relations also suggests that a mother's confidence in caring for a small baby is linked to her experience, the baby's temperament and the extent to which mothers can 'read' the baby and anticipate their baby's needs (see Chapters 8 and 9).

The quality of women's support networks also need to be considered. Western psychological theories emphasize the exclusivity of the mother–child relationship and the mother's responsibility for the baby, with the result that the role of support from others is less frequently considered. Some mothers draw on a wide network of support from the family and community, although fathers are the most frequent source of support (Tulman and Fawcett, 1991; Nicolson, 1990; White and Woollett, 1991). Some women encourage fathers and others to care for infants more than others. Relatives provide more care in extended and close knit families. Fathers care for infants less in cultures where female relatives are involved in caring for children (Brannen and O'Brien, 1995; Woollett, Dosanjh and Nicolson, et al., 1995).

Mothers' feelings and experiences

A range of feelings and experiences have been examined: these include women's embodied experiences, 'baby blues' and post-natal depression, tiredness and exhaustion, mother–baby relations and being a 'good mother'. They are discussed with reference to current constructions of and diversity in women's feelings and experiences.

Women's embodied experiences

Physical recovery after childbirth can be slow, calling into question current medical emphasis on new mothers as 'fit and well' (DiMatteo, Kahn and Berry, 1993). Glazener, Abdalla, Russell and Templeton (1993), for example, found that 87 per cent of women reported one problem in the first eight weeks, mainly perineum pain and breast problems. These were somewhat more likely amongst first time mothers and women who had caesarean sections and assisted deliveries. And Tulman and Fawcett (1991) found that by six months, a quarter of the women said they had not recovered physically, with just under half saying they had found their physical recovery more difficult than they anticipated. Women's recovery was improved if their babies were sleeping through the night and mothers felt less tired.

Pain and discomforts following childbirth together with women's concerns about their bodies and body shape may influence women's feelings about their bodies (their embodied experiences). Women (and their partners) sometimes report finding their bodies unattractive after delivery, and such feelings (and cultural preoccupations with thinness as attractive) may put pressure on women to 'get back into shape' (Ussher, 1989; Parr, 1996). Women's feelings about their bodies may also be related to and influenced by their sexual feelings and sexual relationships. Perineum pain, exhaustion, and the hormonal changes associated with childbirth and breastfeeding may reduce sexual desire and activity in the post partum (Alder, 1994; Reamy and White, 1987; Raphael-Leff, 1991; Ussher, 1989). Women's sexual feelings may also be affected by their experience of medical examinations and loss of privacy in pregnancy and delivery. Some women may experience a reduction in sexual feelings because being a mother may interfere with their view of their body as 'sexual'. This may be exaggerated if women experience their relationship with their baby as cutting across other feelings including those towards a 'sexual partner' (Nicolson, 1998; Raphael-Leff, 1991; Ussher, 1989; Alder, 1994). However, women's feelings vary considerably: some women feel that giving birth and being a mother has heightened their sexual feelings and sense of being a 'real woman' (Alder, 1994).

Women's emotions

During the first post-natal weeks women report a variety of intense and conflicting feelings, ranging from tiredness, tearfulness, anxiety, 'low spirited', to proud, excited and 'high as a kite'. These feelings are reported by women whose birth went well and who are thrilled with their baby as well as by those whose births were difficult and who take longer to get to know and feel love for their babies (Green, Coupland, Kitzinger, 1990; Astbury, 1994). Women's moods and feelings change rapidly and unpredictably for reasons which women often cannot explain, often adding to a sense of bewilderment and being 'out of control' (Niven, 1992).

'Baby blues' and post-natal depression

Medical and psychological research into women's feelings has emphasized problems and negative feelings, such as 'baby blues', post-natal depression and post-partum psychoses (see Chapter 6). This is not surprising given that women who feel depressed are more likely to seek help from professionals. 'Baby blues' (and post-natal depression) are often linked with hormonal changes and hence viewed as 'normal' in the post partum. While 'baby blues' are usually seen as short term and transitory, for some women they may be linked to post-natal depression. Feminist and social science approaches to women's depression place greater emphasis on women's circumstances to account for such feelings, for example their tiredness, pain and soreness following childbirth, and their new situation of caring for a small baby, as well as being in hospital with unknown people (Niven, 1992; Nicolson, 1986; Green, 1995).

When women are experiencing emotional upheavals, it is perhaps not surprising that relations between mothers and health professionals may be tense. These may also be exacerbated by opposing ideas and expectations about women's feelings and the 'needs' of mothers and babies. Providing care which is sensitive and appropriate to women who are in pain and discomfort and experiencing emotional and physical upheavals is a challenging task. This is especially the case with a short post-partum hospital stay which means that staff have little opportunity to get to know women and hence provide individualized care. The introduction of team midwifery should improve this situation.

Women's accounts, however, suggest that they are less likely than psychologists and health professionals to account for their depression and negative emotions in terms of individual problems and pathology. They seem rather to relate their accounts to anxieties around childcare, for example knowing what the baby wants when they cry or being able to settle them effectively, and to the hard and relentless work of mothering. They also link their feelings to the constraints motherhood brings, for example to their lack of autonomy and 'feeling trapped' and 'out of control', or not having enough 'time for themselves' (Oakley, 1979; Woollett and Parr, 1997; Green, Coupland and Kitzinger, 1990; DiMatteo, Kahn and Berry, 1993; Astbury, 1994). McIntosh (1993) argues that because women view depression as related to their experiences of motherhood, they do not consider it amenable to medical and other individualized forms of treatment and hence rarely seek help.

Women's experiences of the post partum can also be understood in terms of their expectations and how closely these match their experiences. Green, Coupland and Kitzinger (1990) found that women were more likely to experience their post-partum experiences positively when their expectations were high. When women's expectations are high they may focus more on the positive aspects of childbirth and post-partum experiences and seek out ways to improve things.

Interest in 'baby blues' and post-natal depression has increased awareness, and linking them with hormonal changes means that they are viewed as 'normal' experiences rather than as indications of failure or 'unnaturalness' on the part of individual mothers. However, there is also a risk that in normalizing 'baby blues' and post-natal depression, intolerable situations for which women do need help may be dismissed as transitory problems which will 'go away' with time.

Tiredness and exhaustion

As Niven (1992) argues, exhaustion may characterize better than depression the experiences of many women in the post partum. Of major concern for many women are their feelings of tiredness and exhaustion, and how under these circumstances they can cope with the relentless demands of childcare (DiMatteo, Kahn and Berry, 1993; Tulman and Fawcett, 1991; Nicolson, 1993). When women are delivered at night, they often lose a night's sleep. This, their excitement after delivery, and a strange hospital environment in which they are likely to be disturbed by other people combine to make sleep difficult in the immediate post-partum days and to disrupt women's sleep routines (Niven, 1992). Once they come home feeding and caring for a small baby at frequent intervals at night as well as during the day makes it difficult for women to rest and catch up on sleep. How long their exhaustion lasts depends on how quickly babies settle into a regular/predictable sleeping routine (see Chapter 9) and whether other people help with childcare (Small, Brown, Lumley and Astbury, 1994; Anderson, Fleming and Steiner, 1994).

Tiredness may also serve to increase women's anxiety and to decrease their sense of competence and confidence in themselves as mothers. Feelings of exhaustion and depression often come as a shock and may overwhelm feelings of relief at having given birth successfully, excitement and joy about the new baby and with being a mother, and mean that the early post-partum weeks are often a difficult time.

Mother–baby relations

A key aspect of women's experiences after childbirth concerns their feelings about their babies (Astbury, 1994). These feelings are complex and varied: some women experience an immediate sense of love and feel that they get to know their babies quickly. But for other women this is a slower process and even at six months post partum some women are still learning to know and to love their babies (Anderson, Fleming and Steiner, 1994). The baby may also influence women's feelings: when the health or weight of babies are a cause for concern, mothers may be extremely anxious and may question their skills and confidence as mothers. Other characteristics of the baby such as their gender, temperament, and their 'readability' all influence mothers' pleasure and confidence in the early days (Stratton, 1982, and see Chapters 8, 9 and 10).

Psychological accounts with their emphasis on 'attachment' and establishing close relations between mothers and babies provide a powerful context within which women evaluate their feelings for and experiences with their baby. Women sometimes appreciate the opportunity to 'get to know' their babies and establish feeding patterns in the labour and post-partum wards without the pressures of other responsibilities. Although there is little information about women's ideas about 'bonding' and the establishment of early relationships, some women appear to be aware of 'bonding theory' and this has an impact on how they view their early contact with their babies and their baby's emotional development. Other women, however, seem to place less emphasis on the establishment of a relationship with the baby at this stage. This may be because they take loving their baby and having a close relationship for granted, and focus instead on aspects of their experiences which they find more problematic (Nicolson, 1991/2). Yet other women, however, resist the 'bonding theory', arguing instead that the mother–baby relationship develops gradually in a wider social context which may involve the baby's father, and the wider family and social network (Woollett, Dosanjh, Nicolson et al., 1995; Woollett and Dosanjh-Matwala, 1990b).

Being a 'good' mother

The nature and intensity of mothers' feelings often come as a shock to women (DiMatteo, Kahn and Berry, 1993). While they may have given considerable thought to their childbirth plans or how to feed their babies, women often find it difficult to anticipate their feelings for their babies and about being a mother. A discrepancy between women's expectations and the reality of mothering is perhaps not unexpected given the emphasis on motherhood as romantic and 'natural' (Marshall, 1991). Viewing it as 'natural' implies that mothering will be 'easy' (see Chapter 1) and encourages women to see any problems they experience in terms of individual failure or pathology rather than as the understandable impact of exhaustion or the complexity of getting to know and care for a baby.

Sometimes concerns about whether their feelings are 'normal' may excerbate women's worries and negative feelings (Nicolson, 1986; Nicolson, 1991/2; Ussher, 1989). So, for example, if women do not immediately feel love towards their baby they may interpret this as a sign that their feelings are 'unnatural', and if they feel weepy and unfulfilled by their experience of giving birth, they may worry about whether they are 'real' women. Those working with new mothers need to help mothers to acknowledge their feelings and challenge unhelpful stereotypes about how they 'ought' to feel.

Current ideas about 'good mothering' in western cultures also emphasize the need for mothers to be sensitive and 'child-centred' by putting their baby's 'needs' before their own (Woollett and Phoenix, 1996). Women who do not quickly feel 'attached' to their babies or find it difficult to be 'sensitive' to their babies may be concerned about their feelings and their 'normality' as women and mothers. Some women, including those with more traditional approaches to gender roles, may cope better with this loss of control, in the early weeks at least (Grossman, Eichler and Winickoff, 1980). However, this may add to the loss of autonomy and control some women experience in the post partum and may discourage them from trying to ensure that they can rest and do things 'for themselves'.

Diversity in women's post-partum experiences

Medical and psychological approaches to the post partum tend to consider mothers in universal terms, emphasizing common aspects of their experiences. Diversity and variability in women's experiences and feelings are less frequently researched and so there is little systematic evidence about the range of women's feelings. However, as we have already suggested, research which takes women's perspectives reports that women's experiences vary considerably: the feelings of individual women change over time and, as they become more familiar with their babies, women's confidence in their parenting skills increases (Walker, Crain and Thompson, 1986; Niven, 1992). Factors which seem to be associated with women's experiences include those to do with women themselves, their health and well-being, and their expectations of motherhood based on current ideas about what are 'normal' and 'natural' feelings and ways of coping in early motherhood (Simkin, 1991; Nicolson, 1993).

One source of diversity which has been explored is parity. First time mothers have somewhat different medical experiences of childbirth and the post partum because they are more likely than women having second and subsequent children to be induced and they stay in hospital longer (Woollett, Dosanjh, Nicolson et al., 1995; Niven, 1992). In addition first time mothers are more likely to report painful perineum and breast problems (Glazener, Abdalla, Russell and Templeton, 1993). Women with children already are more confident and positive than first time mothers (Walker, Crain and Thompson, 1986), although the satisfaction of first time mothers increases over the early weeks (Grace, 1993). Women with experience of parenting, including women who are bringing up children from a partner's previous relationship, may be better able to cope with their feelings because they know from their previous experiences that babies do settle into a routine and parents are able to take up again other activities and relationships (Alexander and Higgins, 1993). Parity is also related to life changes: the birth of a first child brings greater changes in identity, status and life style than does the birth of subsequent children, although there are changes for the parents of second and subsequent children, not least those involving relationships with the older children (White and Woollett, 1992; Munn, 1991).

Women's experiences also relate to their age, and their social and economic circumstances. Women who are older or younger than the 'norm' are considered more 'at risk', but the impact of age is largely influenced by other factors, such as parity, the support of fathers and the wider family, women's housing and economic situation, and women's self-esteem and confidence as parents (Phoenix, 1991; Berryman, Thorpe and Windridge, 1995, and see Chapter 4). It also needs to be remembered that 'older' and 'younger' mothers are not homogeneous groups but vary considerably. While some younger mothers may not have a partner or be living in difficult economic circumstances, others are well supported (by parents or/ as well as the baby's father) and living in stable financial and social situations. Age and employment are confounded: older women tend to have been in paid employment longer than younger women, and older women are somewhat more likely to be in relationships with less traditionally gendered roles (Berryman, Thorpe and Windridge, 1995).

Different cultures and communities have somewhat different ideas about post-partum feelings and experiences. Those most commonly reported relate to ideas about the need for rest and recovery, the vulnerability of mothers and babies, and ideas about the involvement of other family members in childcare. In some cultures the post partum is associated with seclusion, dietary and contact taboos, and sometimes by ritual purification ceremonies before women are reintroduced into their social world (Raphael-Leff, 1991). This is the case for some Asian women giving birth in the UK and is explained by them in terms of 'vulnerability' of themselves and their babies, especially by those women who considered themselves to be more traditionally Asian and those who have not been brought up in the UK (Woollett and Dosanjh-Matwala, 1990a; Dobson, 1988).

Non-Asian women living in the UK also refer to constraints on their activities in the post partum (for example not going out often or not cooking), but these are explained in terms of lack of time or interest rather than cultural or religious practices. They may, however, serve a similar function of segregating newly delivered women from their community and day-to-day responsibilities while they 'get to know' the new baby and while breastfeeding and other routines are established (Woollett and Dosanjh-Matwala, 1990a; Raphael-Leff, 1991).

While some differences in ideas about the post partum are reported amongst Asian women, there is no straightforward association with 'race' and ethnicity. Knowing a woman's 'race' and ethnicity does not allow health professionals to predict her ideas about the management of the post partum. Health professionals need to ensure that they avoid stereotypical ideas and that they recognize differences *within* as well as those *between* cultures. This means going beyond 'cultural accounts' to acknowledge that variations between women within ethnic and social groups may be as wide as those between groups (Department of Health: Changing Childbirth, 1993) and to seek information directly from women about their ideas and preferences (Marshall, 1992).

Fathers' experiences

The emphasis of research is on mothers and mother–child relations. In recent years there has been greater recognition of the role of fathers in child-birth in Europe and USA as fathers regularly accompany women in delivery (Lewis, 1986; Woollett, White and Lyon, 1982; White and Woollett, 1991; Nicolson, 1990). However once babies are delivered fathers do not have a clearly defined role. Their main task seems to be to inform people of the birth and organize visits to hospital, but they are purely 'visitors' on the post-natal wards and are rarely involved in the care of their babies (Lewis, 1986; White and Woollett, 1991). In contrast to the emphasis on the establishment of mother–child relations, there is little consideration of the value of fathers 'getting to know' their babies in the early days (Moss, Bolland, Foxman and Owen, 1987a; Eiser and Eiser, 1985; Woollett and Dosanjh-Matwala, 1990a). As Niven (1992) argues, this means that by the time mothers and babies come home, mothers know their babies better and have more experience of caring for them.

Frequently fathers who are in employment take time off work when the baby comes home, although there is no paid paternity leave in the UK and Ireland in contrast with Germany and other European countries. Fathers' presence in the early days enables them to get involved and develop their childcare skills. There are now expectations (from mothers, fathers and more generally) that fathers will be involved with their babies and their care, but there is little evidence that fathers are substantially involved (Niven, 1992; Lewis, 1986; White and Woollett, 1991). Women take most responsibility for childcare, regardless of what was the established pattern of responsibility for household tasks prior to the baby's birth and parents' expectations that tasks would be shared (Oakley, 1979; Ruble, Fleming, Hackel and Stangor, 1988).

Mothers report that fathers are their main source of support (Lewis, 1986; Nicolson, 1990). There is little evidence about the factors which influence fathers' involvement, although one factor which seems to be important is the availability of support: fathers participate more in childcare when other family members are not available (Lewis, 1986; Woollett, Dosanjh, Nicolson et al., 1995). When other people are not available fathers may feel a greater need and mothers may encourage their involvement. There are also some indications that fathers' involvement is influenced by their own ideas about gendered roles and those of the wider culture (Wetherell,

1995). Thorpe, Dragonas and Golding (1992) for example, found that Greek parents had more traditional ideas about the role of fathers, and that men were more distanced, emotionally and physically, from their partners than British fathers. However, Asian fathers living in East London seem to be no less involved than non-Asian fathers (Woollett, Dosanjh, Nicolson et al., 1995).

When fathers are involved, mothers benefit from the support they provide and they are able to sustain their belief in a 'fair' division of labour through, for example, recognizing that while fathers may not spontaneously care for their babies, they will do so 'if asked' (Oakley, 1979). The support fathers offer is somewhat different to that offered by female relatives: fathers provide emotional support (someone with whom to 'talk things through') in contrast to the more practical support (childcare or housework) offered by female relatives (Beail, 1985; Lewis, 1986; Niven, 1992).

Fathers' lives and identities are less changed by parenthood than are those of mothers. Whereas motherhood brings substantial changes in women's employment, men's employment roles remain largely unchanged by fatherhood (Alexander and Higgins, 1993). Fathers may try to compensate for reductions in family income resulting from women's withdrawal from paid employment outside the home by working longer, or by becoming more committed to their jobs, further reducing the practical support they can provide for mothers (Moss, Bolland, Foxman and Owen, 1986). In comparison with mothers, there is little research which examines men's feelings about being a father or about how they incorporate fathering into their other roles and identities (Wetherell, 1995; Nicolson, 1990).

Research on fathers also indicates the need to examine the ways in which becoming parents and coping with the hard work of parenting in the early weeks influences the relationship between parents and their satisfaction in their relationship. Most studies suggest a reduction in satisfaction in the first year of parenting (Tomlinson, 1987; Moss, Bolland, Foxman and Owen, 1986). This would seem to be associated with a reduction in the time couples have to spend with one another (and especially 'child-free time') and in their level of intimacy, including their sexual intimacy (Raphael-Leff, 1991; Parr, 1996).

But marital satisfaction after childbirth is also associated with renegotiation of the couple relationship and incorporation of the baby into the family. It has been suggested that how effectively this is done depends in part on the nature of a couple's relationship: couples with traditional ideas about men's and women's roles may experience fewer tensions if women give up paid employment outside the home and make motherhood their central role than is the case for couples committed to shared roles and activities. Couples who have enjoyed going out a great deal may need to deal with the restrictions which parenting entails (Fitzpatrick, Vangelisti and Firman, 1994; Alexander and Higgins, 1993; Tomlinson, 1987; Grossman, Eichler and Winickoff, 1980). Couples with good communication skills, who have empathy for one another's feelings, and a history of dealing successfully with conflicts prior to becoming parents may manage this renegotiation more effectively than those without such skills and experience (Tomlinson, 1987; Moss, Bolland, Foxman and Owen, 1987b; Belsky and Kelly, 1994; Fitzpatrick, Vangelisti and Firman, 1994). Men and women becoming parents for a second or subsequent time may experience fewer changes in their relationship, but they may need to renegotiate their relationships with older child(ren). This sometimes takes the form of fathers getting closer to older children, while mothers are very involved in the care of a new baby (White and Woollett, 1992; Munn, 1991).

Relations with others: the wider family and support networks

There is relatively little research which considers the role of the wider family and community in the early weeks after childbirth. Relationships with the extended family change with the birth of a child: a new baby in the family is an exciting event for grandparents, uncles and aunts, cousins, etc. as well as for parents. Sometimes the birth of a baby is associated with increased closeness and support from grandparents, most commonly in the form of financial assistance and childcare (Smith, 1991; Lewis, 1986). In most cultures the safe arrival of a new member of the family and community is marked by ceremonies and celebrations. In western societies these take the form largely of christenings and naming ceremonies (Woollett and Dosanjh-Matwala, 1990a).

Other relationships may change in the post partum, including those with friends and work colleagues, but the nature and extent of these changes often depends on women's circumstances. Women becoming mothers at an early age, for example, may find themselves isolated because their friends are not parents and so do not share their interests and activities (Phoenix, 1991). For older women becoming a mother may mean becoming closer to friends who are already parents, being able to share concerns about parenting and offer one another support. For the increasing number of women who are having babies on their own, friends and families may provide a major source of support (Phoenix, 1991).

Tasks and issues in the post partum

In this chapter we have examined the medical, psychological, social and cultural significance of the early post-partum weeks. There is increasing recognition of the complexity and diversity of women's experiences and feelings as they become parents, and the ways in which partners, families and key professionals may impact upon those experiences and feelings. Some key tasks and issues raised in this chapter include:

- **Recovery from childbirth:** although it has received little attention in medical and psychological accounts, a major task for women in the early post-partum weeks is recovery from childbirth both physically and psychologically. This is not necessarily a straightforward process of 'getting back to normal' but is often a gradual and complex process which involves coming to terms with and making sense of the emotions aroused by childbirth and being a new parent, especially if their experiences did not match their expectations (DiMatteo, Kahn and Berry, 1993; Green, Coupland and Kitzinger, 1990; Raphael-Leff, 1991).

- **Women's well-being and adjustment:** women make sense of their experiences in complex and diverse ways. The complexity of women's feelings can be seen in studies which take women's perspectives and draw on their accounts (e.g. Astbury, 1994; Oakley, 1979; Nicolson, 1998). These indicate, for example, that tiredness and exhaustion are as important to women as depression which is a main concern in research and professional accounts (Stoppard, 1995; Nicolson, 1996). In addition, women's sense of their well-being and adjustment seems to be influenced by social constructions of 'normal' and 'natural' adjustments in the post partum.

  For first time parents, childbirth marks the start of new identities, feelings and experiences. In the post partum women begin the process of adjustment to motherhood with its comcomitant losses and gains. Examples of losses are the identities they have given up (including those associated with employment), their autonomy and their pre-pregnancy bodies. The gains of motherhood include new identities and status as a mother, a close relationship with the baby, shared interests and companionship with other mothers, and if they have a partner, shared feelings and purpose (Nicolson, 1998; Parr, 1996; Niven, 1992; Chapters 9 to 12).

- **Establishment of mother–child relations:** constructions of the post partum based on 'bonding' and attachment theories view the key task to be the establishment of mother–child relations, often portrayed as a rapid and straightforward process. This underestimates the complexity and variability of the processes by which mothers and babies get to know and adapt to one another. From the early days babies are interested in and responsive to their social worlds but their competence is limited (e.g. Fogel, 1993) and it is mothers who take the lead, coordinating their activities with their child's state, mood, etc. (Simkin, 1991).

- **Role of health professionals:** research has failed to show simple relationships between the management of delivery and post-partum care and women's experiences and adjustments (e.g. Oakley, 1979; Murray and Cartwright, 1993). Some women have clear plans for their delivery, for example in terms of how important it is to maintain 'control' and their involvement in decisions about their own and their baby's care. However, what may be of most importance to women is whether they feel that their birth experience was a 'good' one, and health professionals were supportive and caring.

  The provision of mother-centred care, for example as specified by Changing Childbirth (1993), requires health professionals to take account of the diversity of women's ideas and expectations. When there is a discrepancy between the ideas of women and health professionals, women may be concerned that health professionals will judge them in terms of their own definitions of 'good/normal' adjustment and, for example, view them as 'too' emotional or as 'not bonded with' their baby. To ensure the provision of mother-centred post-partum care, health professionals need to acknowledge and respect women's ideas and preferences and, taking into account the highly charged emotional context of the early post-partum weeks, to negotiate ways of reducing the potential for tensions and to ensure that the advice they offer is related to women's personal circumstances.

Applications

1. Women's physical recovery from childbirth varies considerably. While some women are 'fit and well' and able to look after themselves and their babies very quickly after childbirth, others (and especially those whose deliveries involved interventions) experience physical problems.

2. Women's feelings in the post partum also vary. While health professionals need to be concerned about 'baby blues' and post-natal depression, they also need to recognize and provide help for women for whom tiredness and exhaustion are a problem and women who are not finding it easy to renegotitate relationships with a partner.

3. While mothers and babies are their main concern in the post partum, health professionals also need to be aware of mothers' wider social context and the impact this might have for women's well-being, recovery and their ability to care for their babies.

4. The provision of individualized care requires that health professionals relate their practice and advice to mothers' ideas about 'good/normal' adjustment in the post partum. These are drawn in complex ways from women's experiences, coping strategies, relationships, religion and culture.

Acknowledgements

We would like to acknowledge the assistance of Patsy Fuller in preparing this chapter.

Further reading

Department of Health (1993). *Changing Childbirth: Report of the Expert Maternity Group*. London: HMSO.

Niven, C. A. (1992). *Psychological Care for Families: Before, During and After Birth*. Oxford: Butterworth–Heinnemann.

Raphael-Leff, J. (1991). *The Psychological Processes of Childbearing*. London: Chapman and Hall.

Woollett, A. and Nicolson, P. (eds) (1997). Post partum care and experiences of mothering. *Journal of Reproductive and Infant Psychology*. Special Issue. **15** (2).

References

Alder, B. (1994). Postnatal sexuality. In *Female Sexuality, Psychology, Biology and Social Context* (P. Y. L. Choi and P. Nicolson, eds). Hemel Hempstead: Harvester Wheatsheaf.

Alexander, M. J. and Higgins, E. T. (1993). Emotional trade-offs of becoming a parent: how social roles influence self-discrepancy effects. *Journal of Personality and Social Psychology*, **65**, 1259–69.

Anderson, V. N., Fleming, A. S. and Steiner, M. (1994). Mood and the transition to motherhood. *Journal of Reproductive and Infant Psychology*, **12**, 69–78.

Astbury, J. (1994). Making motherhood visible: the experience of motherhood questionnaire. *Journal of Reproductive and Infant Psychology*, **12**, 79–88.

Beail, N. (1985). Fathers and Infant Caretaking. *Journal of Reproductive and Infant Psychology*, **3**, 54–63.

Belsky, J. and Kelly, J. (1994). *The Transition to Parenthood: How a First Child Changes a Marriage*. London: Macmillan.

Berryman, J., Thorpe, K. and Windridge, K. (1995). *Older Mothers: Conception Pregnancy and Birth After 35*. London: Pandora Press.

Botting, B. J., Macfarlane, A. J. and Price, F. (1990). *Three, Four or More: A Study of Triplets and Higher Order Births*. London: HMSO.

Brannen, J. and O'Brien, M. (eds) (1995). *Childhood and Parenthood*. London: Institute of Education.

Clulow, C. (1982). *To Have and To Hold*. Aberdeen: Aberdeen University Press.

Davis-Floyd, R. E. (1994). The technocratic body: American childbirth as cultural expression. *Social Science and Medicine*, **38**, No. 8, 1125–40.

Department of Health (1993). *Changing Childbirth: Report of the Expert Maternity Group*. London: HMSO.

DiMatteo, M. R., Kahn, K. L. and Berry, S. H. (1993). Narratives of birth and the postpartum: analysis of the focus group responses of new mothers. *Birth*, **20** (4), 204–11.

Dobson, S. M. (1988). Transcultural Health Visiting: caring in a multi-cultural society. *Recent Advances in Nursing*, **20**, 61–80.

Eiser, C. and Eiser, J. R. (1985). Mothers' experiences on the postnatal ward. *Child: Care, Health and Development*, **11**, 349–54.

Fitzpatrick, M. A., Vangelisti, A. L. and Firman, S. M. (1994). Perceptions of marital interactions and change during pregnancy: a typological approach. *Personal Relationships*, **1**, 101–22.

Fogel, A. (1993). *Developing Through Relationships: Origins of Communication, Self, and Culture*. Hemel Hempstead: Harvester Wheatsheaf.

Garel, M., Lelong, N. and Kaminsky, M. (1987). Psychological consequences of caesarean childbirth in primiparas. *Journal of Psychosomatic Obstetrics and Gynaecology*, **6**, 197–209.

Glazener, C., Abdalla, M., Russell, I. and Templeton, A. (1993). Postnatal care: a survey of patients' experiences. *British Journal of Midwifery*, **1**, 67–74.

Grace, J. T. (1993). Mothers' self-reports of parenthood across the first 6 months postpartum. *Research in Nursing and Health*, **16**, 431–9.

Green, J. (1995). 'Postnatal depression': Is it postnatal, is it depression? Paper presented at Annual Conference, Society for Reproductive and Infant Psychology, September 1995. University of Leicester.

Green, J. M., Coupland, V. A. and Kitzinger, J. V. (1990). Expectations, experiences, and psychological outcomes of childbirth: a prospective study of 825 women. *Birth*, **17**, 15–24.

Grossman, F. K., Eichler, L. S. and Winickoff, S. A. (1980). *Pregnancy, Birth and Parenthood: Adaptation of Mothers, Fathers and Infants*. San Francisco: Jossey-Bass.

Jones, A. D. and Doughtery, C. (1982). Childbirth in a scientific and industrial society. In *The Ethnography of Fertility and Birth* (C. P. MacCormack, ed.). London: Academic Press.

Kitzinger, S. (1978). *Women as Mothers*. London: Fontana.

Klaus, M. H. and Kennell, J. H. (1982). *Parent–Infant Bonding*. Second edition. St Louis: C.V. Mosby.

Lewis, C. (1986). *Becoming a Father*. Milton Keynes: Open University Press.

Lomax, H. (1995). What's your loss like love? An analysis of midwife–client interaction during the post-natal examination. Paper presented at British Psychological Society Annual Conference, University of Warwick, April 1995.

Marshall, H. (1991). The social construction of motherhood: an analysis of childcare and parenting manuals. In *Motherhood: Meanings, Practices and Ideologies* (A. Phoenix, A. Woollett and E. Lloyd, eds). London: Sage.

Marshall, H. (1992). Talking about good maternity care in a multi-cultural context: a discourse analysis of midwives and health vistors. In *The Psychology of Women's Health and Health Care* (P. Nicolson and J. Ussher, eds). London: Methuen.

McHaffie, H. E. (1990). Mothers of very low birthweight babies: how do they adjust? *Journal of Advanced Nursing*, **15**, 6–11.

McIntosh, J. (1993). Postpartum depression: Women's help seeking behaviour and perceptions of cause. *Journal of Advanced Nursing*, **18**, 178–84.

Moss, P., Bolland, G., Foxman, R. and Owen, C. (1986). Marital relations during the transition to parenthood. *Journal of Reproductive and Infant Psychology*, **4**, 57–68.

Moss, P., Bolland, G., Foxman, R. and Owen, C. (1987a). The hospital inpatient stay: the experience of first time parents. *Child: Care, Health and Development*, **13**, 153–67.

Moss, P., Bolland, G., Foxman, R. and Owen, C. (1987b). The division of household work during the transition to parenthood. *Journal of Reproductive and Infant Psychology*, **5**, 71–86.

Munn, P. (1991). Mothering more than one child. In *Motherhood: Meanings, Practices and Ideologies* (A. Phoenix, A. Woollett and E. Lloyd, eds). London: Sage.

Murray, L. and Cartwright, W. (1993). The role of obstetric factors in post partum depression. *Journal of Reproductive and Infant Psychology*, **11**, 215–19.

Nicolson, P. (1986). Developing a feminist approach to depression following childbirth. In *Feminist Social Psychology* (S. Wilkinson, ed.). Milton Keynes: Open University press.

Nicolson, P. (1990). A brief report of women's expectations of men's behaviour in the transition to parenthood: contradictions and conflicts for counselling psychology practice. *Counselling Psychology Quarterly*, **3** (4), 353–61.

Nicolson, P. (1991/1992). Explanations of post natal depression: structuring knowledge of female psychology. *Research on Language and Social Interaction*, **25**, 75–96.

Nicolson, P. (1993). The social construction of motherhood. In *Introducing Women's Studies, Feminist Theory and Culture* (D. Richardson and V. Robinson, eds). London: Macmillan.

Nicolson, P. (1998). *Post-natal Depression: Psychology, Science and the Transition to Motherhood*. London: Routledge.

Niven, C. A. (1992). *Psychological Care for Families: Before, During and After Birth*. Oxford: Butterworth–Heinemann.

Oakley, A. (1979). *Becoming a Mother*. Oxford: Martin Robertson.

Parr, M. (1996). Support for couples in the transition to parenthood. Unpublished PhD Thesis. University of East London.

Phoenix, A. (1991). *Young mothers?* Cambridge: Polity.

Raphael-Leff, J. (1991). *The Psychological Processes of Childbearing*. London: Chapman and Hall.

Reamy, K. J. and White, S. E. (1987). Sexuality in the puerperium: a review. *Archives of Sexual Behaviour*, **16**, 165–86.

Ruble, D. N., Fleming, A. S., Hackel, L. S. and Stangor, C. (1988). Changes in the marital relationship during the transition to first time motherhood: effects of violated expectations concerning division of household labor. *Journal of Personality and Social Psychology*, **55**, 78–87.

Savage, J. (1987). *Nurses, Gender and Sexuality*. London: Heineman in Nursing.

Simkin, P. (1991). Just another day in a woman's life? Women's long-term perceptions of their first birth experience, Part 1. *Birth*, **18**, 203–10.

Small, R., Brown, S., Lumley, J. and Astbury, J. (1994). Missing voices: what women say and do about depression after childbirth. *Journal of Reproductive and Infant Psychology*, **12**, 89–104.

Smith, P. K. (1991). *The Psychology of Grandparenthood*. London: Routledge.

Stoppard, J. M. (1995). A social constructionist analysis of Brown and Harris' 'Social origins of depression': implications of experts' discourses for research on women and depression. Paper presented to BPS Psychology of Women Section Conference, Leeds, July.

Stratton, P. (ed.) (1982). *Psychobiology of Human Newborn*. Chichester: Wiley.

Svedja, M. J., Campos, J. J. and Emde, R. R. (1980). Mother–infant bonding: a failure to generalise. *Child Development*, **51**, 775–9.

Thorpe, K., Dragonas, T. and Golding, J. (1992). The effects of psychosocial factors on the mothers' emotional well-being during early parenthood: a cross-cultural study of Britain and Greece. *Journal of Reproductive and Infant Psychology*, **10**, 205–18.

Tomlinson, P. S. (1987). Spousal difference in marital satisfaction during transition to parenthood. *Nursing Research*, **36**, 239–43.

Tulman, L. and Fawcett, J. (1991). Recovery from childbirth: looking back six months after delivery. *Health Care For Women International*, **12**, 341–50.

Ussher, J. M. (1989). *The Psychology of the Female Body*. London: Routledge.

Walker, L. O., Crain, H. and Thompson, E. (1986). Mothering behaviour and maternal role attainment during the postpartum period. *Nursing Research*, **35**, 352–5.

Wetherell, M. (1995). Social structure, ideology and family dynamics: the case of parenting. In *Understanding the Family* (J. Muncie, M. Wetherell, R. Dallos and A. Cochrane, eds). London: Sage.

White, D. G. and Woollett, A. (1991). The father's role in the neonatal period. In *Becoming a Person* (M. Woodhead, R. Carr and P. Light, eds). London: Routledge.

White, D. and Woollett, A. (1992). *Families: A Context for Development*. Basingstoke: Falmer Press.

Woollett, A., White, D. and Lyon, L. (1982). Observations at birth. In *Fathers: Psychological Perspectives* (N. Beail and J. McGuire, eds). London: Junction Books.

Woollett, A. and Dosanjh-Matwala, N. (1990a). Asian women's experiences of childbirth in East End: the support of fathers and female relatives. *Journal of Reproductive and Infant Psychology*, **8**, 11–22.

Woollett, A. and Dosanjh-Matwala, N. (1990b). Asian women's experiences on the post natal wards. *Midwifery*, **6**, 178–84.

Woollett, A., Dosanjh, N., Nicolson, P., Marshall, H., Djhanbakhch, O. and Hadlow, J. (1995). A comparison of the experiences of pregnancy and childbirth of Asian and non-Asian women in East London. *British Journal of Medical Psychology*, **68**, 65–84.

Woollett, A. and Phoenix, A. (1996). Motherhood as pedagogy: developmental psychology and the accounts of mothers of young children. In *Feminisms and the Pedagogies of Everyday Life* (C. Luke, ed.). New York: State University of New York Press.

Woollett, A. and Parr, M. (1997). Psychological tasks for women and men in the post partum. *Journal of Infant and Reproductive Psychology*, **15**, 159–83.

6

The well-being of mothers

Karen Thorpe and Sandra A. Elliott

> Following on from Chapter 5, Karen Thorpe and Sandra Elliott consider the well-being of mothers in the months following the birth of a child. Most of the research in this area has been concerned with the phenomenon of 'post-natal depression' post-natal depression which affects around 10–15 per cent of mothers. As well as discussing the various theories about causes and treatments for post-natal depression, this chapter also puts post-natal depression into perspective by discussing the full range of emotional experiences in the early years after the birth of a child. How do personal circumstances and social support influence emotional well-being? When do women's personal feelings become a legitimate target for professional intervention? What can health services do to help women who experience emotional difficulties? Is it only the responsibility of health professionals to 'care' for women with young children – or of the wider society?

There can be no doubt that the birth of a child is an event which imposes significant change on a woman's life. It inevitably affects a woman's social and personal identity. Motherhood for some women marks a change of role, particularly for those who leave paid employment, while for others it requires the assumption of an additional role. For all women the birth of a child presents new emotional challenges which are potentially stressful and likely to impact on emotional well-being.

The majority of women maintain mental health after the birth of a child. It is estimated that 10–15 per cent of women experience depression or more serious mental illness in the year following the birth of a child. Although this is a significant minority, this means that 85–90 per cent are emotionally well. However, the range of reactions to motherhood vary enormously. Some women simply manage to cope with the early years of motherhood while for others this time is a source of contentment, fulfilment and enjoyment. The first part of this chapter examines the emotional well-being of women in the early years after the birth of a child. It examines women's reactions to motherhood and the factors that influence how happy they are in the early years of their child's life. The second part of this chapter examines the difficulties which a small but significant minority of women experience in the early years following childbirth and particularly focuses on depression. It considers the role of the professional in assisting women to overcome these difficulties.

Social and personal images of motherhood

Motherhood has been a shock to me. The first baby I have ever held was my own and I was not sure that it was what I wanted . . . how could I know . . .

Becoming a mother is perhaps the hardest thing I have ever done but undoubtedly my greatest achievement. There is no comparable experience.

It is so odd . . . one minute I am Dr B a woman with status who has authority both within my surgery and to the outside world . . . the next I am at the school and I am Mrs B, Joshua's mum, without my own identity and treated as if I didn't have a brain. Isn't it odd how motherhood and intelligence are treated as mutually exclusive.

In modern western societies women become mothers against a background of mixed messages about the value of motherhood. On the one hand motherhood is seen as mandatory and synonymous with adult identity (Salmon, 1985; Woollett, 1991). Studies of young women suggest that even in their teens the majority see motherhood as part of their life plan and expect to have at least two children (Beckett, 1986; Sharpe, 1976; Wallach and Maitlin, 1992). The model of their own mothers and other women is a potent one. Failure to become a mother can be socially isolating. Women who are childless by choice are often characterized as self-centred or unfulfilled (Stewart and Robinson, 1989; Woollett, 1991) while women who experience involuntary childlessness report feelings of failure and a sense of exclusion from the 'club of womanhood' (Oakley, 1981; Berryman, 1993). On the other hand motherhood represents, for many, a loss of social status. In western societies this is intimately bound with economic value and for the majority of women motherhood marks a reduction or cessation of paid work and hence economic contribution (Brannen and Moss, 1988). The unpaid work of child-rearing, while seen as essential, is not accorded an equivalent status to that of paid work (Oakley, 1981). However, society on the other hand does not encourage or enable the return of women to the work force if they should so choose after the birth. This is evident in the failure to provide childcare facilities and prevailing non-acceptance of non-parental care. Mothers bear the financial and emotional cost of their decisions about paid work alone (Brannen and Moss, 1988; Berryman, Thorpe and Windridge, 1995).

Women's personal views and experiences also convey a mixed reaction to motherhood. Women from a diverse range of backgrounds quite clearly voice joys and frustrations associated with being a mother. In studies exploring the reactions of women to becoming a mother, the tangible effects – loss of career advancement, financial cost, change in relationship with partner – are clearly evidenced. However, much greater emphasis is placed on the personal and psychological impact of motherhood. In a study of the timing of motherhood (Thorpe and Cinnamon, unpublished data) for example, in which 140 women were questioned about their experiences of motherhood, these intensely personal and psychological themes predominated regardless of the age at which the woman questioned had become a mother.

The major losses associated with becoming a mother described by these women were those of personal freedom and individual identity:

When I was pregnant I thought that I would do lots of new projects – I was only going to work part-time. What is so difficult and frustrating is that not only can I not do these things but I can't do the things I used to do. Jobs are never finished. I never get time to myself.

Mother of child aged 9 months

Juxtaposed against these comments were those expressing the emotional gains women felt they derived from the unique mother–child relationship:

. . . just the love and affection I receive from my child (is so rewarding) and also the feelings it brings with being a family. I love watching our son change and grow and the funny things he does . . . I enjoy sharing this with my partner.

Mother of child aged 12 months

Being a mother has allowed me to 'do childhood' again . . . I can have fun, joke – be a kid too . . . its a sense of freedom . . . I enjoy being involved in her busy life.

Mother of child aged 4 years

Against the background of mixed social messages about the value of the role of motherhood and the personal experiences of intense frustration and joy resulting from this role, there are a range of factors which have been found to influence the impact of motherhood on an individual woman's well-being by either supporting her or increasing her experience of stress. The following section examines three groups of variables which might influence individual reactions to pregnancy, childbirth and early parenthood: experience of stressful life circumstances and events, social environment and personal characteristics. It examines key factors which have been found to affect women's emotional well-being in the early years after having a child. Before turning to this section, however, it is important to make some notes about the nature of research concerning emotional well-being of mothers.

Studies examining the emotional well-being of mothers most commonly focus on the problems associated with motherhood and are concerned with *depression* or *poor emotional well-being*. These studies use quantitative methods in which standard assessments of mental health are administered. To assess emotional well-being the woman is asked a range of questions about symptoms using either an interview or questionnaire format. These may include questions about energy levels, crying, anxiety, coping, sleep and thoughts of suicide. From this interview a score is calculated (based on the number and/or severity of symptoms). This score is then used in one of two ways. First, it may be used to define clinically significant depression. If the woman reports sufficient symptoms to score above a defined cut-off point then she may be designated a 'case' of depression. Second, the scores may be viewed relative to each other across the continuum of high to low. Those women with higher scores (more symptoms) would be seen as having poorer emotional well-being than those with lower scores but no one point is specified which defines a clinically significant state. This approach is concerned with a range of well-being, but it is important to note that because the assessments are typically focused on symptoms it does not equate to a measure of happiness through to depression. The measures do not typically focus on feelings of positive well-being.

Sources of stress and emotional well-being among mothers

Social circumstance

A common finding in the studies examining the relationship between mental health and social circumstance is that across the general population, women with lower social status (measured either by classification of occupation or educational level) are more likely to experience poor emotional well-being. Thus Brown and Harris (1978) report a one-year period prevalence rate of depression of 17 per cent in their sample of working class women–a two-fold increase in population prevalence compared with other published prevalence figures for general populations of women (e.g. Ryle, 1961; Myers, Weissman, Tischler, 1984). The implication drawn from findings such as this is that living in circumstances of social adversity predisposes to poor emotional well-being. An important question is whether social circumstance underlies experience of emotional well-being of women in the early years after child-birth.

The range of studies which have examined the relationship between social status and the emotional well-being among child-bearing women present inconsistent findings. Thus while some studies report an increase risk of depressive symptomology among those with lower social status (Thorpe, Golding, MacGillivray and Greenwood, 1991; Thorpe et al., 1995a,b; Gjerdingen and Challoner, 1994; Feggetter and Gath, 1981; Playfair and Gowers, 1981; O'Hara, Neunaber and Zekoski, 1984) others find no such relationship (Green 1990; O'Hara and Zekoski, 1988). O'Hara and Zekoski's (1988) review of 13 papers specifically examining post-natal depression found only two which reported associations with social status. These inconsistencies in findings are likely to reflect differences in methodology and particularly the timing of the study. The studies vary markedly in the size and composition of study populations, the measure of social status (occupation of partner, occupation of woman herself, educational status), measure of depression/emotional well-being (standard versus non-standard, self-report versus independent diagnostic interview) and approach (continuous versus caseness) to defining emotional well-being and time points of measurement. A key issue is that the salience of particular factors to experience of emotional well-being varies across the transition to parenthood and the early years after the birth of a child. Thus Thorpe, Golding, MacGillivray and Greenwood (1991), in a representative population sample of 13,135 British women five years after the birth of a child, found that double the proportion of women in social classes IV and V reported symptoms of depression than their counterparts in non-manual social class (categories I, II, III-NM) while Green (1990) found no effect in the post-partum period in a similarly representative sample of 825 British women. It would seem that social class is least likely to predict emotional well-being in the immediate post-partum period.

Another major issue is that indices of social status may be too crude a measure of social circumstance and that research should actually focus directly on specific social circumstance and living conditions. There is certainly evidence that women living on low incomes (Gjerdingen and Challoner, 1994); in poorer housing conditions (Kitamura, Shima, Sugawara and Toda, 1993; Millar, 1994; Richman, Stevenson and Graham,

1982; Littlewood and Tinker, 1981) who are themselves not working (Zelkowitz and Milet, 1995) whose partner is unemployed (Baker and Taylor, submitted) or who do not have a partner (Thorpe, Golding, MacGillivray and Greenwood, 1991; Webster, Thompson, Mitchell and Werry, 1994) are more likely to report symptoms of depression. There is some possibility that this finding reflects a reporting bias with women living in poorer social conditions being more willing to report depressive symptomology than those living in more affluent conditions (Baker and Taylor, submitted) but it may also be the case that adverse social circumstances is one underlying factor which increases vulnerability to depression. Women living in socially adverse conditions do not have material resources to buffer the impact of negative life events and are more likely to encounter other situations that themselves predispose to depression such as poor physical health (Graham, 1984).

Life events

Brown and Harris' (1978) studies suggest that significant life events are the catalyst for the onset of depression and consistent with this finding is a solid group of studies reporting an association between life events and poor emotional well-being in the early years after the birth of a child (Paykel, Emms, Fletcher and Rassaby, 1980; Playfair and Gowers, 1981; O'Hara, Rehm and Campbell, 1982, 1983; Cutrona, 1983, 1984; Thorpe, Dragonas and Golding, 1992a,b). There is also evidence that life events in pregnancy may adversely affect emotional well-being in the post-natal period (Thorpe, Dragonas and Golding, 1992; O'Hara, Rehm and Campbell, 1982, 1983; O'Hara, Neunaber and Zekoski, 1984). Two studies which specifically studied postnatal depression did not find an association between life events and post-natal depression (Pitt, 1968; Kumar and Robson, 1984).

A range of events which bring either temporary or permanent changed life circumstances are included in inventories of life events: death or illness of family member or close friend, onset of personal conflict, accident, moving house and bad news are commonly included. Some studies have specifically examined events related to child-bearing. The Avon Longitudinal Study of Pregnancy and Childhood, an ongoing study of 14,000 families, includes among its inventory of life events: the impact of antenatal screening tests, medical complications (e.g. bleeding) or the news of twins, a negative reaction of the partner to the pregnancy, and returning to work after the birth. Preliminary findings from this study suggest negative events and life change (e.g. moving house) are stressful and have an adverse effect on emotional well-being. The greater the number of such events, the more likely a woman is to experience depressive symptoms (Thorpe, Golding, MacGillivray and Greenwood, 1991; Thorpe, Greenwood and Goodenough, 1995).

Antenatal well-being

An increasing body of evidence suggests that emotional well-being in the antenatal period is predictive of post-natal emotional well-being (Fergusson, Horwood and Thorpe, 1996; Green and Murray, 1994; Green, 1990; Thorpe, Golding, MacGillivray and Greenwood, 1991; Dennerstein et al., 1989). Two clear findings emerge from studies of emotional well-being across the transition to parenthood. First, rates of depressive symptomology tend to be higher in the antenatal period than in the post-natal period (Green and Murray, 1994; Fergusson, Horwood and Thorpe, 1996). Second, though reporting of depressive symptoms decreases for the population as a whole after childbirth, the group of women who are more likely to experience depressed mood post-natally are those who have experienced poor well-being antenatally. In a recent study of approximately 9000 women in which emotional well-being was measured at 18 and 32 weeks gestation and 8 and 32 weeks post partum, for example a high continuity of emotional well-being was found across the two antenatal time points with a marked decrease in reports of depression after the birth of the child. Thirty-eight per cent of women who scored above the 12 cut-off points on the EPDS antenatally had fallen below this criterion for 'depressed' status at 8 weeks post partum. The authors conclude that while childbirth may be the catalyst for onset of depressed mood in a small group of women, for many birth is a positive event which reduces the incidence of poor emotional well-being. Green (1990) and Green and Murray (1994) both suggest that antenatal well-being is an important but under-researched factor in the emotional well-being of mothers and that attention should focus on the question of what makes women unhappy during pregnancy. The large scale study reported by Fergusson, Horwood and Thorpe (1996) certainly supports this view.

Physical health of mother and baby

Both pregnancy and childbirth may alter a woman's sense of physical well-being and are associated with the development of new somatic symptoms (Thorpe, Greenwood and Goodenough, 1995; MacArthur, 1991; MacArthur, Lewis and Knox, 1991). In pregnancy a range of symptoms particularly nausea and vomiting and raised blood pressure are more common but there is great individual variation in the experience of these (Thorpe, Greenwood and Goodenough, 1995). After the birth of a child incidence of physical symptoms not previously experienced, particularly backache, headache, haemorrhoids and problems of bladder control, have been found to increase (MacArthur, 1991; MacArthur, Lewis and Knox, 1991). Again there is great individual variation. The mode of delivery of the child will affect the physical health of the mother, with those experiencing assisted deliveries (caesarean section, forceps and ventouse deliveries) experiencing more physical ill health particularly in the early weeks following delivery (MacArthur, Lewis and Knox, 1991).

Though currently there is little research in this area, intuitively, poor physical health will have an impact on the emotional well-being of mothers. A study comparing the physical and emotional health of women carrying a twin pregnancy with those carrying a single child found a significant association between ratings of physical health and emotional well-being though this relationship was less evident among women with a twin pregnancy (Thorpe, Greenwood and Goodenough, 1995). It is likely that the support received by women carrying twins and expectations of health had a modifying effect on the relationship between physical health and emotional well-being for the women expecting twins. Evidence that physical ill health influences emotional well-being following delivery is less conclusive. MacArthur, Lewis and Knox (1991) in their study *Health after Childbirth* found that the incidence of new onset both of physical and emotional symptoms increased following childbirth but did not specifically investigate the possibility of a causal relationship. They did however indicate an association between fatigue and depressive symptoms at this time. Depression is reported by the authors to be associated with features of the delivery, particularly a long first stage of labour and caesarean section. The adverse psychological effects of caesarean section have been previously noted (Green, 1990; Garel, Lelong, Marchand and Kaminski, 1990). An important finding from the study of Green (1990) is that, with the exception of women who delivered by caesarean section, the mode of delivery was not in itself related to poor emotional well-being. For women who had intervention at delivery other than caesarean section the sense of having appropriate information about the procedure and control in decision-making about the course of intervention was important. It was not intervention per se but the feeling of whether this was appropriate or not which influenced emotional well-being for these women.

The physical health of the baby after delivery also impacts upon maternal well-being. Mothers whose children are born pre-term, at low birthweight and/or are admitted to special care initially face the crisis of dealing with their sick child and the disappointment of not having had a 'perfect child' and in the longer term experience fatigue associated with caring for their baby in hospital and anxiety about returning home with their sick child (McHaffie, 1989, 1990; Redshaw and Harris, 1995). A higher proportion of these mothers will themselves have had operative deliveries and may, as a result, experience their own physical ill health (Redshaw, Harris and Ingram, 1996). To date there are no published studies specifically examining the incidence of depression among women whose children are very ill following birth, though Kumar and Robson (1984) note an association between pre-term delivery and post-natal depression and both Hopkins, Campbell and Marcus (1986) and Gjerdingen and Challoner (1994) report an association between infant illness and maternal depression. Most available data relate to the emotional well-being of mothers of children who have disabilities and these studies suggest that it is not the disability per se but behavioural characteristics of the child and the associated demands of parenting which affect maternal well-being (Harris and McHale, 1989).

Childcare burden

The number of children for whom a woman has to care has been consistently found to relate to depression. Brown and Harris (1978) found that women who had more than three children under the age of 14 were more vulnerable to depression. Similarly Thorpe, Golding, MacGillivray and Greenwood (1991) found an increased risk of depression for mothers with three or more children and present figures which suggest almost a two-fold increase in depression for those with four or more children compared with those who have no more than two children.

It is not only the number of children which relates to maternal depression, but also the configuration of the family. Two analyses based on large cohort studies have examined the impact of spacing of children on the emotional well-being of mothers. These provide evidence of an inverse relationship between spacing of children and maternal emotional well-being (Thorpe, Golding, MacGillivray and Greenwood, 1991; Thorpe, Greenwood and Goodenough, 1995a). In these studies, one conducted in the first year post partum the other at five years after the birth of a child, mothers of twins and of closely spaced single children (less than two years apart) were found to be at risk of experiencing depression compared with mothers of widely spaced and only children. Five years after the birth of twins mothers were found to have a two-fold increase in symptoms of depression compared with mothers of widely spaced or only children (Thorpe, Golding, MacGillivray and Greenwood, 1991). The age of children also may affect a mother's emotional well-being. The demands of caring for young children is high and having a number of preschool aged children may limit mobility and be socially isolating. Certainly reports from mothers who have twins or higher order multiples suggest this is the case (Thorpe, Golding, MacGillivray and Greenwood, 1991; Botting, MacFarlane and Price, 1990; Price, 1991). Contrary to the expectation that the childcare burden is greatest in the preschool years however is the finding from the preliminary analysis of the Avon Longitudinal Study of Pregnancy and Childbirth where the major effects on maternal well-being were found for the total number of children under the age of 18 (compared with under 5, 5–10 and over 10 years) suggesting that other stages of child development may place different pressures on the mother and affect her well-being (Thorpe et al., 1995a).

Studies comparing children with and without disability (reported above) suggest that the individual demands of the child are key predictors of maternal emotional well-being, and in all populations as well as those with disability the temperament and behaviour of the child will be associated with different levels of maternal stress. With young babies for example sleeping and crying behaviour are likely to impact upon a mother's physical and emotional health. Cutrona (1983) reports an association between the number of childcare stresses (e.g. problems quieting babies cries, problems with breastfeeding, not enough support from partner) and depression at 2 weeks and 8 weeks post partum. Fergusson, Lynskey and Horwood (1993) point to the problems of reporting bias, with depressed mothers being more likely to report their child's behaviour as problematic, but also found that an increase in child behaviour problems independently predicted poor maternal emotional well-being. Similar findings are reported by Sheeber and Johnson (1992) and Wallander, Pitt and Mellins (1990).

Sources of support and emotional well-being among mothers

Social networks and social support

An increasing body of research documents the importance of an individual's social environment to their physical and emotional health.

Degree of social contact is one aspect of social environment which has been studied. Studies of women in pregnancy and the early years post partum present a picture in which their social network serves as a buffer against poor emotional well-being. Certainly, family and friends can be a source of functional support for the mother and relieve some of the burdens of caring for a young child. However, there is also some evidence that the frequency and availability of social contact does not always have a positive impact on emotional well-being. A study of Greek and British couples across the transition to parenthood for example found that contact with family could be a source of stress (Thorpe, Dragonas and Golding, 1992a,b). In particular those parents who lived in close contact with parents or parents-in-law found that they were a source of stress. Similarly, studies of families who have twins or higher order multiples found that the assistance from family or health professions for the functional care of their children was not necessarily valued by the parents and indeed could be a source of stress because of organizational demands and loss of personal space (Botting, MacFarlane and Price, 1990).

These findings highlight the need to define the social environment more clearly and identify the elements that influence emotional well-being the most (Cutrona, 1984). One important distinction is that between social network and social support. It is not only the availability of social contact and functional support (network) but also the availability of someone in whom to confide and share experiences (social support) which have a bearing on emotional well-being (Parr, 1996).

The role of the partner in providing functional support has been examined as a potential mediator of emotional well-being. Studies have particularly focused on the value of the presence of a partner at delivery and their participation in functional care of the child and household tasks. Evidence from these studies does not present a clear picture in which provision of functional support alone facilitates good maternal emotional well-being. It is likely that a rather more complex picture in which the couple's individual role definitions and expectations about division of labour influence the relationship between functional support and emotional health (Thorpe, Golding, MacGillivray and Greenwood, 1991).

Emotional support

The availability of emotional support would appear to be far more directly linked to maternal emotional well-being. Measures of social support have consistently been found to be better predictors of emotional well-being and associated behaviours than social network (Cutrona, 1984; Thorpe, Golding, MacGillivray and Greenwood, 1991; Greenwood and Thorpe, 1993). The feeling of being understood and having someone in whom one can confide are important protective factors which buffer the effects of stressors which may adversely affect emotional well-being.

For a woman in the early years after the birth of her child the most important source of emotional support is her partner, especially in modern western societies where individuals are often geographically separated from their families (Parr, 1996). A consistent finding in research studies is that mothers who do not have a partner have a considerably higher risk of experiencing depression than those who do (Webster, Thompson, Mitchell and Werry, 1994). Similarly women who rate their marriages as dysfunctional are more likely to experience depression (Kumar and Robson, 1984; O'Hara, 1986;

Schweitzer, Logan and Stassberg 1992). Schweitzer, Logan and Stassberg (1992) for example, report that women in marriages characterized by high levels of control and low levels of emotional support are at greatest risk of experiencing post-natal depression. In contrast a supportive relationship will positively affect maternal well-being (Parr, 1996). Emotional support from a partner has also been found to benefit health related behaviours, for example in the reduction of alcohol consumption during pregnancy (Greenwood and Thorpe, 1995; Lelong et al., 1995).

Paid work

Although returning to the environment of paid employment can be a source of stress for mothers of young children, it is also a source of identity independence and social contact (Malley and Stewart, 1988). Paid work is typically assigned a higher social status than full-time motherhood and is potentially an important source of social contacts and emotionally supportive friendships. Though returning to paid work brings with it the stress of separating from a young child (Parr, 1996; Berryman, Thorpe and Windridge, 1995; Brannen and Moss, 1988) and adds additional demands on a mother, there is an increasing body of evidence which suggests that paid work has a positive impact on emotional well-being (Malley and Stewart, 1988; Rodin and Ickovics, 1990). Women who return to work after having a child have been found to have better general health. An important issue here is the mother's attitude to paid work and her reasons for returning to work. Women who return to work under the pressure of financial necessity and who would prefer to be full-time mothers tend not to experience the positive benefits of returning to paid work (Hock and Demeiss, 1990).

Personal qualities and emotional well-being among mothers

Studies of emotional well-being of mothers have focused primarily on sources of stress which might increase vulnerability and on a range of factors in the social environment which might increase resilience to poor emotional well-being. However an important issue is whether the personal characteristics of the mother might also influence her emotional reaction to pregnancy, childbirth and the stresses of early parenthood. Are some women inherently more likely to experience poor emotional well-being when they become mothers?

Personality and emotional well-being of mothers

A range of studies have examined the relationship between scores on standardized assessments of personality and emotional well-being of mothers in the early years following the birth of a child. Some studies are methodologically limited because they measure emotional well-being and personality concurrently. Hence distortions in personality assessment may occur as a result of mental state (particularly depression). A consistent finding is that individuals who obtain high scores on measures of neuroticism and/or trait anxiety are more prone to experience poor emotional well-being following the birth of a child (Todd, 1964; Pitt, 1968; Watson, Elliott and Rugg, 1984;

Dalton, 1971; Playfair and Gowers, 1981; Boyce, Parker, Barnett et al., 1991). Of seven papers reviewed, only one, Kumar and Robson (1984), failed to find such an association though it is important to note that this study assessed personality prospectively and therefore is less likely to confound emotional well-being and personality assessment. In contrast however, the prospective study of Boyce, Parker, Barnett et al. (1991) found that women who scored high on measures of neuroticism had a three-fold increased risk of experiencing depression in the first six months post partum. This study also utilized a new measure of personality, the Interpersonal Sensitivity Scale (Boyce and Parker, 1989) and found that individuals with high interpersonal sensitivity (measured prospectively) had a ten-fold increased risk of experiencing depressive symptoms in the first six months post partum. It provides convincing evidence that some aspects of personality increase vulnerability to poor emotional well-being in the post-partum period. Much less is known about the relationship of personality and emotional well-being for mothers outside this first year.

Psychiatric history and emotional well-being of mothers

Previous experience of psychiatric problems, particularly previous depressive episodes, have been found to increase a woman's vulnerability to depression following the birth of a child (O'Hara, Rehm and Campbell, 1983; O'Hara, 1986; Watson, Elliott and Rugg, 1984) though this was not found in the study of Kumar and Robson (1984). There is also some evidence that those with a family history of psychiatric problems have a higher risk of themselves experiencing depression after the birth of a child (Nilsson and Amgren, 1970a,b; O'Hara, 1986) though again this is not consistently reported (Kumar and Robson, 1984).

Pattern of cognition and emotional well-being of mothers

A range of studies have demonstrated that the way an individual explains an event may vary and that this reflects an individual's world view – their characteristic way of perceiving events – and relates to depression (Alloy, 1988). Thus while one mother may perceive a baby's persistent crying as a sign of their failure as a mother and feel helpless and unable to respond in a directed way, another may focus on the crying as a communication from the child and take a problem-solving approach in identifying and removing the source of the baby's discomfort. These styles of cognition are undoubtedly affected by poor emotional well-being (Alloy, 1988) but it may also be the case that pre-existing styles of cognitive attribution, measured before the birth of a child, affect the likelihood of experiencing depression after the birth. Two studies do report such an association (O'Hara, Rehm and Campbell, 1982; Cutrona, 1983) however two others have failed to find such an association (O'Hara, Neunaber, Zekoski, 1984; Manly, McMahon, Bradley and Davidson, 1982). Currently, the amount of research concerning cognitive style and emotional well-being is limited. It warrants further consideration because cognitive therapies have been found to be an effective approach to the treatment of depression.

When things go wrong: theoretical frameworks for intervention

. . . I enjoyed my pregnancy and I enjoyed having him, it was the greatest thing I have ever experienced until I came home. And then I thought, God, I don't want you . . . I felt as if I was inside this box, all by myself, with nobody to help me, or to help me understand why I was like this . . . I have been sad before and I have been unhappy, but never like after I had Thomas, to the point where I just didn't want to live any more.

Holden, Elliott and Gerrard, 1992, p. 11

Things can, and do, go wrong for any of us at any time. Sometimes we feel anxious, depressed and unable to cope. Whilst the previous section shows that some women are more vulnerable than others, none of us are immune to misadventure and misery. This section will explore the types of problems women experience when they slide to the poor well-being end of the emotional well-being continuum. The dominant model which describes such difficulties as 'Post-natal Disorders' is explained but not adopted as the only viable descriptive framework. This section also considers the relative merits of other frameworks through which such experiences may be viewed and responded to. The section will, therefore, reflect the complexity of the moral, ethical, philosophical and practical issues faced by health professionals working in community health settings (Orford, 1992) and primary care (Marzillier, 1992).

If negative emotions are normal then what constitutes a problem and when do a woman's personal feelings become a legitimate target for interventions by health professionals? There are almost as many ways of answering this question as there are interested parties wanting to help mothers.

The field of post-natal mental health was initially dominated by the specific medical perspective exemplified by Dalton (1971, 1980) who used the term Post-natal Depression (PND) to refer to all episodes of psychiatric disorder occurring for the first time in a woman's life with onset within the first six months following childbirth. She attributed all such disorders to the sharp drop in progesterone after childbirth.

The opposing position was then taken up by sociological writers who argued that depression after childbirth was not pathological but a reasonable response to an unreasonable social role change dictated by a society designed by and for men. Oakley for example claimed that 'Science, responding to an agenda of basically social concerns, has provided the label "postnatal depression" as a pseudoscientific tag for the description and ideological transformation of maternal discontent' (Oakley, 1980, p. 277).

There ensued what Ballinger (1996) terms the sterile debate on raised rates of depression in women post-natally, characterized by the question 'Are our hormones or our husbands to blame?' As she points out hormones are easier to do something about! Seeing an obstetrician for hormone therapy is also less stigmatizing than seeing a psychiatrist and financially more adaptive than throwing out the baby's father.

Before any such treatment choices are exercised someone must reach the conclusion that a woman's mental state constitutes a problem, rather one of the many responses which make up the rich tapestry of maternal experience illustrated at the beginning of the chapter. Most women with poor emotional well-being are aware that something is amiss though they may not know what to call their problem and whether or where to seek help or may disagree with professionals who offer help as to the appropriate description or help for their problems (Nicolson, 1989; Small, Brown, Lumley and Astbury, 1994; Whitton, Appleby and Warner, 1996). A personal account can illustrate the distancing which can occur when health professionals employ a discourse helpful to their own decision making, typically a diagnostic framework, which has no meaning in the discourse of the recently delivered mother. When asked to describe her experience of motherhood Alibhai (1989) began with 'a long drawn out silent scream' prompted by her problem of communicating distress and experiences when 'we have not evolved composite concepts, a language in common, or status equality which are the prerequisites for genuine understanding' (pp. 24–25). To convey her experience of motherhood she wanted to explain why she cried for two weeks after the birth of her son. 'In the hospital they called it post-natal depression' (p. 36). This diagnostic label obviously meant nothing, and explained nothing for her. Instead it conveyed how out of touch with her needs and experience the professionals were. Alibhai cried 'firstly because I had not wanted to want him so badly – in spite of my love and desire to have him, and "optimum" childbirth conditions – the never-had-it-so-good feelings were constantly being overshadowed by a deep sense of sorrow. It felt like Ari had arrived into a no man's land, an orphanage. These feelings were so powerful they actually knocked against my ribs, for a fortnight. Now they just quietly tremble within, every time his security is threatened.' (p. 27). Alibhai goes on to describe her own mother's post-natal tears, the life which was the context for this, then her own life in Uganda, the turmoil for Ugandan Asians after Amin ordered them out and her first six years in Britain. She concludes that 'This background is essential to understand the feelings of loss and fear I experienced when my son was born. Especially in terms of what Britain had begun to mean to me then. That had been another psychological earthquake. In the hospital they called it post-natal depression. I think it was a watershed time when my past identity, personal and political, had crashed into the new bits and pieces that had begun to grow since I had arrived here...' (p. 36). It is important to remember that no post-natal experience can be meaningfully understood without an understanding of the personal context provided by background and current circumstances, whether as dramatic as Alibhai's or apparently mundane. Qualitative research aims to avoid the trap Oakley attributes to scientific diagnosis by describing mothers' problems from the personal experiential perspective and in their own terms rather than by diagnostic labels (e.g. Mauthner, 1995; Nicolson, 1989). This research will permit the development of detailed psychological models of post-natal experience but the very nature of these complex contextual personal accounts provides no simple means for busy health professionals to recognize women in need of help. It is this failure of rich personal accounts and qualitative research to meet the practical needs of primary care professionals which probably accounts for the poor response to Oakley's call to reject terms such as post-natal depression for poor maternal emotional well-being.

Despite the fact that only a minority of women experiencing distress after childbirth ever reach a psychiatrist, reports of post-natal distress in the research and lay literature alike have tended to use psychiatric frameworks and terminology, with all the advantages and disadvantages this implies (Clare, 1980; Davison and Neale, 1996). Clarity is not helped by inconsistency in the use of terms, particularly 'Post-natal Depression'. This term has been used to refer to any psychiatric illness with its first onset in the six months after childbirth or to include psychosis, depression and the 'Blues' in the puerperium, regardless of time of onset, or more narrowly to refer to Depression in the puerperium which meets standardized diagnostic criteria, including earlier as well as post-natal onsets. Current thinking in perinatal psychiatry considers the distinction between psychotic and non-psychotic disorders to be meaningful (Appleby, Kumar and Warner, 1996) and does not include the common, time-limited experiences known as the 'Blues' in the list of psychiatric disorders. The following text uses upper case to denote diagnostic labels and lower case to denote mood or symptoms because of the similarity of terms used in diagnostic and emotional continuum models.

Puerperal Psychoses typically have rapid onset within the first two weeks after delivery and are characterized by perplexity and confusion as well as one or more of the classic signs of psychosis such as delusions and hallucinations. This may be accompanied by depressive stupor in Psychotic Depression, alternating with Mania in Bipolar (i.e. Manic Depressive) Disorder, or characterized by thought disorder in Schizophrenia or may include a confusing mix of symptoms characteristic of more than one traditional category. The debate continues as to whether there is a subgroup of psychotic depressions which is specific to the puerperium or whether all are manifestations of a life long vulnerability to psychoses which may reappear at other times (Kendell, Chalmers and Platz, 1987; Kumar, 1989; Riley, 1995). The speed and timing of onset of puerperal psychoses leads most clinicians to suspect a biological aetiology specific to childbirth, at least for a subgroup (Brockington and Cox-Roper, 1988) though again the nature of such underlying pathology has still to be identified (Riley, 1995).

Post-natal Depression is a more common problem with a less dramatic onset. The diagnostic category of Non-psychotic Clinical Depression (as recognized by psychiatrists) is distinguished from depressed mood after childbirth (the broader category of those experiencing post-natal depression), by judgements on duration (usually more than two weeks) and severity (usually including four or more additional symptoms, such as sleep, appetite or psychomotor disturbance, anxiety, fatigue, guilt, inability to cope, poor concentration or suicidal thoughts). The grey area of depressive symptomatology between transient depressed mood and Clinical Depression is typically referred to as Subclinical Depression or borderline caseness. Between 10 and 15 per cent of women interviewed two to three months after childbirth will report depression sufficient to meet diagnostic criteria and over 20 per cent will experience Clinical Depression at some time in the first post-natal year (Watson, Elliott, Rugg and Brough 1984). The prevalence of Depression in the first post-natal year is similar to the one year period prevalence in other community samples (Watson, Elliott and Rugg, 1984) and comparison groups of mothers (Cooper, Campbell, Day et al., 1988; Cox, Murray and Chapman, 1993; O'Hara, Zekoski, Philipps and Wright, 1990; O'Hara, Schelchre, Lewis and Jarner, 1991). However onsets are not evenly spread across the year and peak in the first post-natal month, with half the onsets by three months and three-quarters by six months (Cooper, Campbell, Day et al., 1988). High rates of Depression would usually be associated with high suicide rates. In fact the suicide risk in mothers is low (Appleby, 1996) which is consistent with the notion that concern about the effect on their children prevents women from opting for this solution to their depression.

O'Hara and Swain (1996) used a meta-analysis of putative risk factors measured in pregnancy to produce a tentative composite of the prototypical pregnant woman at risk for post-natal depression. 'She is most likely to occupy a lower social stratum but women representing middle and upper social strata will also be abundantly represented. She is very likely to have experienced stressors during pregnancy and may have had a more difficult than normal pregnancy or delivery. She will be experiencing marital difficulties and experience her partner as providing little in the way of social support. Compounding the life stress she is experiencing and her poor marital relationship will be her perception that others in her social network are not particularly supportive of her. Finally, her history will show evidence of psychopathology, in most cases major depression or dysthymia, and she will show evidence of being at least mildly depressed and anxious, and excessively worried' (p. 46).

Currently the most widely used classifications of depression are ICD-10, the tenth revision of the World Health Organisation's International Classification of Diseases (1992) and DSM-IV, the fourth edition of the American Psychiatric Association's Diagnostic and Statistical Manual of Mental Disorders (1994).

Unfortunately, neither of these classify puerperal disorders as they are understood by psychiatrists specializing in motherhood and mental illness, represented by their international society, the Marcé Society (Brockington and Cox-Roper, 1988; Kumar, 1989). The ICD-10 is preferred because it has at least reinstated a specific category for puerperal mental disorders, albeit with instructions to use this category only if sufficient information has not been obtained in order to accurately place it elsewhere (Cox, 1994). The absence of a primary classification hinders research in the field, including that which could answer the very question as to whether some, or all, categories of mental health problems experienced post partum differ from those at other times in their symptom profiles, phenomenology, predisposing factors, precipitants, maintaining factors or consequences. Riley therefore requests that 'whatever the clinical coding given to puerperal patients, a further coding should be made under ICD-10, category 099.3 – "Mental disorders and diseases of the nervous system complicating pregnancy, childbirth and the puerperium" – so that future researchers can easily identify puerperal admissions.' (Riley, 1995, p. 110).

Since Pitt's (1968) paper on depression after childbirth which surprised the psychiatric community by finding formerly unrecognized psychiatric morbidity, Post-natal Depression has been the focus of research and media attention so it has become necessary to remind researchers and health professionals that all the other problems which occur at other times are also present in the post-natal period including alcohol and drug abuse, eating disorders and psychological problems associated with physical disorders (Riley, 1995). Anxiety is common after the birth of a child, especially the first, or if baby or mother has health problems, or indeed if the mother is depressed and having difficulty coping. For most, these are transient or minor worries. In some women the birth leads to the onset of problems severe enough to meet the criteria for an Anxiety Disorder. There have been recent clinical descriptions of post-natal onset Panic Disorder and stress reactions resembling Post-traumatic Stress Disorder following traumatic labour and delivery experiences (Bloor and Jones, 1988; Metz, Sichel and Goff, 1988; Moleman, van der Hart and van der Kolk, 1992, reported in Riley, 1995).

Primary care and obstetric staff tend to look to the diagnostic systems of psychiatry as the framework for dealing with people with emotional problems, partly because they are familiar with applying medical models to physical health. Most will use this as a guide for determining what constitutes a problem to be referred to psychiatric services, since they are used to providing services for 'illness'. However, diagnostic systems were designed for classifying patients known to have a mental health problem, and, in the days of Kraepelin, presumed to have a mental illness. They were not designed for the purpose of making an ill/well judgement. Systems have been refined so that by default someone who does not meet criteria for any disorder on the list can be deemed not ill and not requiring psychiatric treatment. However diagnostic systems do not necessarily indicate which of the lesser (subclinical) levels of distress non-psychiatric health professionals could, or should, meaningfully provide help with to alleviate current distress or to prevent deterioration to clinical levels. Severity of 'illness' in a psychiatric classification is not synonymous with level of need for health and social care (Fernando, 1995) nor does the application of a diagnostic label necessarily confirm 'illness' in the narrow sense of indicating primary, biological pathology. Primary care and maternity staff continue to rely on their own professional experience as much as their education in perinatal psychiatry to determine their level of input with each client which may leave them vulnerable to demand manipulation by more vocal attention-seeking clients whilst missing the quietly depressed, 'smiling' depressed and non-attending depressed mothers. To put it another way, many health visitors faced with unhappy mothers have realized the limitations of the diagnostic framework since the question 'can I help her or not?' is not fully answered by determining whether she has Postnatal Depression or not.

Psychologists may use concepts such as 'abnormal psychology' and 'abnormal behaviour' which have strong parallels with the medical terminology of 'Psychiatry' and 'Mental Illness' but without the implicit assumption of an underlying disease process. These terms do reasonably well in conveying the speciality of the psychologist but founder on the dichotomy abnormal/normal when applied to behaviour and experience in order to determine problems and classify individuals as 'abnormal'. Normality is socially defined and is the result of lack of agreement as to what constitutes abnormality. With specific reference to the experience of new mothers, Bennett (1981) argues that 'The attempt to identify and understand abnormal reactions at this time, in the absence of any delineation of what is normal, seems unlikely to be entirely successful'. This is consistent with abnormal psychology texts which conclude that 'no current definition of abnormal behaviour is satisfactory' (Davison and Neale, 1990, p. 58), so the health professional cannot rely on indices of abnormality to determine what constitutes a problem.

An alternative which acknowledges the need to respond to and research expressions of distress in the individual whilst avoiding the pathology labels of abnormal psychology and psychiatry, is the use of continuum models (e.g. Bennett, 1981; Green, 1990; Mauthner, 1995; Windridge and Berryman, 1996). These may use global labels of the extremes (such as positive emotional well-being to poor emotional well-being) or several more specific labels of the negative poles (such as anxiety and depression), or even present a continuum for each individual item in the form of a visual analogue scale. Complex multifactorial models of experience can be constructed. Complex models have the potential to more closely describe reality than do simplistic dichotomies such as Depressed versus Normal with artificial and arbitrary cut-off points (Elliott, 1984). However, these models are harder to sustain the closer the theorist comes to the practical issues of service provision since they do not provide answers to the questions of purchasers and managers who must make the decisions on 'how much of what service for how many?'

Evolutionary perspectives portray negative emotions as a normal part of human existence. They go further than portraying negative emotions as understandable responses to adversity and part of the normal range. They claim that negative emotions are essential, constructive parts of the human repertoire. To take a more familiar analogy, the pain we experience when touching a kettle is unpleasant but prompts us to remove ourselves from a situation which could cause increasing damage. People who are unable to feel pain are in danger. They are at a disadvantage compared to those of us who have this unpleasant experience 'pain' in our repertoire. Evolution has retained fatigue to prompt us to rest, fear to make us fight or flee and anxiety to indicate the need to prepare or avoid. It seems reasonable to assume that depression has also been retained within our emotional repertoire because it serves some positive adaptive purpose, although controversy remains as to what the evolutionary function might be (Birtchnell, 1995; Gilbert, 1995). Whilst negative emotions sometimes lead to personal growth and purposive life style change, few would recommend emotional pain as the preferred route to such goals. Obviously, we do even better if we realize that the kettle will be hot and do not touch it in the first place! This is the philosophy which underlies psychosocial antenatal prevention programmes for post-natal distress. Not all negative emotions will be prevented, however. In common with the other models which reject 'illness' and 'abnormality' dichotomies, the evolutionary perspective does not offer any clear guidelines as to where the divide falls between negative emotions which are part of an informative and constructive process and those which are serving no useful purpose and constitute a problem in their own right. This perspective is therefore less helpful for post-natal staff confronted with the need to decide which distressed mothers require their intervention.

It is apparent that no simple answer can be found to the question 'what constitutes a problem?' It can not be addressed without consideration of the further question 'for whom is the mother's psychological status a problem?' In most circumstances it is the mother herself and it would be inappropriate to remove the mother's right to define her own problems. The personal experiential perspective is *always* present and will be a powerful determinant of help seeking and acceptance. The role of the health professional would therefore be in facilitating the mother in recognizing, and constructing a descriptive framework for her difficulties and enabling her to communicate this to appropriate sources of help. Unfortunately, many depressed women do not come to the attention of health professionals who can alleviate their distress (Cox, Connor and Kendell, 1982).

At what point should a shift from the woman's own perspective of her problems to a medical perspective of her 'pathology' be made? Is it necessary to supply a label which brings her suffering into a diagnostic framework in order to justify the deployment of *health* service resources and personnel in her assistance?

From an anti-psychiatry perspective the problem is seen to reside in social position and role, and the solution is assumed to be sociopolitical not medical. Labelling a problem as an individual health problem requiring health care is, in this view, adding to the problem not benefiting the individual (Szasz, 1987). The implication is that the shift from the woman's to the medical perspective medicalizes her experiences at best and stigmatizes them at worst. The fear is that any mental health care is inherently destructive – a view reflected in some mothers' own fears (Whitton, Appleby and Warner, 1996). This raises ethical dilemmas, for example, should health professionals refrain from intervening with the depressed mother whom they believe to be at risk of suicide or infanticide?

In contrast psychiatrists generally advocate the use of the diagnostic, or 'illness', framework for all post-natal mental health concerns. A problem which requires the help of a health professional is one which fits one of the diagnostic descriptions (syndrome criteria). In some instances the risks and fears of labelling are recognized and addressed by efforts to destigmatize the labels. In particular the term Post-natal Depression is seen as legitimizing help giving and help seeking without having stigmatizing connotations. It is a psychiatric label that is not intended to arouse fears of being labelled as mentally ill and unfit to care for children (Whitton, Appleby and Warner, 1996). Psychiatrists make the assumption that mental health services can successfully treat post-natal mental health problems (Oates, 1994), so the low detection rate for post-natal emotional problems represents a cause for concern (Cox, Connor and Kendell, 1982; Cox, Holden and Sagovsky, 1987; Small, Brown, Lumley and Astbury, 1994; Wickberg-Johansson, Erlandsson and Hwang, 1996) and requires explanation (Holden, 1996, Whitton, Appleby and Warner, 1996). From this perspective it is the *failure* to label which is destructive. The solution to the low detection rate is seen to lie in taking the psychiatric diagnostic framework as far into the community as possible via the maternity and primary care services (Cox, Holden and Sagovsky, 1987; Oates, 1996; Whitton, Appleby and Warner, 1996).

Cox (1994) criticizes what he terms the 'normalization' approach and argues that this introduces a risk of missing organic causes of depression, such as thyroid dysfunction or even cerebral tumour. On the basis of his experience of a specialist psychiatric day unit for parents and babies he argues that most of those attending 'are not only "clients" or "customers" but also patients – they suffer, and most seek informed medical help' (Cox, 1994, p. 5). This is an uncontroversial position to adopt in a post-natal mental health facility such as the day unit in Stoke-on-Trent, since those attending will have already identified themselves as having a problem in the mental health sphere (or at least agreed to consider their GP's proposal of framing of their problems as a mental health issue in order to institute a mental health assessment referral). However, the case for the universal adoption of the diagnostic systems of psychiatry to all health settings concerned with perinatal care is not clear. Most midwives and health visitors will occasionally find themselves assessing a woman who undoubtedly has a severe perinatal mental disorder. However, most of their contacts will be with perinatal women experiencing a variety of 'problems with living'. They will not have had the opportunity, experience or need to develop the specialist skills for the subclassification of perinatal mental illness required of staff in perinatal mental health facilities. Should they improve their familiarity with the diagnostic approach by applying it to all their contacts with new mothers? Even if the label chosen for the mild end can simultaneously be viewed as non-stigmatizing in the mother's networks yet avoid dismissal as the 'worried well' not entitled to mental health services by psychiatrists, there may be risks attached to medicalizing problems which may otherwise be viewed as problems of living.

So research demonstrating that many women avoid the diagnostic labels preferred by health professionals and chose not to seek health care (McIntosh, 1993; Nicolson, 1989; Small, Brown, Lumley and Asbury, 1994) can be construed either as confirming the limitations of the diagnostic approach which should be abandoned (Nicolson, 1989) or the limitation of women's understanding which demands antenatal education in puerperal disorders and the value of diagnostic labelling (Whitton, Appleby and Warner, 1996). Maternity and primary care staff *could* be trained to apply the diagnostic approach of psychiatry to all problems of emotional well-being they encounter for fear of missing a problem of medical origin but *should* they?

The non-labelling, humanistic, sociocultural perspective can, in fact, co-exist with the diagnostic medical framework if a suitable filtering system can be found through which only those who would benefit from a medical label would pass. An example of such a filter is the Edinburgh Postnatal Depression Scale (EPDS), a short simple screening questionnaire for routine use with all post-natal women developed by Cox, Holden and Sagovsky (1987). Their validation study reported a split half reliability of 0.88 and standardized alpha co-efficient of 0.87. Adopting a 12/13 cut-off produced a sensitivity of 86 per cent, specificity of 78 per cent and positive predictive value of 73 per cent. Sensitivity was increased to 94 per cent by lowering the cut-off to 9/10 but with a resultant reduction in specificity to 51 per cent and positive predictive value to 58 per cent. Subsequent studies with differently constructed samples and diagnostic criteria obtained sensitivities ranging from 64 to 95 per cent, specificities ranging from 82 to 93 per cent and positive predictive values from 39 per cent to 75 per cent (Harris, Huckle, Thomas et al., 1989; Murray and Cox, 1990; Murray and Carothers, 1990). A further interview to consider health service intervention would then be required only for those indicating distress on the questionnaire or during routine contacts. Whilst this process provides an explicit structure where little existed before, it is not simple. For example the choice of cut-off depends on consideration of the population and nature and availability of interventions (Elliott, 1994; Gerrard, Elliott and Holden, 1994). The authors of the scale have now produced a book outlining the uses and abuses of the screening tool (Cox and Holden, 1994) and training programmes are available (Gerrard, Holden, Elliott et al., 1993).

This section has provided some insight into the controversy surrounding importing issues of emotional well-being into the health care framework. Few non-medical primary care staff adopt either of the extreme positions – diagnostic framework for everyone or for no-one. The task becomes one of understanding the potential risks and benefits of the medical and social constructionist positions when developing systems to identify those whom the health care programme may help. The key point to be made here is that both primary screening systems to eliminate those with positive emotional well-being and secondary screens leading to a 'decision to treat' should utilize methods and cut-off points which balance the risks of false positives (labelling someone with a problem inappropriately/unhelpfully/expensively) versus the risks of false negatives (failing to recognize a problem which leads to deterioration in mother and/or risk to mother or baby).

Interventions

Prevention is rarely as *feasible* as it is with post-natal depression. Post-natal depression follows a major life event which can be predicted well in advance. Throughout that phase women are in regular contact with health professionals and educators in non-stigmatizing contexts. Potential opportunities are high whilst potential costs are low. Prevention is also *plausible* and a variety of strategies have been suggested, e.g. progesterone prophylaxis (Dalton, 1980), change at the macro-environmental level (Oakley, 1980; Welburn, 1980), antenatal psycho-educational strategies addressing beliefs about parenthood, emotions and coping strategies and individual psychotherapeutic help in pregnancy (Elliott, 1989a,b). Evidence that prevention is *possible* is hard to find. Despite some convincing individual case reports on progesterone, no satisfactory scientific evidence has been produced for its effectiveness (Harris, 1996). Prevention programmes from psychosocial perspectives have had some success with antenatal education for emotional well-being (Gordan and Gordan, 1960; Cowan and Cowan, 1987) but less encouraging results with individual psychotherapy (Shereshefsky and Lockman, 1973). One study utilized a psychosocial intervention combining social support, continuity of care and psycho-education in monthly group meetings during pregnancy and the first post-natal six months plus an antenatal visit by the health visitor. Vulnerable first-time mothers invited to take part in this programme produced significantly higher well-being scores on questionnaires and a significantly lower proportion were diagnosed as Depressed or Borderline Depressed during the first three post-natal months at psychiatric interview (Elliott, Sanjack and Leverton, 1988). Even the sociocultural and evolutionary perspectives of emotional states, which portray negative emotions as appropriate responses allow that it is *preferable* to avoid unpleasant emotions. This may be particularly important at key times of personal experience and development. For example, depression after childbirth may lead not only to long-term personal distress about 'missing' the first months of baby's life but to problems for the developing child itself (Murray, 1992; Murray and Cooper, 1996; Murray, Kempton, Woolgar and Hooper, 1993).

However, things do not always go to plan. The best we can expect is that half of the cases of post-natal depression can be prevented (Elliott, Sanjack and Leverton, 1988; Elliott, 1989a). A variety of interventions have therefore been developed for post-natal distress.

At the mildest end of poor emotional well-being, interventions will be provided by health visitors, midwives and self-help groups. It would be inappropriate for these psychosocial interventions to be termed 'treatment' or indeed 'therapy'. Although grounded in the counselling philosophy (Cox, 1986; Holden, Cox, Sagovsky, 1989), practitioners of this approach prefer to use terms like 'sensitive emotional support' by midwives and 'active listening' or 'postnatal depression visits' by health visitors to avoid creating the impression that they are qualified 'counsellors' (Gerrard, Elliott and Holden, 1994). Finally, volunteer agencies describe their interventions as crisis helplines, self-help groups and befriending (Elliott, 1989a; Riley, 1995). Some volunteer services such as Home Start and New Pin are facilitated by health professionals but utilize non stigmatizing settings and prioritize peer support. New Pin has provided a model of providing health care without healthcare labels or an alienating professional culture (Mills and Pound, 1986; Pound and Mills, 1985).

As with prevention, primary care interventions are not successful in alleviating all post-natal distress. Around one third will require referral for specialist help (Holden, Cox and Sagovsky, 1989), so primary care staff have to decide who to refer on, when and to whom.

A variety of secondary mental health care professionals accept health visitor or GP referrals of post-natal women. However, in many instances the level and type of help required is not immediately apparent to the health visitor. Research into psychotherapy and counselling has made little progress in addressing the key question posed by Paul in 1969 'What treatment, by whom, is most effective for this individual with what specific problem, under which set of circumstances and how does it come about?' (Paul, 1969, p. 44). There is also the question of which approaches are acceptable to which women, since effective treatments have no value if women refuse the referral offered or fail to attend the appointment with the mental health specialist (Robinson and Young, 1982).

A number of interventions have been described which do not use medical treatments or the illness/cure terminology unacceptable to some. These may be described as 'therapeutic interventions'; for example, cognitive behaviour therapy (Brierley, 1988 and cited in Elliott, 1989a), Rogerian client-centred/non-directive counselling (Holden, Cox and Sagovsky, 1989; Hunter, 1994), cognitive behavioural counselling (Whitton, Appleby and Warner, 1996), 'professional intervention' by a social worker (Barnett and Parker, 1985), interpersonal psychotherapy (Stuart and O'Hara, 1995), psychoanalytic psychotherapy (Daws, 1989), psychodynamic psychotherapy and psychodrama (Morris, 1987). Such interventions are generally seen as quite distinct by their practitioners, but may not differ in their effectiveness. Only a few have so far been compared to 'untreated' controls receiving routine care. Barnett and Parker (1985) found that highly anxious first-time mothers receiving professional support from a social worker were significantly less anxious than untreated controls and than those who had received non-professional support from an experienced mother by 12 month follow-up. Holden, Cox and Sagovsky (1989) reported a significantly higher recovery rate from Post-natal Depression for women receiving weekly 'listening visits', utilizing an approach based on non-directive counselling, than for women receiving routine care (67 per cent versus 38 per cent).

In the most sophisticated design to date, Cooper and Murray (1997) compared three interventions with routine primary care. The interventions were designed to be quite distinct in theoretical basis, presumed mode of action and primary target of intervention. To ensure purity of approach a specialist was employed for each therapy. However, to test if the approaches could be adapted for use in the British NHS, three generalists (including two health visitors) were also recruited. Non-directive counselling was chosen in order to replicate the findings of Holden, Cox and Sagovsky (1989). Cognitive behaviour therapy was used in the context of an appropriately modified form of interaction guidance treatment so that the focus of treatment would not be maternal depression but on the problems identified by the mother in the management of her infant as well as on observed problems in the quality of the mother–infant interaction. Finally the dynamic therapy used was a 'brief mother–baby psychotherapy' in which the mother's relationship with the baby was considered in the light of her own early childhood attachments. Despite all the efforts to promote differences, the three therapies proved equally effective in reducing the duration of depression and the rate of maternal reports of relationship problems. Furthermore early remission from depression was associated with a reduced rate of insecure attachments regardless of which, if any, therapy was used to alleviate depression. It appears from this study that, although treatment can have a positive effect on the mother's relationship with her child separate from, and in addition to, any improvement in the relationship due to reduction in depression, reduction in the duration of depression per se can reduce the level of infant problems associated with depression. It would seem that it is not only the woman herself who would benefit from preventing the occurrence of the depression in the first place, since 'infant problems associated with depression, in particular infant behaviour problems and insecure attachment, would themselves be prevented' (Cooper and Murray, 1997).

Few controlled trials of medical treatments have been undertaken in the puerperium, possibly because doctors share the reluctance to use drugs with breastfeeding women. Appleby, Warner, Whitton and Faragher (in press) recently compared an antidepressant, fluoxetine, to cognitive counselling and found them equally effective with no added benefit from using both. This study did, however, appear to confirm the reduced acceptability of medical care since the main reason given for refusing to take part in the trial, which more than half the 188 depressed women invited to take part did, was 'reluctance to take medication'.

Whilst some reject any approaches which medicalize their problems others find it socially acceptable to attribute their coping problems to their hormones, thereby implying a gynaecological rather than a psychiatric disorder. Research is beginning to clarify the relationship between ovarian hormones, cognitive functions and mood (Weick, 1996). However, studies have so far failed to identify any hormonal cause for post-natal mental health problems (Harris, 1994; O'Hara, Schlechre, Lewis and Jarner, 1991), with the possible exception of depression which accompanies other symptoms of thyroid disorder (Harris, 1996). There is recent evidence that oestrogen can speed up the recovery from severe depression after childbirth (Gregoire, Kumar, Everitt et al., 1996; Henderson, Gregoire, Kumar et al., 1991) but it is unclear whether this is via non-specific psychotropic properties or via the 'cure' of an oestrogen deficiency.

Despite the absence of controlled trials for traditional psychiatric interventions for the severe end of the continuum of post-natal distress, perinatal psychiatrists are confident in their interventions. For example, Oates writing about post-natal mental illness services states that 'As is usual for acute-onset major affective illness, treatment is effective. Indeed, it may be that puerperal affective disorders, in particular, are more responsive to treatment and are of briefer duration than non-puerperal illnesses' (1994, p. 11). In relation to Puerperal Psychosis, Riley notes that 'few authors comment in any systematic way on their methods of treatment, reflecting the difficulty of applying a standard regimen to such a polymorphous syndrome' (1995, p. 123). Plans are now being made for collaboration across many centres and countries in order to find sufficient similar cases for systematic evaluation of drugs such as lithium for manic or bipolar (manic-depressive) states. The lack of research evidence for psychiatric treatments is unlikely to be the first concern of a husband or health visitor faced with a psychotic or suicidally depressed mother. They will prioritize a safe setting with 24-hour care and consider it a bonus if it has the conducive environment, experienced staff and place for the baby provided by specialist mother and baby units.

Emotional well-being of mothers: a summary

Society portrays motherhood as a necessity and yet for the majority of women motherhood is associated with a devaluation of their role in society. Women's personal reactions to becoming a mother reflect this ambivalence articulating both intense frustration and joy. Though it is possible to describe general patterns in the reaction to becoming a mother there is great individual variation in how a woman responds emotionally. Her personal circumstances will undoubtedly bear upon her emotional well-being at this time and those women who experience greatest stress and do not have a supportive environment are those most likely to encounter depression. Antenatal programmes can facilitate women in reducing demands and avoidable stressors as well as increasing support during the transition to parenthood in order to promote positive emotional well-being. Unfortunately, many factors which increase the risk of psychological problems lie outside the control of prospective parents and any available services. Services need to explore cost-effective systems to alleviate emotional problems in parents and to prevent secondary problems in the children and their families. Services should be proactive to maximize primary and secondary prevention. Providers should be alert to the potential for serious problems including suicide and infanticide but wary of designing intrusive systems driven by anxiety about missing these rare conditions.

Applications

- Discovery of women requiring additional emotional support post-natally cannot be left to chance. Systematic procedures for early identification and follow-up are needed.
- Screening programmes for post-natal depression in primary care settings need to be developed in consultation with mental health professionals in local secondary care services to establish referral criteria and procedures for post-natal disorders which cannot be managed in primary care.
- Health professionals, particularly health visitors, need to develop and use active listening skills in post-natal care.
- Primary care staff need to have an explicit awareness of the advantages and disadvantages of diagnostic labelling in order to make offers of additional help in a manner sensitive to the needs of the individual woman.
- Severe mental illness, especially with psychotic features, clearly requires referral for specialist psychiatric care.
- The match of problem with intervention is less clear for non-psychotic conditions. The rough rule of thumb for primary care professionals remains to offer only that which they feel they can cope with and to consult with secondary care colleagues or general practitioners whenever they feel a problem is not within their capacity and capability.
- Post-natal women have special experiences and special needs, so secondary care professionals should consider additional training in perinatal mental health if they plan to act as facilitators to primary care screening and intervention programmes.

References

Alibhai, Y. (1989). Burning in the cold. In *Balancing Acts: On being a mother* (K. Gieve, ed.). London: Virago.

Alloy, L. B. (ed.) (1988). *Cognitive Processes in Depression*. New York: Guilford Press.

American Psychiatric Association (1994). *Diagnostic and Statistical Manual of Mental Disorders*. APA.

Appleby, L. (1996). Suicidal behaviour in childbearing women. *International Review of Psychiatry*, **8**, 107–16.

Appleby, L., Kumar, C. and Warner, R. (1996). Perinatal psychiatry. *International Review of Psychiatry*, **8**, 5–7.

Appleby, L., Warner, R. W., Whitton, A. L. and Faragher, B. (1997). A controlled trial of Fluoxetine and cognitive-behavioural counselling in the treatment of postnatal depression. *British Medical Journal*, **314**, 932–6.

Baker, D. and Taylor, H. (submitted). Postnatal depression and primary health care: Is the need for treatment being met? Manuscript submitted for publication.

Ballinger, C. B. (1996). Aetiological factors related to development of postpartum mood disorders. Perinatal Depression Symposium. Dundee Healthcare.

Barnett, B. and Parker, G. (1985). Professional and non-professional intervention for highly anxious primiparous mothers. *British Journal of Psychiatry*, **146**, 289–93.

Beckett, H. (1986). Adolescent identity development. In *Feminist Social Psychology* (S. Wilkinson, ed.). Milton Keynes: Open University Press.

Bennett, E. A. (1981). Coping in the puerperium: the reported experience of new mothers. *Journal of Psychosomatic Research*, **25**, 13–21.

Berryman, J. C. (1993). Who wants egg donation? *Issue*, Winter, 13–14.

Berryman, J. C., Thorpe, K. J. and Windridge, K. C. (1995). *Older Mothers: Conception, Pregnancy and Birth after 35*. London: Pandora.

Birchnell, J. (1995). Exercising caution in applying animal models to humans: a replay to Price and Gardner. *British Journal of Medical Psychology*, **68**, 207–10.

Bloor, R. N. and Jones, R. A. (1988). Post-traumatic stress disorder and sexual dysfunction. *British Journal of Sexual Medicine*, **15**, 170–72.

Botting, B. J., MacFarlane, A. J. and Price, F. V. (1990). *Three, Four or More: A study of Triplets and Higher Order Births*. London: HMSO.

Boyce, P., Parker, G., Barnett, B., Cooney, M. and Smith, F. (1991). Personality as a vulnerability factor for depression. *British Journal of Psychiatry*, **159**, 106–14.

Boyce, P. and Parker, G. (1989). Development of a scale to measure interpersonal sensitivity. *Australian and New Zealand Journal of Psychiatry*, **23**, 341–51.

Brannen, J. and Moss, P. (1988). *New Mothers at Work*. London: Unwin.

Brierley, E. (1988). A cognitive-behavioural approach to the treatment of postnatal distress. *Marcé Bulletin*, **1**, 27–41.

Brockington, I. and Cox-Roper, A. (1988). The nosology of puerperal mental illness. In *Motherhood and Mental Illness 2* (R. Kumar and I. F. Brockington, eds). London: Wright.

Brown, G. W. and Harris, T. (1978). *Social Origins of Depression: A Study of Psychiatric Disorder in Women*. London: Tavistock.

Clare, A. (1980). *Psychiatry In Dissent*. London: Routledge.

Cooper, P. J. and Murray, L. (1997). The impact of postnatal depression on infant development: a treatment trial. In *Postpartum depression and child development* (L. Murray and P. J. Cooper, eds). Guilford Press.

Cooper, P. J., Campbell, E. A., Day, A., Kennerly, H. and Bond, A. (1988). Non-psychotic psychiatric disorder after childbirth: a prospective study of prevalence, incidence, course and nature. *British Journal of Psychiatry*, **152**, 799–806.

Cowan, C. P. and Cowan, C. P. (1987). A preventive intervention for couples becoming parents. In *Research on Support for Parents and Infants in the Postnatal Period* (C. F. Z. Boukydis, ed.). Ablex.

Cox, J. L. (1986). *Postnatal Depression: a guide for health professionals*. Edinburgh: Churchill Livingstone.

Cox, J. L. (1994). Introduction and classification dilemmas. In *Perinatal Psychiatry* (J. L. Cox and J. M. Holden, eds). Gaskell.

Cox, J. L. (1996). Perinatal Mental Disorder – a cultural approach. *International Review of Psychiatry*, **8**, 9–16.

Cox, J. L. and Holden, J. M. (eds) (1994). *Perinatal Psychiatry*. Gaskell.

Cox, J. L., Connor, Y. M. and Kendell, R. E. (1982). Prospective study of the psychiatric disorders of childbirth. *British Journal of Psychiatry*, **140**, 111–17.

Cox, J. L., Holden, J. M. and Sagovsky, R. (1987). Development of the 10 item Edinburgh Postnatal Depression Scale. *British Journal of Psychiatry*, **150**, 782–6.

Cox, J. L., Murray, D. and Chapman, G. (1993). A controlled study of the onset, duration and prevalence of postnatal depression. *British Journal of Psychiatry*, **163**, 27–31.

Cutrona, C. E. (1983). Causal attributions and perinatal depression. *Journal of Abnormal Psychology*, **92**, 161–72.

Cutrona, C. E. (1984). Social support and stress in the transition to parenthood. *Journal of Abnormal Psychology*, **93**, 378–90.

Dalton, K. (1971). Prospective study into puerperal depression. *British Journal of Psychiatry*, **118**, 689–92.

Dalton, K. (1980). *Depression After Childbirth*. Oxford University Press.

Davison, G. C. and Neale, J. M. (1990). *Abnormal Psychology* (5th edition). Chichester: John Wiley and Sons.

Davison, G. C. and Neale, J. M. (1996). *Abnormal Psychology* (revised 6th edition). Chichester: John Wiley and Sons.

Daws, D. (1989). *Through the night: helping parents and sleepless infants*. Free Association Books.

Dennerstein, L., Lehert, P. and Riphagen, F. (1989) Post partum depression: risk factors. *Journal of Psychosomatic Obstetrics and Gynaecology.*, Suppl. **10**, 53–65.

Elliott, S. A. (1984). Pregnancy and After. In *Contributions to Medical Psychology* (S. Rachman, ed.) Vol. 3, 93–116 Pergamon.

Elliott, S. A. (1989a). Psychological Strategies in the Prevention and Treatment of Postnatal Depression. In *Bailliere's Clinical Obstetrics and Gynaecology*, Vol. 3, 879–903.

Elliott, S. A. (1989b). Postnatal Depression: Consequences and Intervention. In *Premenstrual, Postpartum and Menopausal Mood Disorders* (L. M. Demers, J. L. McGuire, A. Phillips and D. R. Rubinow, eds). Urban & Schwarzenberg Inc.

Elliott, S. A. (1990). Commentary on 'Childbirth as a life-event'. *Journal of Reproductive and Infant Psychology*, **8**, 147–59.

Elliott, S. A. (1990). Postnatal depression: implications for clinical research and practice. *Clinical Psychology Forum*, **25**, 48.

Elliott, S. A. (1994). Uses and misuses of the E.P.D.S. in primary care. In *Perinatal Psychiatry* (J. L. Cox and J. M. Holden, eds). Gaskell.

Elliott, S. A., Rugg, A. J., Watson, J. P. and Brough, D. I. (1983). Mood Changes During Pregnancy and After the Birth of a Child. *British Journal of Clinical Psychology*, **22**, 295–308.

Elliott, S. A., Sanjack, M. and Leverton, T. J. (1988). Parent Groups in Pregnancy: A Preventive Intervention for Postnatal Depression. In *Marshalling Social Support: Formats, Processes and Effects*. (B. H. Gottlieb, ed.). Sage.

Feggetter, P. and Gath, D. (1981). Non-psychotic psychiatric disorders in women one year after childbirth. *Journal of Psychosomatic Research*, **25**, 369–72.

Fergusson, D. M., Horwood, L. J. and Thorpe, K. J. (1996). Changes in depression during and following pregnancy. *Paediatric and Perinatal Epidemiology*, **10** (in press).

Fergusson, D. M., Lynskey, M. T. and Horwood, L. J. (1993). The effect of maternal depression on maternal ratings of child behaviour. *Journal of Abnormal Child Psychology*, **21**, 245–69.

Fernando, S. (1995). *Mental Health in a Multi-ethnic Society*. London: Routledge.

Garel, M., Lelong, N., Marchand, A. and Kaminski, M. (1990). Psychosocial consequences of caesarean childbirth: A four year follow-up study. *Early Human Development*, **21**, 105–14.

Gerrard, J., Holden, J. M., Elliott, S. A., McKenzie, P. and Cox, J. L. (1993). A Trainer's Perspective of an Innovative Training Programme to Teach Health Visitors about the Detection, Treatment and Prevention of Postnatal Depression. *Journal of Advanced Nursing*, **18**, 1825–32.

Gerrard, J., Elliott, S. A. and Holden, J. M. (1994). The management of postnatal depression: A manual for mental health trainers of primary care staff. Unpublished manuscript.

Gilbert, P. (1995). Power, social rank and depression: comments on Price and Gardner. *British Journal of Medical Psychology*, **68**, 211–15.

Gjerdingen, D. K. and Challoner, K. M. (1994). The relationship of women's postpartum mental health to employment, childbirth and social support. *Journal of Family Practice*, **38**, 465–72.

Gordan, R. E. and Gordan, K. K. (1960). Social factors in prevention of postpartum emotional problems. *Obstetrics and Gynaecology*, **15**, 433–8.

Graham, H. (1984). *Women, Health and Family*. Brighton: Wheatsheaf.

Green, J. M. and Murray, D. (1994). The use of the Edinburgh Postnatal Depression Scale in research to explore the relationship between antenatal and postnatal dysphoria. In *Perinatal Psychiatry* (J. Cox and J. Holden, eds). London: Gaskell.

Green, J. M. (1990). "Who is unhappy after childbirth?": Antenatal and intrapartum correlates from a prospective study. *Journal of Reproductive and Infant Psychology*, **8**, 175–83.

Greenwood, R. and Thorpe, K. J. (1993) Emotional well-being, life stress and women's consumption of alcohol. Paper presented at SRIP conference, Bristol.

Gregoire, A. J. P., Kumar, R., Everitt, B., Henderson, A. F. and Studd. J. W. W. (1996). Transdermal oestrogen for treatment of severe postnatal depression. *The Lancet*, **347**, 930–33.

Halonen, J. S. and Passman, R. H. (1985). Relaxation training and expectation in the treatment of postpartum distress. *Journal of Consulting and Clinical Psychology*, **53**, 839–45.

Harris, B. (1994). Biological and hormonal aspects of postpartum depressed mood. *British Journal of Psychiatry*, **164**, 288–92.

Harris, B. (1996). Hormonal aspects of postnatal depression. *International Review of Psychiatry*, **8**, 27–36.

Harris, B., Huckle, P., Thomas, R., Johns, S. and Fung, H. (1989). The use of rating scales to identify postnatal depression. *British Journal of Psychiatry*, **154**, 813–17.

Harris, V. S. and McHale, S. M. (1989). Family life problems, daily caregiving activities and the psychological well-being of mothers of mentally retarded children. *American Journal on Mental Retardation*, **94**, 231–9.

Henderson, A. F., Gregoire, A. J., Kumar, R. et al. (1991). Treatment of severe postnatal depression with oestradiol skin patches. *Lancet*, **38**, 816–17.

Hock, E. and Demeiss, D. K. (1990). Depression in mothers of infants: the role of maternal employment. *Developmental Psychology*, **26**, 285–91.

Holden, J. M. (1996). The role of health visitors in postnatal depression. *International Review of Psychiatry*, **8**, 79–86.

Holden, J. M., Cox, J. L. and Sagovsky, R. (1989). Counselling in a General Practice setting: A controlled study of Health Visitor interventions in the treatment of postnatal depression. *British Medical Journal*, **298**, 223–6.

Holden, J. M., Elliott, S. A. and Gerrard, J. (1992). The management of postnatal depression. Unpublished original manual for health visitors.

Hopkins, J., Campbell, S. B. and Marcus, M. (1986). The role of infant-related stressors in postpartum depression. *Journal of Abnormal Psychology*, **96**, 237–41.

Hunter, M. (1994). *Counselling in Obstetrics and Gynaecology*. BPS Books.

Kendell, R. E., Chalmers, J. C. and Platz, C. (1987). Epidemiology of puerperal psychoses. *British Journal of Psychiatry*, **150**, 662–73.

Kitamura, T., Shima, S., Sugawara, M. and Toda, M. A. (1993). Psychological and social correlates of the onset of affective disorders among pregnant women. *Psychological Medicine*, **23**, 967–75.

Kumar, R. (1989). Postpartum psychosis. In *Bailliere's Clinical Obstetrics and Gynaecology*, Vol. 3, pp. 823–38.

Kumar, R. and Robson, K. M. (1984). A prospective study of emotional disorders in childbearing women. *British Journal of Psychiatry*, **144**, 35–47.

Lelong, N., Kaninskir, M., Chwalow, J. et al. (1995). Attitudes and behaviour of pregnant women and health professionals to alcohol and tobacco consumption. *Patient Education and Counselling*, **25**, 39–40.

Littlewood, J. and Tinker, A. (1981). *Families in Flats*. London: HMSO.

MacArthur, C. (1991). Health after childbirth. *British Journal of Obstetrics and Gynaecology*, **98**, 1193–204.

MacArthur, C., Lewis, M. and Knox, E. G. (1991). *Health after Childbirth*. London: HMSO.

Malley, J. E. and Stewart, A. J. (1988) Women's work and family rules: sources of stress and sources of strength. In *Handbook of Life Stress, Cognition and Health* (S. Fisher and J. Reason, eds). Chichester: John Wiley and Sons.

Marzillier, J. (1992). Clinical Psychology and primary health care. In *What is Clinical Psychology?* (J. Marzillier and J. Hall, eds). Oxford: Oxford University Press.

Mauthner, N. S. (1995). Postnatal depression: the significance of social contacts between mothers. *Women's Studies Int. Forum*, **18**, 311–23.

McHaffie, H. E. (1990). Mothers of very low birthweight babies: How do they adjust? *Journal of Advanced Nursing*, **15**, 6–11.

McHaffie, H. E. (1989). Mothers of very low birthweight babies: who supports them? *Midwifery*, **5**, 113–21.

McIntosh, J. (1993). Postpartum depression: women's help-seeking behaviour and perceptions of cause. *Nursing*, **18**, 178–84.

Manly, P. C., McMahon, R. B., Bradley, C. F. and Davidson, P. O. (1982). Depressive attributional style and depression following childbirth. *Journal of Abnormal Psychology*, **91**, 245–54.

Metz, A., Sichel, D. A. and Goff, D. C. (1988). Postpartum panic disorder. *Journal of Clinical Psychiatry*, **49**, 278–9.

Millar, H. F. (1994). Housing Conditions and Maternal Health. Unpublished MSc thesis. University of Bristol.

Mills, M. and Pound, A. (1986). Mechanisms of change. The New Pin project. *Marce Bulletin*, **2**, 3–7.

Moleman, N., van der Hart, O. and van der Kolk, B. A. (1992). The partus stress reaction: A neglected aetiological factor in postpartum psychiatric disorders. *Journal of Nervous and Mental Diseases*, **180**, 271–2.

Morris, J. B. (1987). Group psychotherapy for prolonged postnatal depression. *British Journal of Medical Psychology*, **60**, 279–81.

Murray, L. (1992). The impact of postnatal depression on infant development. *Journal of Child Psychology and Psychiatry*, **33**, 543–61.

Murray, L. and Carothers, A. D. (1990). The validation of the EPDS on a community sample. *British Journal of Psychiatry*, **157**, 288–90.

Murray, D. and Cox, J. L. (1990). Screening for Depression during pregnancy with the EPDS. *Journal of Reproductive and Infant Psychology*, **8**, 99–107.

Murray, L. and Cooper, P. J. (1996). The impact of postpartum depression on child development. *International Review of Psychiatry*, **8**, 55–64.

Murray, L., Kempton, C., Woolgar, M. and Hooper, R. (1993). Depressed mothers' speech to their infants and its relation to infant gender and congnitive development. *Journal of Child Psychology and Psychiatry*, **34**, 1083–101.

Myers, J. K., Weissman, M. M., Tischler, G. L. (1984). Six month prevalence of psychiatric disorders in three communities. *Archives of General Psychiatry*, **41**, 959–67.

Nicolson, P. (1989). Postnatal depression: implications for clinical research and practice. *Clinical Psychology Forum*, **19**, 15–18.

Nicolson, P. (1990). The meaning of postnatal depression: a further comment. *Clinical Psychology Forum*, **25**, 48–9.

Nilsson, A. and Amgren, P. E. (1970a). Para-natal emotional adjustment: a prospective study of 165 women, Part 1. *Acta Psychiatrica Scandinavica Supplementum*, **220**, 1–61.

Nilsson, A. and Amgren, P. E. (1970b). Para-natal emotional adjustment: a prospective study of 165 women, Part 2. *Acta Psychiatrica Scandinavica Supplementum*, **220**, 62–141.

O'Hara, M. W. (1986). Social support, life events and depression during pregnancy and the puerperium. *Archives of General Psychiatry*, **43**, 569–73.

O'Hara, M. W., Neunaber, D. J. and Zekoski, E. M. (1984). A prospective study of postpartum depression: prevalence, course and predictive factors. *Journal of Abnormal Psychology*, **93**, 158–71.

O'Hara, M. W., Rehm, L. P. and Campbell, S. B. (1982). Predicting depressive symptomology: Cognitive behavioural models and postpartum depression. *Journal of Abnormal Psychology*, **91**, 457–61.

O'Hara, M. W., Rehm, L. P. and Campbell, S. B. (1983). Postpartum depression: A role for social network and life stress variables. *Journal of Nervous and Mental Disease*, **171**, 336–41.

O'Hara, M. W., Schlechre, J. A., Lewis, D. A. and Jarner, M. W. (1991). Controlled prospective study of postpartum mood disorder; psychological, environmental and hormonal variables. *Journal of Abnormal Psychology*, **100**, 63–73.

O'Hara, M. W. and Swain, A. M. (1996). Rates and risk of postpartum depression – a meta-analysis. *International Review of Psychiatry*, **8**, 37–54.

O'Hara, M. W. and Zekoski, E. M. (1988). Postpartum depression: A comprehensive review. In *Motherhood and Mental Illness 2: Causes and Consequences* (I. F. Brockington and R. Kumar, eds). London: Wright.

O'Hara, M. W., Zekoski, E. M., Philipps, L. H. and Wright, E. J. (1990). Controlled prospective study of postpartum mood disorders: Comparison of Childbearing and non childbearing women. *Journal of Abnormal Psychology*, **99**, 3–15.

Oakley, A. (1980). *Women Confined: Towards a Sociology of Childbirth*. Martin Robertson.

Oakley, A. (1981). *From Here to Maternity: Becoming a Mother*. Harmondsworth: Penguin.

Oates, M. (1994). Postnatal mental illness: organisation and function of services. In *Perinatal Psychiatry* (J. L. Cox and J. M. Holden, eds). Gaskell.

Oates, M. (1996). Psychiatric services for women following childbirth. *International Review of Psychiatry*, **8**, 87–98.

Orford, J. (1992). *Community Psychology Theory and Practice*. Chichester: Wiley.

Parr, M. A. (1996). Support for British Couples in the Transition to Parenthood. Unpublished doctoral thesis. University of East London.

Paul, G. (1969). Behaviour modification research: design and tactics. In *Behaviour therapy: appraisal and status*. (C. M. Franks, ed.). New York: McGraw-Hill.

Paykel, E. S., Emms, E. M., Fletcher, J. and Rassaby, E. S. (1980). Life events and social support in puerperal depression. *British Journal of Psychiatry*, **136**, 339–46.

Pitt, B. (1968). Atypical depression following childbirth. *British Journal of Psychiatry*, **114**, 1325–35.

Playfair, H. R. and Gowers, J. I. (1981). Depression following childbirth – a search for predictive signs. *Journal of the Royal College of General Practitioners*, **31**, 201–8.

Pound, A. and Mills, M. (1985). A pilot evaluation of NEWPIN: home visiting and befriending scheme in South London. *Association of Child Psychiatry and Psychology Newsletter*, **7**, 13–15.

Price, F. V. (1991). Extraordinary circumstances: coping with triplets, quads and more. In *The Stress of Multiple Births* (D. Harvey and E. Bryan, eds). London: Multiple Births Foundation.

Redshaw, M. and Harris, A. (1995). Maternal perceptions of neonatal care. *Acta Paediactrica*, **84**, 593–8.

Redshaw, M. and Harris, A. and Ingram, J. (1996). *Delivering Neonatal Care*. London: HMSO.

Richman, N., Stevenson, J. and Graham, P. (1982). *Preschool to School: a Behavioural Study*. London: Academic Press.

Riley, D. (1995). *Perinatal Mental Health*. Abingdon: Radcliffe Medical Press.

Robinson, S. and Young, J. (1982). Screening for depression and anxiety in the postnatal period: acceptance/rejection of a subsequent treatment offer. *Australian and New Zealand Journal of Psychiatry*, **16**, 47–51.

Rodin, J. and Ickovics, J. R. (1990) Women's health: review and research agenda as we approach the 21st century. *American Psychologist*, **45** (9), 1018–35.

Ryle, A. (1961). The psychological disturbances associated with 345 pregnancies in 137 women. *Journal of Mental Science*, **107**, 279–86.

Salmon, P. (1985). *Living in Time: a New Look at Personal Development*. London: Dent.

Schweitzer, R. D., Logan, G. P. and Stassberg, D. (1992). The relationship between marital intimacy and postnatal depression. *Australian Journal of Marriage and the Family*, **13**, 19–23.

Sharpe, S. (1976). *Just Like a Girl*. Harmondsworth: Penguin.

Sheeber, L. B. and Johnson, J. H. (1992). Child temperament, maternal adjustment and changes in family lifestyle. *American Journal of Orthopsychiatry*, **62**, 178–85.

Shereshefsky, P. M. and Lockman, R. F. (1973). Comparison of counselled and not counselled groups. In *Psychological aspects of a first pregnancy* (P. M. Shereshefsky and L. J. Yarrow, eds). Raven Press.

Small, R., Brown, S., Lumley, J. and Astbury, J. (1994). Missing voices: what women say and do about depression after childbirth. *Journal of Reproductive and Infant Psychology*, **12**, 89–104.

Stewart, D. E. and Robinson, G. E. (1989). Infertility by choice or by nature. *Canadian Journal of Psychiatry*, **34**, 866–71.

Stuart, S. and O'Hara, M. W. (1995). Interpersonal psychotherapy for postpartum depression: a treatment programme. *Journal of Psychotherapy Practice and Research*, **4**, 18–29.

Szasz, T. S. (1987). Justifying coercion through theology and therapy. In *The evolution of psychotherapy* (J. K. Zeig, ed.). Brunner Mazel.

Teasdale, J. D. (1985). Psychological treatments for depression: How do they work? *Behaviour Research and Therapy*, **23**, 157–65.

Thorpe, K. J., Golding, J., MacGillivray, I. and Greenwood, R. (1991). A comparison of the prevalence of depression in the mothers of twins and the mothers of singletons. *British Medical Journal*, **302**, 875–8.

Thorpe, K. J., Dragonas, T. and Golding, J. (1992a). The effects of psycho-social factors on the mother's emotional well-being in pregnancy: a cross-cultural study of Britain and Greece. *Journal of Reproductive and Infant Psychology*, **10**, 191–204.

Thorpe, K. J., Dragonas, T. and Golding, J. (1992b). The effects of psycho-social factors on the mother's emotional well-being during early parenthood: a cross-cultural study of Britain and Greece. *Journal of Reproductive and Infant Psychology*, **10**, 205–17.

Thorpe, K. J. and Cinnamon, J. (1992). The Timing of Motherhood. Unpublished research report. University of Queensland, Australia.

Thorpe, K. J., Greenwood, R. and Goodenough, T. (1995a). The emotional well-being of mothers of twins in the first year postpartum: a comparison of mothers of singletons by number and spacing of children. Paper presented at the Society for Reproductive and Infant Psychology Conference, Leicester, September 1995.

Thorpe, K. J., Greenwood, R. and Goodenough, T. (1995b). Does a twin pregnancy have a greater impact on physical and emotional well-being than a singleton pregnancy? *Birth*, **22**, 148–52.

Todd, E. D. M. (1964). Puerperal depression: A prospective epidemiological study, *Lancet*, **ii**, 1264–6.

Wallach, H. R. and Maitlin, M. W. (1992). College women's expectations about pregnancy, childbirth and infant care: A prospective study. *Birth*, **19**, 202–7.

Wallander, J. L., Pitt, L. C. and Mellins, C. A. (1990). Child functional independence and maternal psychosocial stress as risk factors threatening adaption in mothers of physically and sensorially handicapped children. *Journal of Consulting and Clinical Psychology*, **58**, 818–24.

Watson, J. P., Elliott, S. A., Rugg, A. J. and Brough, D. I. (1984). Psychiatric disorder in pregnancy and the first postpartum year. *British Journal of Psychiatry*, **144**, 453–62.

Webster, M. L., Thompson, J. M. D., Mitchell, E. A. and Werry, J. S. (1994). Postnatal depression in a community cohort. *Australian and New Zealand Journal of Psychiatry*, **28**, 42–9.

Weick, A. (1996). Ovarian hormones, mood and neurotransmitters. *International Review of Psychiatry*, **8**, 17–26.

Welburn, V. (1980). *Postnatal Depression*. Fontana.

Whitton, A., Appleby, L. and Warner, R. (1996). Maternal thinking and the treatment of postnatal depression. *International Review of Psychiatry*, **8**, 73–8.

Wickberg-Johansson, B., Erlandsson, B. and Hwang, C. P. (1996). Primary healthcare management of postnatal depression in Sweden. *Journal of Reproductive and Infant Psychology*, **14**, 45–56.

Windridge, K. C. and Berryman, J. C. (1996). Maternal adjustment and maternal attitudes during pregnancy and early motherhood in women of 35 and over. *Journal of Reproductive and Infant Psychology*, **14**, 69–76.

Woollett, A. (1991). Having Children: Accounts of childless women and women with reproductive problems. In *Motherhood: Meanings, Practices and Ideologies* (A. Phoenix, A. Woollett and E. Lloyd, eds). London: Sage.

World Health Organisation (1992). The ICD-10 Classification of Mental and Behavioural Disorders. WHO.

Zelkowitz, P. and Milet, T. H. (1995). Screening for postpartum depression in a community sample. *Canadian Journal of Psychiatry*, **40**, 80–86.

7

Mothers, fathers and early sex roles

Charlie Lewis and Jo Warin

The early chapters in this book were concerned predominantly with the experiences of parents, while the later ones are concerned with infants. In this chapter and the next, the dynamic relationship between infants and parents is considered. Lewis and Warin in this chapter focus on the always contentious area of sex roles. Gender and gender roles are fundamental concepts in reproductive and infant psychology, and were introduced by Gerda Siann in the first chapter of Volume 1 of the series. In this chapter, Lewis and Warin consider the possibility of a dynamic interaction between the changing gender roles and identities of mothers and fathers as they negotiate the transition to parenthood and the developing gender identity of their young children. How does the presence of a baby change the sex-role related behaviour of parents? What is the impact of parental behaviour on the development of gender roles in infants? Are parental sex-role stereotypes transmitted to children in a simple one-way process – or do children influence adults too?

Families with infants have received much research attention over the past thirty years. However, the literature seems to be somewhat fragmented, as there are many family members to study, issues to address and ways of considering the changes that occur. As the previous chapters in this volume show, many interested in the psychology of reproduction have studied mothers' and fathers' experiences as parents. Yet the bulk of research in the area concentrates upon the near miraculous neonatal capabilities and rapid acquisition of skills in infancy, as shown in the major reviews of this literature (see e.g. Bremner, 1994). The remaining chapters in this book adopt this focus upon infants. As an attempt to form a bridge between these two diverse literatures, and the surrounding chapters of this volume, the aim of this chapter is to focus upon one area of infant development, the acquisition of sex-role behaviour and understanding. It will examine this single 'outcome' of family processes to consider whether changes in parents' roles and identities can be seen to have an influence upon the changes which become apparent in the child's understanding. The development of gender roles will be portrayed as the outcome of dynamic and reciprocal family processes.

The chapter will start with a brief summary of the literature on men's and women's transition to parenthood. On the one hand the research literature portrays a difference in the responsibilities and domestic duties undertaken by both partners and in this respect the experience of each partner is separate. Yet, on the other hand, the literature also portrays the transition to parenthood as a shared experience and suggests that the mutual nature of the parental relationship is a key predictor of the infant's adjustment.

The rest of the chapter will then examine the impact of parental behaviour on the development of gender roles in infants. It explores three contrasting theoretical perspectives. The first is biological and is based upon evidence which reveals very early gender preferences and understandings. We will argue that this evidence does not only show innate tendencies in infants, but also suggests that children start to absorb gender related information from their environment at a very early stage. Clearly parents are the most significant and available sources of such information and so we will move on to the second broad theoretical perspective: the psychoanalytic. This section will focus on the arguments put forward by post Freudian psychoanalyst Nancy Chodorow. She suggests that gender roles are perpetuated as a result of the different ways in which boys and girls need to establish independence from their mothers and develop an individual identity. This process is known as individuation. The third approach is concerned with the more direct forms of parental influences on sex-role socialization within the family. Here we will discuss the means by which information and values concerning gender are developed in the infant through the rewarding and the modelling of appropriate gender behaviour. The aim will be to show that each of the above perspectives contributes to our understanding of early family development as a complex pattern of influences, involving the child's innate capabilities, the parents' relationship and the cultural pressures upon them to rear their infants in sex-stereotypical ways.

The transition to parenthood: A separate yet shared experience

Normally woman lives through her children, man lives through his work.
New York Times, 5 September 1915

Forty years ago E. E. Le Masters (1957) published a provocative article which set in motion a debate that continues to this day. He argued that the arrival of a child disrupts the parent's lifestyle and identity so much that the period should be depicted as a 'crisis' in that individual's development. The paper had the effect of focusing attention upon early parenting as a problematic experience, with some arguing that the term crisis is appropriate (e.g. Dyer, 1963), while others failed to find extensive stress in new parents (e.g. Hobbs, 1965). Since the 1960s the debate has changed its orientation towards searching for normative changes in the 'transition to parenthood', to use the term coined by Alice Rossi (1968). Two issues have dominated the discussion:

1. Do men and women go through the same experiences? By discussing parenthood, as opposed to motherhood or fatherhood, the literature has often included men's experiences, albeit not originally in an explicit attempt to compare women's and men's experiences.
2. What influences the transition to make it either a joyful and uplifting experience or a stimulus for depression and identity crisis? These issues tend to be addressed together.

Unlike other areas in which men have been relatively neglected, comparisons between the transitions to motherhood and fatherhood have continued to generate much fruitful discussion in the literature. Before we briefly review this literature we must emphasize that, with a few welcome recent exceptions, the research has tended to focus upon a limited section of the populations of highly industrialized countries – almost exclusively white and largely middle or even upper-middle class. There is relatively little data on new fathers who do not live with their babies, or parents in a variety of family forms which do not conform to the nuclear family stereotype. So with this caution in mind what do the studies tell us about men's and women's experiences? What has been the effect of studying fathers, while centuries of discussion has focused on mothers (see Chapter 1)?

The literature reveals an apparent contradiction. In the first place men's and women's experiences seem to be fundamentally different, yet secondly many couples describe the transition to parenthood as a shared venture which consolidates the ties of equality and reciprocity in their relationship. Obviously only one partner goes through the pregnancy and delivery and there are social patterns which conform to the pattern of eighty years ago, described in the quotation at the start of this section. In his very detailed observation of Pennsylvania family life over the infant's early months Jay Belsky (e.g. Belsky and Volling, 1987) recorded that the only activity in the home which fathers carried out was the category of behaviour labelled 'read/watch TV'. When both parents were at home together mothers devoted more time to caring for the baby and to interacting with and responding to him/her. As with most other studies Belsky found that early parenting is a highly gendered activity in households where the parents live together. The accumulated research shows that mothers become more involved and skilled at caring for the infant as they spend more time over the early months with the baby, leaving fathers feeling less competent and involved (Parke and Tinsley, 1981). The above patterns hold within African American households (Hossain and Roopnarine, 1994). As Cowan and Cowan (1988) report, fathers tend to concentrate their activities within specific yet constantly changing domains. Within the first six months of parenthood they do less clothes washing than before, but contribute more to cooking, cleaning the house and shopping, presumably while their partners care for the baby. Between six and eighteen months fathers do less meal preparation and house cleaning, while their shopping activity increases (Cowan and Cowan, 1988).

The division of 'tasks' to do with caring for the baby and running the house seems to become accentuated after the arrival of the baby. This does not mean to imply that the division of labour is equal in most couples before parenthood, as there are clear gender differences in what teenagers are prepared to do in the home (Emler and Hall, 1994). Nor does the literature simply focus upon the numbers of nappies changed or bottles fed. It also examines the psychological experiences associated with parenting. Many simply assume that the man must be less psychologically involved as a result of his diminished practical participation (e.g. Grossman, Eichler and Winickoff, 1980). Such assumptions perhaps underestimate the intensity of the experience for many men (see e.g. Lewis, 1986). Research which has concentrated longitudinally upon fathers' and mothers' reactions to the arrival of a child show qualitative differences. For example, Feldman (1987) found that mother's reports of: adjustment problems six months post partum were predicted by their feelings (and their perceptions of marital stress) during the pregnancy. Both maternal and paternal 'strain' were predicted by the father's general stress (often work related) before the child arrived. As men tend to be more embedded in their careers and/or their role as economic providers, their preoccupation with work spills over into family relationships. Since most mothers cut down their work at the time of the first child's arrival, their concerns are centred around the home and family.

The second and on the surface contradictory picture which emerges from the literature on parents over the transition is that they share many experiences. Images of spousal relationships since the 1930s have stressed their 'companionate' nature (Mowrer, 1930) and couples in a variety of studies have subscribed to such a belief, irrespective of whether they are describing sharing the symptoms of nausea in pregnancy or the joys of nappy changing (Lewis, 1986). Despite the unequal division of labour, couples produce explicit accounts of these shared, equal experiences (e.g. Backett, 1987). To some extent these stories of shared parenting are shown in empirical investigations. As the research of Feldman (1987) reported above showed, the best predictor of adjustment to parenthood before the baby arrives is the relationship between the parents. This is replicated in other studies (e.g. Cox, Owen, Lewis and Henderson, 1989). Indeed Belsky (1990) has argued that marital adjustment is an even better predictor of paternal relationships than is maternal involvement with infants.

It seems that the ability to overcome the demands of coping with a new baby is largely correlated with quality of the spousal relationship and the feeling of joint involvement. Just what causes this is nearly impossible to tease apart, but the strength of the association is evident under a variety of circumstances. For example, when a baby arrives prematurely and requires special care (see Chapter 13), mothers and fathers adopt similar styles when interacting with the baby (Levy-Shiff, Sharrir and Mogilner, 1989) and mothers state that their ability to cope with the baby is related to their husbands' ability to do likewise (Chatwin and MacArthur, 1993). But the frame of reference for understanding the transition to parenthood should not be restricted to the support which parents give to one another. Research has long indicated that wider social support networks are important. For example, satisfaction with the transition to parenthood is correlated with perceived support from the new grandparents (Hansen and Jacob, 1992).

In summary, the research on the transition to parenthood (in the limited range of family types which have been studied) shows that there is a feeling of joint suffering and enjoyment of the early months of parenthood. While most couples experience a decline in their relationships, one-fifth report an improvement (Cowan and Cowan, 1992) and adjustment to the baby seems to reflect the state of the parents' relationships, particularly that between one another. While 12 per cent of couples split up in the first eighteen months of the child's life in Cowan and Cowan's study, this was lower than comparable families without children in the same geographical area.

At the same time the transition to parenthood is marked by a series of changes which divide what parents do with their children. Even where mothers go back to work they still take the major responsibility for childcare in all but a few families. Surveys of large populations of fathers reveal that the proportion of 'highly involved' men is less than 10 per cent (Russell and Radojevic, 1992). Meanwhile the rest do much less than their spouses. For example, 60 per cent of these fathers had never looked after their children alone (Russell, 1983). What does this imply for the child's development? The rest of this chapter addresses this issue by considering one aspect of children's development – the acquisition and knowledge of their own and others' gender gender-roles.

Three perspectives upon early sex-role development

Research over the past thirty years has demonstrated a consistent picture. As Eleanor Maccoby (1988) suggests, by the age of two when observed in public settings involving peers (like play groups) the child's social world is clearly segregated along lines of gender. In other words within 24 months children gain an understanding of roles and relationships which is highly sex stereo-typed. In popular discussion there exist three contrasting belief systems about how such sex-role stereotypes develop, which will be discussed in turn below.

The first has much in common with the vast amount of literature which focuses upon the amazing range of skills which the infant appears to possess at birth. This view holds that there is something 'natural' or innate in the way children adopt beliefs about what dress or behaviour are appropriate for each sex. Many parents still look on at their preschool sons running riot in the play group or their daughters engaging in doll play and trot out familiar adages, like 'boys will be boys'.

The other two popular beliefs are based on the assumption that parents somehow instil a value system into their children. Given that the literature on the transition to parenthood, discussed above, the second shows that parents perform different roles within the family, particularly when their children are young. Perhaps such styles have a major influence upon the child's unfolding understanding of gender? Psychoanalysts have long argued that the very system of differentiated roles adopted by men and women reproduces itself from one generation to the next, through the unconscious, or preconscious, transmission of complex meanings about others and the 'self'. This perspec-tive provides the most comprehensive, but perhaps least 'testable', account of early sex differences which an understanding of the transition to parenthood might lead us to.

The third account is that their differing styles of interaction are transmitted in a much more straightforward way as a result of explicit attempts by parents to channel the infant's sex-appropriate behaviour.

Infant sex-role differences: a biological prerogative?

It is clear that children's sex-role behaviours are influenced by their physio-logical make-up. In very early life boys have been shown to be less attentive to stimuli (Lewis, 1972) and more fussy (Moss, 1967) or at least to produce more intense bursts of fussiness, even when other factors like the effects of circumcision are controlled for (Rosenthal, 1983). Of course not all boys are circumcised, but in most studies some are and the effects need to be taken into account. The research of Money and Erhardt (1972) long ago estab-lished that there is a physiological basis to some of these differences and that such effects can be lasting. They showed that females who receive high levels of testosterone in the uterus are more likely to become tomboys and appear more 'masculine' throughout childhood.

That such biological factors affect early behavioural sex differences is beyond doubt. However, it is very difficult to establish just how widely such factors exert their influence on the child's emerging sex-role understanding and behaviour. It is clear that during the first two years of life children become very aware of what is appropriate for their sex, but just why this is so remains unspecified. For example, some time in the first year of life children come to distinguish between male and female 'stimuli' (e.g. Leinbach, 1991). Studies utilizing techniques of visual preference (looking more at one of a pair of presented stimuli) or habituation (how long it takes to get used to a novel stimulus) show that by their first birthdays children become adept at discriminating the sexes. In the visual world, for example, when shown a succession of photographs of adults of one sex, some five-month-olds will look longer at a new picture of an adult of the opposite sex than one of a member of the same sex. This occurs even when there are large individual differences between photographs of men or women (Leinbach, 1991). Similarly, seven-month-olds will attend longer to the voice of an adult of one sex if they have previously listened to a member of the opposite sex (Miller, 1983). There is evidence to suggest that such a skill is present as early as two months (Jusczyk, Mullinnex and Pisoni, 1992). The implication is that even young babies can differentiate between the distinctive auditory features of male and female voices. In keeping with the wave of research showing the very early emergence of perceptual skills in infancy, such studies indicate that from a very young age babies show a basic discrimination between men and women.

Even more remarkable is that it seems that by their first birthday children have a firm impression of what gender they should affiliate with. They appear to be able to select an appropriate stimulus from only minimal evidence. For example, Kujawski and Bower (1993) made a film of toddlers walking to and fro across a room, where the toddlers were in the dark and attached to their joints were luminous strips. All that was visible on the film was a patchwork of movement patterns. It is easy for adults to discern that the film is of an infant walking, but *not* the sex of the baby. However, one-year-olds reliably looked longer at other infants of the same sex, at least in first looks at pairs of moving stimuli presented simultaneously. These results suggest that at this age children have some understanding of gender identity, in distinguishing 'like me' and 'unlike me' from crude movement patterns. Such early preferences continue. Over the second year of life, children tend to adopt sex-linked styles of play. Girls specialize in dressing up and soft toy play while boys' play involves manipulation of blocks and pushing trucks and cars around (Goldberg and Lewis, 1969; Smith and Daglish, 1997), while their behaviour is more assertive and vigorous (Fagot, Hagan, Leinbach and Kronsberg, 1985). When strict controls are taken to ensure that their actions are not being stage-managed by their parents, even six-to-twelve-month-old girls are more sociable than boys; they initiate more bids for interaction and are more responsive to maternal initiations of interaction (Gunnar and Donahue, 1980).

While there is no doubt that from around the end of the first year children demonstrate a preference for, and therefore an understanding of, their own gender, the reasons why they do this are not obvious. Researchers who have identified these early competences have often assumed that they have identified only the manifestation of a biological imperative. Kujawski and Bower (1993), for example, assume that the ability to infer movement in same sex children is wired in to the young child. Even though our laboratory has produced concordant findings with younger children (six months of age), this does not allow us to rule out the possibility of early learning. It is conceivable that children might in some way be taught to react to stimuli appropriate to their sex. Stronger claims can be made against a simple biological argument when it comes to the types of toy selected for play, since such artifacts are clearly culturally produced. So it seems that beyond gross patterns of behaviour in very early infancy and a few examples of severe disruption to normal physiological development, the causes behind very early sex differences in behaviour and sex stereotyping cannot be attributed to simple biological forces. We need to understand the child's developing sex roles in terms of other perspectives. Here we return to issues more closely linked to the transition to parenthood.

Parental role differentiation: object relations perspectives

The psychoanalytic tradition has long claimed that family interactions and relationships determine a child's identity as male or female. It suggests that in order to begin to grasp the complexities of these patterns of influence we have to go beyond examining the enactment of such roles. In its detail this is the only approach that can begin to account for the apparently immutable differentiation between the sexes. Freud (1925) explained the acquisition of the male sex role by identifying the Oedipus complex. When the boy represses the desires he feels for his mother and comes to identify with his rival, his father, he internalizes social norms of appropriate behaviour, thereby developing a superego. Thus the process of developing awareness of one's own gender is integral to the process of acquiring a sense of self. Freud's account of the equivalent process by which the female comes to internalize the characteristics of the mother is based on the premise of penis envy, an account that has been criticized and restructured by Horney (1926), Klein (1928) and Mitchell (1974). Freud's emphasis on the supremacy of the libido has been rejected by current psychoanalytic theory but his legacy remains within the psychoanalytic approach in two key ways:

1. That sexual identity is at the core of the self concept.
2. The processes of gender development are unconscious ones.

It is these latter attributes that are both its strength and its weakness; it stresses the immutability of sex roles, but makes this aspect of psychoanalytic theory almost impervious to empirical testing.

Those theorists who have developed, extended and reformulated the original psychoanalytic postulates have provided what appears to be the greatest impetus towards a satisfactory explanation of the development of sex differentiation, in particular those associated with 'object relations theory'. Object relations theorists attempt to explain the processes by which a person comes to experience her/his 'self' in relation to 'others', and the part played by the internalization of 'others' in the development of the 'self'. 'Object' in this sense means the person, or aspect of a person, that comes to form part of the internal psychic make-up of the 'self'. Early relationships are deemed to be crucial in drawing up the ego boundaries that separate self from others and provide the context in which infants attempt to resolve their conflicting needs for dependence and autonomy. D. W. Winnicott (1964) is the most familiar proponent of this approach. More recently, Chodorow (1978) and Dinnerstein (1978) have made significant contributions to our understanding of the asymmetrical development of sexual identity in boys and girls. Chodorow's theory, in particular, helps to explain why sex roles appear to be so resistant to change. It stresses continuity, or their 'reproduction', across generations. It may also explain the early manifestations of gender understanding and affiliations described above, since the differential process for boys and girls is rooted in infancy.

Chodorow argues that the source of the different psychic make-up of boys and girls can be traced to the fact that mothers are the primary caretakers and primary 'love-objects' of their new born infants. She claims that it is this single factor that has hitherto escaped analysis. She redresses this omission by examining the possibility that women's mothering not only brings about a different psychology in men and women, but moreover creates the self-perpetuation of that difference. Mothering, as exclusive or at least primary caregiving, develops the needs and desires of girls to 'mother' the next generation. The starting point for male and female infants is the symbiotic relationship with the mother, who is initially experienced as merged and fused with the infant. The process of individuation and differentiation from the mother is experienced differently by boys and girls. In order for boys to develop a separate and autonomous identity they have to establish themselves as being different from their mothers. Given that fathers are absent to a greater or lesser degree from primary childcare, the boy has difficulty in defining himself as male. His sense of maleness is constructed negatively, by what it is not. This has three implications:

1. In the search for knowledge of masculinity the boy has to be especially alert to any available information from the world outside the domestic sphere which will contribute to his understanding of the male world.
2. Because the son is less involved, less 'merged' with his father than his mother, he has a more objective perspective from which to view 'maleness'. However, because the father may only be present for brief periods, the knowledge of masculinity that the child gains is necessarily limited, and therefore likely to be much more stereotyped than the girl's equivalent sense of femininity derived from her mother.
3. The boy has to resort to active rejection of the female as the most available strategy for discovering and asserting his sexual identity as male.

The process of individuation is very different for girls. Chodorow explains that although girls may seek out their fathers as a means of breaking away from the symbiotic relationship with their mother, they will nevertheless look to their mother for an understanding of femininity. By this account the girl does not have the same strong need as the boy does for repressing the sense of 'oneness' with the mother. In the interests of his masculinity, so Chodorow argues, the boy has to repudiate the female. This is entrenched further by incoming cultural information which asserts the superiority of male activities. He develops the need to devalue the power of women, denying his first symbiotic relatedness to his mother. In doing this he is repressing his desire for dependence, and the source of his relational capacities. Chodorow sees this process of repression at this early age as responsible for the difficulties men may later experience in accessing their emotions. The thesis is extended further to explain women's capacities and desires to raise children in order to regain their earliest primary identification with their own mother. Men, she maintains, have repressed those aspects of their make-up that would seek fulfilment in child rearing – a major reason why so many fail to care for infants.

Richards (1982) and Jalmert (1993) have elaborated Chodorow's thesis with regard to the psychology of masculinity. They point out that, whereas a girl's gender identity develops out of personal identification with the mother, boys are concerned with the abstract and non personal aspects of male stereotypes and cultural norms – with what it is to be male rather than with the specific attitudes of an individual with whom they are closely involved. This, Richards (1982, pp. 69–70) points out, leads to a suppression of their nurturing skills: 'Men's socialisation prepares them for a world of male superiority in which they will strive in the world of work and remain withdrawn from the emotional world of family and children'. Further, the suppression of relational capacities affects relationships between men which become motivated by competition rather than support. Men invest in primary heterosexual relationships in which they are also likely to experience the contradictory feelings of fear of dependence leading to hostility and contempt. Richards explains the man's wish for a child as the need to adopt a positional rather than a personal identification with the father. It is the wish to assume the role of the father rather than the wish for a personally gratifying relationship with a son or daughter.

Analysis of the object relations account
The implication of the approach expressed most clearly by Chodorow is that a change in the sexual division of parenting would bring about a transformation of male and female psychology and halt the seemingly endless perpetuation of sex roles. It would also facilitate the greater psychological health of both men and women: 'Personal connection to and identification with both parents would enable a person to choose those activities she or he desired, without feeling that such choices jeopardised their gender identity' (Chodorow, 1978, p. 218). As such, Chodorow's thesis is an idealized one. It can be criticized on two related counts. In the first place (see Siann, 1995), Chodorow bases her arguments upon case examples from psychotherapy rather than empirical investigations. So neither does she provide supportive research evidence for her claims, nor does she fully address the wider economic, social and political issue of sexual inequality. She mentions that it is the social and economic aspects of parenting and the overall sexual division of labour which produce a distinct differentiation between parents (Chodorow, 1978, pp. 212–19), but her primary objective is to speculate about the psychological effects of such differentiation. Such speculation needs to tie in with data from other areas of the child's psychosocial functioning, which show the effects of mothers and fathers performing different family functions.

The background to the second argument emerges from a debate about role differentiation itself. Initial concern focused on Chodorow's assumption that women do actually provide the primary childcare (Bart, 1983; Young, 1983). In one respect, this aspect of her thesis is not in doubt, since whilst nearly all men play with their infants (see Lamb, 1997 for a review), studies over the past forty years have shown that the daily graft, like nappy changing, is largely undertaken by women (Lewis, 1986; Newson and Newson, 1963). Nevertheless, this division of labour is not exclusive. In the first section of the chapter we highlighted the *shared* as well as sex differentiated aspects of early parenting – most men do some tasks and even if the figure of highly involved fathers is less than 10 per cent, it still leaves a large number of available men who could be studied to test the thesis.

There is sufficient literature from two areas of psychosocial functioning which allows us to search for any effects of the parental role differentiation on children's development. The first concerns the attachments they form (see Melhuish, Chapter 11 of this volume, for a fuller discussion). As Melhuish suggests, infants develop close attachments with their main caregivers over the second year of life, the security of which has great implications in terms of the infant's confidence, independence and feelings of self-worth – otherwise known as their 'inner working model'. For Chodorow's thesis to hold we would expect at the very least a closer attachment between the mother and infant, as opposed to the father and infant. Perhaps more importantly we should expect a closer link between mothers and daughters, particularly in terms of the predictions from mother–infant relationships to the child's later psychological adjustment.

The two above 'predictions' should be treated with some caution as they are not made explicit in Chodorow's work and her scope extends beyond the very early years of life. Nevertheless, they enable us to reflect upon how her theory might be tested. Only the first prediction receives any support from the accumulated evidence. The quality of attachments between infant and caregiver is measured in a standardized procedure known as the 'strange situation' (Ainsworth and Wittig, 1969). Following a stressful experience (separation from the parent), the ease at which the parent can placate the infant when they are reunited is assessed using criteria which distinguish secure attachment relationships from insecure ones (the specific types of relationship are outlined in Chapter 9). A number of studies have compared attachment patterns between infants and either their mother or their father – usually in two strange situation procedures examined two weeks apart. There is some suggestion that the mother–infant relationship is a little closer (Lamb, 1997), but in general analysis of all the accumulated studies shows a high *concordance* between parents – if the child demonstrates security with one parent s/he will likely have a secure relationship with the other in the strange situation (Fox, Kimmerly and Schafer, 1991). Indeed, in families where the parents demonstrate close affection to one another early in infancy, the infant–parent attachments are significantly likely to be closer around the child's first birthday (Cox, Owen, Henderson and Margland, 1992). So, in keeping with the idea of the transition to parenthood as a shared experience, research on concurrent attachments suggest that there are more similarities between parent–infant attachments than differences that might be predicted from the parents' differentiated roles.

Research on the predictive power of early attachments supports Lamb's (1997) claim that mother–infant links are stronger. Main, Kaplan and Cassidy (1985) showed that infant–mother attachment relationships, but not father–infant attachments, predict how confidently a child performs in a social setting (interaction with a stranger adult) at age five to six. They suggested that the mother stands 'foremost' as an attachment figure in the child's working model of the self. More recent investigations have made the picture more complicated. One study suggests that paternal closeness can have negative effects. The longitudinal investigation by Youngblade and Belsky (1992) of 73 families with children from 13 to 60 months suggested that paternal attachment at the earlier age predicted *less* harmonious inter-action between the child and a friend at age five.

However, more concordant data suggest that paternal and maternal styles display different amounts of the same security. Suess, Grossman and Sroufe (1992) conducted a longitudinal analysis with 29 children in a home observa-tion when they were age five. Strange situation assessments of mother–infant attachments from infancy were stronger predictions of the child's later play, conflict resolution and reduced problem behaviours four years later. Suess et al.'s analyses replicated those of Main et al. in finding that mother–infant attachments correlated more strongly with the child's later functioning. However, they also found that the best predictions of the child's adjustment at age five were derived from mother– *and* father–infant attachment com-bined. If children had been securely attached to both parents in the second year they were more likely to be self-reliant at the end of the preschool period. So, we may tentatively conclude that, as secondary parents, fathers do not serve as the same 'secure base' to their infant's developing feelings of self-worth, but the bulk of the evidence suggests that their relationships may *complement* those of their wives/partners (as suggested in the Main et al. and Suess et al. studies above). The mother–father relationship may also be crucial.

The second 'hypothesis' that we might draw from Chodorow is that par-ent–child relationships may influence boys and girls in different ways, since her theory is about parental role differentiation having a differential impact upon boys and girls. The research on attachment seems not to demonstrate different patterns of felt security in boys and girls with either parent, either concurrently or in the longitudinal studies reported above. The latter evi-dence is important as Chodorow's theory speculates that the greatest impact of 'mothering' upon boys and girls should be in the latter preschool years. A similar lack of evidence comes from studies of families where the father is particularly nurturant and involved in childcare. It is the case that their preschoolers appear to attribute adults with fewer sex-role stereotypes (Carlson, 1984). Boys are significantly more gendered in their attributions than girls, but not if their fathers share in their care. However, it must be emphasized that, despite a general increase in maternal employment when their children are young, preschoolers remain highly conservative about sex roles (Smith, Ballard and Barham, 1989) and studies like Carlson's show a minor shift in children's views resulting from their parents' attempt to equal-ize their domestic and employment responsibilities. Longitudinal research on families where the father was the main caregiver early in the child's life shows only minor attitudinal differences about sex differences in employment but not wholesale shifts in teenagers' psychological well-being (Williams, Radin and Allegro, 1992).

Perhaps we should wait until research shows long-term continuities between parents' roles and those adopted by their own children. We would need to find evidence of a difference between men and women in their rationale and desires for bringing up their own children and differences in the quality of the paternal and maternal relationships that are formed. Certainly attachment research shows that expectant mothers' and fathers' descriptions of their attachments predict the patterns of attachments with their own children a year later (Fonagy, Steele and Steele, 1991; Steele, Steele and Fonagy, 1996). But the existing evidence does not find the required continuities to support the specifics of Chodorow's theory.

Socialization influences caused by different parental roles?

Children are usually immersed in a culture which segregates the sexes – it is not just parents who usually adopt different roles. Look at any child's bedroom and you will find clearly sex-stereotypical toys and effects. Rheingold and Cook (1975) took the trouble to quantify the differences. They found that the sort of items available to preschoolers were just those that they play with when observed in the studies cited above. Girls' rooms were decorated in a more 'floral' way and they contained more soft toys like dolls. In contrast boys' bedrooms were significantly more likely to contain toy vehicles, sports equipment, zoo animals and even clocks – the stereotype holds that boys have better spatio-temporal skills, even though there is a wide overlap between the skills of the two sexes (Archer and Lloyd, 1982). The process starts early. Studies in the delivery room have long shown that parents attribute their newborns with sex-stereotypical dispositions even when they have not known the sex of the baby until this time. The classic study was by Rubin, Provenzano and Luria (1974). They asked parents to describe their infants in the delivery room or shortly thereafter. Daughters were described as 'softer' and 'finer featured', while sons were attributed with being 'more alert', 'firmer' and 'stronger'. While these data certainly suggest that the sex-role system imposes strong imperatives upon us to treat boys and girls differently, we must be cautious about making such claims. Many children's bedrooms contain toys which distant relatives give them, not necessarily what they play with. Similarly, what parents say in the delivery room, or anywhere else, may not reflect how they actually interact with their children.

Researchers have therefore resorted to another technique to discern the impact of adult stereotypes on the minutiae of interaction. This is the 'stranger baby' experiment. Here, adults are asked to participate in research on how babies play with unfamiliar adults. Unbeknown to them the infant is introduced with a boy's name in half the cases and with a girl's name in the rest. Thus the adult's sex-role stereotyping can be assessed in interaction without the interference of prior knowledge about the child as an individual. Studies have shown that adults use the gender 'label' given to the child as a cue to how they should interact with infants ranged between three and fifteen months of age. Designated 'females' have been seen to receive more comforting from the adult (Frisch, 1977) and are more likely to be presented with a doll (Seavey, Katz and Zalk, 1975). Labelled 'males' tend to be encouraged to be more active (Frisch, 1977) and to be presented with more 'masculine' toys to play with, like trucks (Smith and Lloyd, 1978).

The stranger baby experiments appear to show the impact of sex stereotyping on adults' behaviour. However, more recent research has complicated the picture and suggested that two factors influence this stereotypical behaviour which were not considered in the studies cited above: the part played by the infant in eliciting such stereotypical actions and the role of the adult's attitudes towards sex roles (Bell and Carver, 1980; Lewis, Scully and Condor, 1992). Both studies have shown that the child's biological sex also has an influence on how the adult acts in these experiments. Bell and Carver (1980) found that passive infants were offered 'feminine' toys, like soft dolls, and were rated by the adult as less 'robust'. Lewis et al.'s (1992) data suggested that girls, irrespective of their gender label, stayed within reach of their mothers four times longer than boys and they made more social bids towards them. Perhaps the most critical feature of this study is that as a result of playing with a boy or a girl the adult's perceptions of her/himself seemed to be influenced in a subtle way, even though in half the cases the adult was given the wrong information about the child's sex. Each filled out Bem's (1974) sex-role inventory in which s/he has to state how much s/he identified with a range of 'masculine', 'feminine' and sex-neutral traits. Having played with a boy adults reported that they felt more positively about the so-called feminine characteristics, particularly being 'shy', 'flatterable' and 'gullible' (according to the research of Bem (1974) adults perceive gullibility as a feminine trait!). Having played with a girl, the adult expressed more positive feelings for the complementary masculine traits, particularly feeling 'dominant' and 'competitive' (Lewis, Scully and Condor, 1992). It thus seems that adult stereotyping does not occur in a vacuum – how the adult acts is partly influenced by the child's contribution to the interaction. The nature of the child's influences upon the adult appear to continue so that at least in the short term how an interaction unfolds seems to influence the adult's self-perceptions. In other words, sex stereotyping may be context dependent.

The data from Lewis et al.'s study serve to highlight a move in theory on early development. It was common in the 1960s to find accounts based upon behaviourist notions, whereby behavioural dispositions are shaped or reinforced by environmental factors, specifically the adult's reward of appropriate action in the child. However, such mechanical influences are now held to be too simple. Children make their own contributions to how interactions unfold, as Bell (1968) pointed out, and how sex-role attitudes are formed in the child and modified within the adult is the product of a negotiation process with several intertwined levels of influence (see Lewis, 1985 for a development of this argument). We cannot therefore claim that parental sex-role stereotypes simply pass from parent to child by a process like diffusion or osmosis. As we shall see, there is much to suggest that parents learn from one another about how to care for their sons and daughters.

Mothers, fathers and facilitation of sex-role differentiation
The possible links between parents' behavioural styles and the infant's sex-role development have been a focus of attention for many decades (Power, 1981). The debate has been dominated by two theoretical perspectives. The first derives from social learning theory and assumes that sex roles are

learned through imitation or reinforcement of sex appropriate behaviours. Block (1976) suggested that mothers and fathers are different agents of socialization. In particular, fathers interact with their sons and daughters in different ways, engaging in more rough and tumble play with their boys and therefore encouraging the development of detached, brusque, masculine 'instrumentality'. Supportive evidence was provided in a longitudinal study by Michael Lamb (1977), who found that during infancy fathers not only engaged in more physical play, they were more likely to do so with their sons. Infant boys in turn were more likely to seek dad out to play. It seemed as if fathers make themselves salient in order to assist their son's sex-role development.

An opposing view was most forcefully expressed over twenty years ago by Maccoby and Jacklin (1974). They examined the existing literature (hundreds of studies) to examine whether men and women treat sons and daughters differently. They concluded that the evidence for differential socialization as the cause of the sex differences in children's behaviour was inconclusive. The debate has continued and developed. Two more recent reviews attempted to demonstrate that the evidence to support a 'paternal socialization' hypothesis is insufficient. Siegal (1987) examined thirty-nine published studies and found only two common themes. In these studies fathers were found consistently to engage in physical play more with sons than daughters and to encourage their children to play with sex-typed toys. Yet in all other respects fathers' styles of interaction were indistinguishable from those of mothers. Lytton and Romney (1991) conducted a larger meta-analysis of 172 studies, involving over 27,000 participants and employing different measures: interviews, observations and questionnaires. Their analysis did not reveal obvious gender-based patterns of mother–child and father–child interaction. For example, in two American reports fathers encouraged sons more than daughters, but in twenty further studies they did not, nor did they when all the difference scores were analysed using a pooled standard deviation. The single factor to emerge from Lytton and Romney's analysis was the finding that *both* parents encourage sex-typed activities in their children, but there was only a marginal difference between sons and daughters. In many respects the debate has shifted to examining the ways in which mothers and fathers might conspire together to encourage their children's sex-appropriate development.

Beverly Fagot (1985) has consistently claimed that late infancy (18–30 months) is a crucial time for sex-role development, since at this time parents impress on males and females just what is appropriate and what is not. In one home-based investigation she studied 92 children over four hours in their homes at 12 months, 18 months and five years (Fagot and Hagan, 1991). Even as early as one year mothers and fathers encouraged boys in their stereotypical male play and assertive behaviour. Parental reactions to the child at 18 months were more accentuated. They continued to reward sex-stereotypical behaviour and assertiveness in sons and even reacted more negatively to their sons' attempts to communicate – conversion is a stereotypically 'feminine' activity. At the same time both parents, particularly mothers, were more rewarding of their daughters' attempts to communicate.

Fagot and Hagan's study suggests that we should be cautious about completely ruling out parental influences, as previous meta-analyses have suggested. How should we interpret such results? Social learning theory cannot provide an adequate explanation as it presumes that mothers and fathers serve as role models for different activities in their sons and daughters. Rather, it seems as if parents jointly agree on what is appropriate for their children and act in unison. The many studies examining parent–infant interaction (e.g. Pedersen, 1980) revealed far more similarities between parents than differences in parents' styles. More recent research has observed a similarity between parents in their nurturance to the child (Bentley and Fox, 1991), their teaching styles (Worden, Kee and Ingle, 1987), and their disciplinary regimes (e.g. Hart, De Wolfe, Wozniak and Burts, 1992). We are therefore left to consider just how sex roles are learned so easily in infancy.

It may be possible to find the answer to this question by turning our attention to the behaviour of parents in public settings rather than in the privacy of home. Many authors have recently turned from home-based observation of children to examining how gender relations are presented in public places like parks, shopping malls or fast food restaurants. In such locations, under the eye of the general public, the underlying child-rearing ideals of parents may be observable since parents may be likely to act with a degree of self-consciousness when interacting with their offspring. For example, Burns and Mitchell have carried out over 1000 observations of family triads (adult male, adult female, toddler) in public parks and zoos. They simply observed the means by which the child was transported through the park and showed that when the social environment is kept constant, patterns of interaction can be identified. Male toddlers were more likely than female toddlers to walk alone. At the same time male caregivers were twice as likely to carry their toddlers (Mitchell, Obradovich, Herring et al., 1992), especially girls (Burns, Mitchell and Obradovich, 1989). Mothers were more likely to push the pushchair, while the father cared for and interacted with the child. For Mitchell, Obradovich, Herring et al. (1992) these patterns make a public display of the transmission of sex roles from one generation to another. It is not by coincidence that in public parks parents touch their infants and toddlers more than they do older children (Sigelman and Adams, 1990).

Conclusion

As this chapter has covered a range of topics and research we will briefly summarize our argument here. We started by reviewing the evidence from studies on the transition to parenthood and suggested that for couples who live together this is a separate yet shared experience. The most consistent areas of difference are in the distribution of domestic labour, with mothers undertaking the greatest proportion of duties related to the care of the infant and fathers reporting more stress related to the increased responsibility for 'bread winning'. Such experiences of daily routine spill over into the developing relationship between each parent and the baby. However, there is also considerable evidence showing similarities between partners in their experiences and in their styles of interaction with their infants. Most couples depict the shared nature of the transition to parenthood and emphasize the significance of the companionate nature of the parental relationship for adjustment to the infant.

The bulk of the chapter examined the impact of parental behaviour on the development of gender roles in infants. In the literature there are three different theoretical perspectives: the biological, the psychoanalytic, and the socialization tradition. Each receives partial support from the evidence. The biological perspective provides evidence of very early gender preferences and understandings. It is clear that infants have the ability to discriminate gender-relevant information at a very early age. However, in addition to revealing a strong biological imperative, the evidence does not close the door on the possibility that social forces are important markers for the infant's biological skills to exploit. Since parents are the most accessible sources of such information the discussion moved on to consider the influences of parents on the development and maintenance of gender roles. Chodorow's is a comprehensive account of gender role development which capitalizes upon the differences in parental roles witnessed in the transition to parenthood and beyond. The evidence from attachment theory tends to reinforce Chodorow's portrayal of the significance of the mother–infant relationship. However, it is necessary to be wary of exaggerating differences in the quality of the maternal and paternal attachment to the infant since some research shows more similarities than differences and suggests that the most secure forms of attachment are with both parents.

The discussion then moved to the third theoretical perspective, considering direct parental influences on infant sex-role socialization. Here we emphasized that parental sex-role stereotypes are not transmitted to children in a simple one-way process and concluded that it is necessary to consider the child's influences upon the adults as part of the process of reciprocal influences in parent–child interactions. There is insufficient evidence for specific gender-based patterns of mother–child and father–child interaction apart from consistent findings regarding fathers' rough and tumble style of play with sons. Clearly parental rewarding and modelling of gender appropriate behaviours is an ingredient in the mixture of influences on the early development of gender roles, but, taken by itself, social learning theory does not provide a complete understanding of early gender role development. The most recent research suggests that we should now turn our attention to finding out how mothers and fathers might conspire together to promote and maintain the development of gender appropriate behaviours. It seems highly plausible that parental values relating to gender roles are transmitted to the infant through implicit and explicit processes of communication between the parents.

Just as the transition to parenthood is a shared yet separate process, so too is the development of the infant's sex-role understanding. We need to add that the shared aspect of the transition is not restricted to the parental relationship but extends to the infant; mother, father and child (and other individuals within the family's social network) work together to reproduce gender roles. Research since the 1960s has stressed the need to consider the infant's own influences on parental behaviours. The child learns from complex processes, which are enacted both within and outside the home. These include both patterns which provide a differentiated model of adult sex roles and it is not surprising that mother–child attachments have the edge on father–child attachments. Yet the child also learns that mother and father encourage gender appropriate behaviour, at least in their interactions in public places. As a result expectations about gender appropriate behaviour become entrenched remarkably early in the child's life and are maintained through the three-way process of interaction between mother, father and infant.

Applications

1. Consider the theoretical issues
How we look at gender development is highly influenced by our theoretical assumptions about development. It is therefore essential that we, as practitioners and researchers, constantly question the beliefs that we have about the influences upon sex-role development.

2. Look at the complexity of the data
The collected studies on early sex roles and parenting show that a range and interaction of factors need to be considered. If the research shows anything it suggests that gender development occurs through being a member of the wider culture as well as within families.

3. Be sensitive to family diversity
Children live, and always have lived, in a diversity of family types. Given that they can learn about appropriate sex-role behaviour in many ways, we should therefore not be judgemental about the effects of particular family patterns upon our children's development.

Further reading

Chodorow, N. (1978). *The Reproduction of Mothering*. Berkeley: University of California Press.
Lamb, M. E. (ed.) (1997). *The Role of the Father in Child Development*. Chichester: Wiley.
Schaffer, H. R. (1996). *Social Development*. Oxford: Blackwell.

References

Ainsworth, M. D. S. and Wittig, B. A. (1969). Attachment and exploratory behaviour of one-year-olds in a strange situation. In *Determinants of Infant Behaviour* (Volume 4) (B. M. Foss, ed.). London: Methuen.

Archer, J. and Lloyd, B. (1982). *Sex and Gender*. Harmondsworth: Penguin.

Backett, K. (1987). The negotiation of fatherhood. In *Reassessing Fatherhood* (C. Lewis and O'Brien, eds). London: Sage.

Bart, P. (1983). Review of the reproduction of mothering. In *Mothering: Essays in Feminist Theory* (J. Treblicott, ed.). London: Rowman and Allenhead.

Bell, N. J. and Carver, W. A. (1980). A reevaluation of the direction of gender effects: expectant mothers' responses to infants. *Child Development*, **51**, 925–7.

Bell, R. Q. (1968). A reinterpretation of the direction of effects in studios of socialization. *Psychological Review*, **75**, 81–95.

Belsky, J. (1990). Parental and nonparental care and children's socio-emotional development: a decade review. *Journal of Marriage and the Family*, **52**, 885–903.

Belsky, J. and Volling, B. (1987). Mothering, fathering and marital interaction in the family triad during infancy: exploring family systems processes. In *Men's Transition to Parenthood* (P. Berman and F. Pedersen, eds). Hillsdale, New Jersey: Lawrence Erlbaum Associates.

Bem, S. (1974). *Sex Role Inventory*. California Consulting Psychologists Press.

Bentley, K. S. and Fox, R. A. (1991). Mothers and fathers of young children: comparison of parenting styles. *Psychological Reports*, **69**, 320–22.

Berman, P. and Pedersen, F. (eds) (1987). *Men's Transition to Parenthood*. Hillsdale, New Jersey: Lawrence Erlbaum Associates.

Block, J. (1976). Issues, problems and pitfalls in assessing sex differences: a critical review of 'The Psychology of Sex Differences'. *Merrill Palmer Quarterly*, **22**, 283–340.

Bremner, J. G. (1994). *Infancy*. Oxford: Basil Blackwell.

Burns, A. L., Mitchell, G. and Obradovich, S. (1989). Of sex roles and strollers: female and male attention to toddlers at the zoo. *Sex Roles*, **20**, 309–15.

Carlson, B. (1984). The father's contribution to child care: effects on children's perceptions of parental roles. *American Journal of Orthopsychiatry*, **54**, 123–36.

Chatwin, S. L. and MacArthur, B. A. (1993). Maternal perceptions of the preterm infant. *Early Child Development and Care*, **87**, 69–82.

Chodorow, N. (1978). *The Reproduction of Mothering*. Berkeley: University of California Press.

Cowan, C. P. and Cowan, P. A. (1988). Who does what when partners become parents: implications for men, women and marriage. *Marriage and Family Review*, **12**, 105–31.

Cowan, C. P. and Cowan, P. A. (1992). *When Couples Become Parents*. New York: Basic Books.

Cox, M. J., Owen, M. T., Henderson, V. K. and Margland, N. A. (1992). Predictions of infant–father and infant–mother attachment. *Developmental Psychology*, **28**, 474–83.

Cox, M. J., Owen, M. T., Lewis, J. M. and Henderson, V. K. (1989). Marriage, adult adjustment and early parenting. *Child Development*, **60**, 1015–24.

Dinnerstein, D. (1978). *The Rocking of the Cradle and the Ruling of the World*. London: Souvenir Press.

Dyer, E. (1963). Parenthood as crisis: a re-study. *Marriage and Family Living*, **25**, 196–201.

Emler, N. P. and Hall, S. (1994). Economic roles in the household system: young people's experiences. In *Justice in Close Relationships: Entitlement and the Affectional Bond* (M. J. Lerner and G. Mikula, eds). New York: Plenum.

Fagot, B. (1985). Beyond the reinforcement principle: another step toward understanding sex role development. *Developmental Psychology*, **21**, 1092–104.

Fagot, B. I. and Hagan, R. (1991). Observations of parent reactions to sex-stereotyped behaviour. *Child Development*, **62**, 617–28.

Fagot, B. I., Hagan, R., Leinbach, M. D. and Kronsberg, S. (1985). Differential reactions to assertive and communicative acts of toddler boys and girls. *Child Development*, **56**, 1499–505.

Feldman, S. (1987). Predicting strain in mothers and fathers of six month old infants. In *Men's Transition to Parenthood* (P. Berman and F. Pedersen, eds). Hillsdale, NJ: Lawrence Erlbaum Associates.

Fonagy, P., Steele, H. and Steele, M. (1991). Maternal representations of attachment during pregnancy predict the organization of infant–mother attachment at one year of age. *Child Development*, **62**, 891–905.

Fox, N. A., Kimmerly, N. L. and Schafer, W. D. (1991). Attachment to mother/attachment to father: a meta-analysis. *Child Development*, **62**, 210–55.

Freud, S. (1925). *Some Physical Consequences of the Anatomical Distinction Between the Sexes.* London: Hogarth Press.

Frisch, H. L. (1977). Sex stereotypes in adult–infant play. *Child Development*, **48**, 1671–5.

Goldberg, S. and Lewis, M. (1969). Play behaviour in the year-old infant: early sex differences. *Child Development*, **40**, 21–31.

Gottman, J. M. and Parker, J. G. (eds) (1988). Conversation of friends. Speculations in affective development. Cambridge: Cambridge University Press.

Grossman, F. K., Eichler, L. S. and Winickoff, S. A. (1980). *Pregnancy, Birth and Parenthood.* San Francisco: Jossey Bass.

Gunnar, M. and Donahue, M. (1980). Sex differences in social responsiveness between six and twelve months. *Child Development*, **51**, 261–5.

Hansen, L. B. and Jacob, E. (1992). Intergenerational support during the transition to parenthood: issues for new parents and grandparents. *Families in Society*, **73**, 471–9.

Hart, C. H., De Wolfe, D. M., Wozniak, P. and Burts, D. C. (1992). Maternal and paternal disciplinary styles: Relations and preschoolers' playground behavioral orientation and peer status. *Child Development*, **63**, 879–92.

Hobbs (1965). Parenthood as crisis: a third study. *Journal of Marriage and Family Living*, **27**, 367–72.

Horney, K. (1926). The flight from womanhood: the masculinity complex in women as viewed by men and women. Reproduced in *Feminine Psychology*. New York: W. W. Norton (1967).

Hossain, Z. and Roopnarine, J. L. (1994). African–American fathers' involvement with infants: relationship to their functioning style, support, education and income. *Infant Behavior and Development*, **17**, 175–84.

Jalmert, L. (1993). The father's role in the child's development. In *Fathers in Families of Tomorrow*. Danish Ministry of Social Affairs: European Commission.

Jusczyk, P. W., Mullinnex, J. and Pisoni, D. B. (1992). Some consequences of stimulus variability on speech processing by 2-month-old infants. *Cognition*, **43**, 253–91.

Klein, M. (1928). Early stages of the Oedipus complex. *International Journal of Psychoanalysis*.

Kujawski, J. and Bower, T. G. R. (1993). Same-sex preferential looking during infancy as a function of abstract representation. *British Journal of Developmental Psychology*, **11**, 201–9.

Lamb, M. E. (1977). The development of mother–infant and father–infant attachments in the second year of life. *Developmental Psychology*, **13**, 637–48.

Lamb, M. E. (1997). The development of father–infant relationships. In *The Role of the Father in Child Development* (3rd edition) (M. E. Lamb, ed.). Chichester: Wiley.

Leinbach, M. D. (1991). The beginning of gender: what's happening before the age of two? Paper presented at the Society for Research in Child Development, Seattle, April.

Le Masters, E. E. (1957). Parenthood as crisis. *Journal of Marriage and Family Living*, **19**, 352–5.

Levy-Shiff, R., Sharrir, H. and Mogilner, M. B. (1989). Mother– and father–preterm infant relationship in the hospital preterm nursery. *Child Development*, **60**, 93–102.

Lewis, C. (1985). Early sex role socialisation. In *The Psychology of Sex Roles* (D. Hargreaves and A. Colley, eds). Milton Keynes: Open University Press.

Lewis, C. (1986). *Becoming a Father*. Milton Keynes: Open University Press.

Lewis, C., Scully, D. and Condor, S. (1992). Sex stereotyping in infants: a reexamination. *Journal of Reproductive and Infant Psychology*, **10**, 53–63.

Lewis, M. (1972). State as an infant–environment interaction: an analysis of mother–infant interaction as a function of sex. *Merrill Palmer Quarterly*, **18**, 95–121.

Lytton, H. and Romney, D. M. (1991). Parents' differential socialisation of boys and girls: a meta-analysis. *Psychological Bulletin*, **109**, 267–96.

Maccoby, E. E. (1988). Gender as a social category. *Developmental Psychology*, **24**, 755–65.

Maccoby, E. and Jacklin, C. (1974). *The Psychology of Sex Roles*. Stanford: Stanford University Press.

Main, M., Kaplan, N. and Cassidy, J. (1985). Security of infancy, childhood and adulthood. In 'Growing Points of Attachment Theory and Research' (I. Bretherton, ed.). Monograph of the Society for Child Development, **50** (12) (Serial No. 209).

Miller, C. L. (1983). Developmental changes in male/female voice classification by infants. *Infant Behavior and Development*, **6**, 313–30.

Mitchell, G., Obradovich, S., Herring, F., Tromborg, C. and Burns, A. L. (1992). Reproducing gender in public places: adults' attention to toddlers in three public locales. *Sex Roles*, **26**, 323–30.

Mitchell, J. (1974). *Psychoanalysis and Feminism*. Harmondsworth: Penguin.

Money, J. and Erhardt, A. A. (1972). *Man and Woman, Boy and Girl*. Baltimore: Johns Hopkins University Press.

Moss, H. (1967). Sex, age and state as determinants of mother–infant interaction. *Merrill Palmer Quarterly*, **13**, 19–36.

Mowrer, E. R. (1930). *The Family: Its Organisation and Disorganisation*. Chicago: University of Chicago Press.

Newson, J. and Newson, E. (1963). *Infant Care in an Urban Community*. London: Allen and Unwin.

Parke, R. D. and Tinsley, B. R. (1981). The father's role in infancy: determinants of involvement in caregiving and play. In *The Role of the Father in Child Development* (2nd edition) (M. E. Lamb, ed.). Chichester: Wiley.

Pedersen, F. A. (1980). *The Father–Infant Relationship: Observational Studies in the Family Setting*. New York: Praeger.

Power, T. (1981). Sex typing in infancy: the role of the father. *Infant Mental Health Journal*, **2**, 226–40.

Rheingold, H. and Cook, K. (1975). The content of boys' and girls' rooms as an index of parents' behavior. *Child Development*, **46**, 459–63.

Richards, M. P. M. (1982). How should we approach the study of fathers? In *The Father Figure* (L. McKee and M. O'Brien, eds). London: Tavistock.

Rosenthal, M. K. (1983). Some variations in the newborn and mother–infant interaction during breastfeeding: some sex differences. *Developmental Psychology*, **19**, 740–45.

Rossi, A. (1968). Transition to parenthood. *Journal of Marriage and the Family*, **30**, 26–39.

Rubin, J. L., Provenzano, F. J. and Luria, Z. (1974). The eye of the beholder: parents' views on sex of newborns. *American Journal of Orthopsychiatry*, **63**, 342–6.

Russell, G. (1983). *The Changing Role of Fathers*. Milton Keynes: Open University Press.

Russell, G. and Radojevic, M. (1992). The changing role of fathers? Current understandings and future directions for research and practice. *Infant Mental Health Journal*, **13**, 296–311.

Seavey, C. A., Katz, F. J. and Zalk, S. (1975). The effect of gender label on adult response to infants. *Sex Roles*, **1**, 103–9.

Siann, G. (1995). Gender and gender identity. In *The Psychology of Reproduction, Volume 1: Reproductive Potential and Fertility Control* (C. A. Niven and A. Walker, eds). Oxford: Butterworth–Heinemann.

Siegal, A. U. (1987). Are sons and daughters more differently treated by fathers than by mothers? *Developmental Review*, **7**, 183–209.

Sigelman, C. K. and Adams, R. M. (1990). Family interactions in public: parent–child distance and touching. *Journal of Nonverbal Behavior*, **14**, 63–75.

Smith, A. B., Ballard, K. D. and Barham, L. J. (1989). Preschool children's perceptions of parent and teacher roles. *Early Childhood Research Quarterly*, **4**, 523–32.

Smith, C. and Lloyd, B. (1978). Maternal behaviour and perceived sex of infants: revisited. *Child Development*, **49**, 1263–5.

Smith, P. K. and Daglish, L. (1997). Sex differences in parent and infant behavior in the home. *Child Development*, **48**, 1050–4.

Steele, H., Steele, M. and Fonagy, P. (1996). Associations among attachment classifications of mothers, fathers, and their infants. *Child Development*, **67**, 541–55.

Suess, G. J., Grossman, K. E. and Sroufe, L. A. (1992). Effects of infant attachment to mother and father on quality of adaptation in preschool: from dyadic to individual organisation of self. *International Journal of Behavioural Development*, **15**, 43–65.

Treblicott, J. (ed.) (1983). *Mothering: Essays in Feminist Theory*. London: Rowman and Allenhead.

Williams, E., Radin, N. and Allegro, T. (1992). Sex role attitudes of adolescents reared primarily by their fathers: an 11-year follow-up. *Merrill Palmer Quarterly*, **38**, 457–76.

Winnicott, D. (1964). *The Family and Individual Development*. London: Tavistock.

Worden, P. E., Kee, D. W. and Ingle, M. J. (1987). Parental teaching strategies with pre-schoolers: a comparison of mothers and fathers within different alphabet tasks. *Contemporary Educational Psychology*, **12**, 95–109.

Young, I. M. (1983). Is male gender identity the cause of male domination? In *Mothering: Essays in Feminist Theory* (J. Treblicott, ed.). London: Rowman and Allenhead.

Youngblade, L. M. and Belsky, J. (1992). Parent–child antecedents of 5-year-olds' close friendships: a longitudinal analysis. *Developmental Psychology*, **28**, 700–713.

8

Parent–infant interaction: interpreting meaning in infants' actions

M. Suzanne Zeedyk

The second chapter which bridges the concerns of infancy and parenthood focuses directly on one aspect of parent–infant communication. Suzanne Zeedyk describes the process by which parents come to make sense of their baby's behaviour. How do parents know when a smile is a smile and not just wind? Do parents project meanings onto infant behaviours until the baby comes to understand that their actions have a particular meaning? Or are babies born with an ability to communicate through meaningful behaviour, which parents learn to recognize? How do parents explain the process of understanding their babies? What implications does this process have for later parent–child relationships? When is it difficult for parents to interpret the actions of their babies? Can professionals help?

The relationship between a parent and an infant begins in the earliest hours and days following birth, as the two partners begin to recognize and respond to each other. From the mother's perspective, the relationship may even have begun before the baby was born, when the kicks of the fetus began to be noticed or a nickname first bestowed. A crucial component of the relationship between parent and baby is the ability of the two to communicate with one another. This chapter will examine how such communication develops. How do infants develop the ability to communicate? How are parents able to understand the meaning of their infant's behaviours? What can cause difficulties in this process, and what are the long-term consequences of such problems? I will begin by outlining the developmental course of parent–infant interactions during the first few years, followed by a discussion of how parents are able to interpret the meaning of infants' actions. Later, I will consider the implications of early interactions for long-term development and examine circumstances in which parent–infant communication becomes problematic.

What is the developmental course of early parent–infant interactions?

The nature of infant actions, and parent–infant interactions, changes in a specific developmental sequence as infants mature. In the earliest months, infants exhibit an early sensitivity and attentiveness to social stimuli, shifting later to an interest in objects in the environment. While developmental research methods have shown that such a sequence exists (see Zeedyk, 1996, for a review), theoretical explanations of it are still being actively debated. The details of this developmental pattern will be described in this section, thereby providing a basis for examining theoretical accounts in the next.

Even in the earliest days and weeks of life, infants exhibit a sensitivity to social stimuli. They prefer vocal, rather than non-vocal, pitches (Eisenberg, 1975) and can identify their mother's voice from those of others at birth (DeCasper and Fifer, 1980). Indeed, fetuses *in utero* also appear to prefer human voices (DeCasper and Fifer, 1980; DeCasper, Lecanuet, Busnel et al., 1994). Within a few days after birth, babies are able to identify their mother by sight (Bushnell, Sai and Mullin, 1989) and by smell (Cernoch and Porter, 1985). Particularly compelling evidence of their early social capacity is their ability, even when only minutes old (Kugiumutzakis, 1985), to imitate adult behaviours such as vocalizations, facial expressions, tongue protrusions, and hand gestures (e.g. Field, Woodson, Greenberg and Cohen, 1982; Kugiumutzakis, 1993; Meltzoff and Moore, 1983; Vinter, 1986). Despite the elusivity with which such behaviours are demonstrated in the earliest weeks, the fact that they exist is sufficient to lead some theorists to argue that infants are innately social in nature.

Around two months of age, infants seem to 'wake up', interacting with others in a more consistent manner. They spend a greater amount of time attending to people, and they exhibit excitement in response to others' attention. If given the choice between social events and those involving objects, they exhibit a preference for social interaction (Kaye, 1982; Trevarthen, 1977; 1979; 1993). The types of games that parents and infants play at this age reflect this partiality; peek-a-boo, song singing and tickling, particularly popular games during this period, are based entirely on social interactions. Such games are possible because infants are already skilled at complex social exchanges.

Indeed, a large amount of mother–infant interaction during this period is spent in 'looking conversations' – exchanges of visual gaze and vocalizations that have a turn-taking quality reminiscent of adult conversations (Beebe, Jaffe, Feldstein et al., 1985). A typical exchange begins with the mother making eye contact with the baby, and he or she returning the gaze. The mother is then likely to smile, followed by the baby smiling. Perhaps the mother speaks to the infant in the standard high-pitched tones known as 'motherese' (Snow and Ferguson, 1977), which produces increased smiling in the baby. The interaction tends to become increasingly emotionally intense, lasting for up to a minute, and usually ending when the baby disengages for a brief time. A new cycle begins when the baby again directs attention to the mother. It is the pattern of shared turn-taking that gives the impression that a genuine conversation is taking place between the two partners and that reinforces the theoretical argument that infants may be innately social in nature.

Between four and five months of age, infants move into a new phase of development, becoming increasingly interested in their environment (Kaye, 1982; Trevarthen, 1977; 1993; Vedeler, 1994). They begin to pay more attention to objects around them, and they spend a greater amount of time playing with toys. Their motor skills have matured substantially by this age, allowing them to reach for and grasp objects very effectively. Parent–infant games now increasingly incorporate objects, such as hiding toys or helping babies to manipulate them. However, infants are not yet able to combine these social and object 'modes.' That is, they can either give their attention to a person or to an object, but it is difficult for them to pay attention to both at the same time.

It is near the age of ten months that they become able to integrate these two modes (Hobson, 1993; Trevarthen, 1979; 1993). They can now use social interaction to communicate about the objects in their world. Parents and infants begin to construct new kinds of games. The mother can point to an aeroplane overhead in the sky and the infant will follow the direction of her finger. Perhaps the mother will comment on some aspect of the plane, and the infant may point to it as well. In this way, the objects surrounding parents and infants are incorporated into their interactions and acquire a particular meaning through that interaction. This aspect of interaction has been labelled 'joint attention' (Moore and Dunham, 1995) because the attention of parent and child is jointly focused on a topic. A ball is not simply a round, red object but is something that parent and infant can share. It can be rolled back and forth in a game of catch. It can feature as a tempting prize when parent and child 'race' to retrieve it across the room. Or it can be used to assist in playing a joke, as when a baby pretends to roll the ball but then holds on to it and laughs at the surprise on his or her partner's face. This shows that infants now understand that parents have expectations about things (i.e. they expect that the ball will be rolled), and the infant can experiment with violating that expectation. Sharing a ball in these ways requires infants to be able to give attention to two things at once (i.e. the object and the parent), and it is not until this point in development that they are able to do that.

Around their first birthday, infants begin to talk. Their use of words is quite limited to begin with, of course, but between the ages of two and six years, they will construct a tremendously large vocabulary. By the time a child begins school, he or she will have learned approximately 14,000 words (Templin, 1957) – approximately nine new words every day for five years! With the use of speech, parents no longer have to guess at the meaning of their infants' actions, for their children can now begin to tell them what they want. This marks a new and more elaborate method of communicating. Indeed, many researchers are reluctant to label the interactions of parents and infants as true communication until infants become able to use words (e.g. Bates, 1979; Camaioni, 1993; Harding, 1984). This brings us to the debate about how parents decide whether a baby is communicating or not. That is, how do parents decide when an infant's actions are meaningful?

How are parents able to interpret the meaning of infants' actions?

Parents spend a tremendous amount of time trying to make sense of their infants' actions, and their spontaneous comments to infants reflect this. For example, when a mother walks into a room and her three-month-old infant smiles at her, she may respond, 'Are you trying to tell me hello?' Or, as a father is preparing a bottle for his screaming child, he might comment, 'I know you're trying to tell me you're hungry. I'm coming with the bottle!' One of the questions that researchers and parents try to answer is whether or not the baby really is trying to tell the parent something. Does the baby *mean* to send the message that he or she is hungry, or is the behaviour an *automatic reaction* to the bodily discomfort of hunger? At some point in development, all people become able to communicate purposely. But because it is impossible to actually ask a baby what he or she means, it is difficult to tell exactly when (and how) purposeful communication begins to occur. Based on parents' comments to their infants, it appears that they believe infants intend to communicate from a young age.

Parents' interpretations about the meaning of infants' actions have been the focus of active debate among developmental researchers. The viewpoints can be separated into two groups. The first set of theorists can be labelled 'as-if' theorists (e.g. Kaye, 1982; Newson, 1978; 1979; Schaffer, 1984; 1989). They contend that parents project meaning onto infant behaviours. According to this view, young infants do not possess the capacity for communication, but parents treat them as if they do. For example, although a mother believes that her infant's smile is intended as a message of greeting for her, these theorists would argue that the baby is not yet capable of communicating and that the mother is only projecting that interpretation onto the behaviours. The actions of young infants are exceedingly organized and coordinated, and parents mistakenly interpret such coordination as meaningful. This mistake is important, though, according to many 'as-if' theorists, for it is only through such parental beliefs, and their accompanying responses, that individual actions eventually do come to have a meaning for the child. Newson (1979, p. 94) offers a particularly clear statement on this point:

> It is thus only because mothers impute meaning to behaviours elicited from infants that these eventually do come to constitute meaningful actions as far as the child himself is concerned.

In summary, Newson and other 'as-if' theorists are arguing that infants are born able to emit complex behaviours but that these are not meaningful. It is only because parents believe they are meaningful and respond accordingly that meaning is able to develop.

The second group of theorists argue, conversely, that infants are born with an innate, if rudimentary, ability to communicate (e.g. Brazelton, 1982; Cohn and Tronick, 1988; Trevarthen, 1977; 1979; 1993; Tronick, 1981; Tronick, Als, Adamson et al., 1978). Within this view, parental beliefs are accorded validity; parents are deemed to be able to recognize the innate meaning within the infant's actions. Their responses to the baby are considered a natural reflection of that recognition. A mother would be considered to be correct in viewing her infant's smile as a message of greeting. Parents can share in the baby's intentions and, through such sharing, help the infant to understand new meaning. Trevarthen's comments (1979, p. 347) summarize this position clearly by comparing it to the 'as-if' position.

> The infant invites [the mother] to share a dance of expressions and excitements. The infant needs a partner but knows the principle of the dance well enough, and is not just a puppet to be animated by a miming mother who 'pretends' her baby knows better.

In effect, Trevarthen and theorists who agree with him contend that the infant is born with an innate capacity to engage in meaningful behaviour.

Parents are able to recognize and share in that meaning. This is a very different theoretical stance from the 'as-if' theorists, who are asserting that parents *create* the meaning.

Once an infant begins to talk, there can be little question that he or she means to communicate. Some theorists (e.g. Bates, 1979; Harding, 1984) view language primarily as a tool that infants use to help them accomplish goals (e.g. they can now ask Mum to get them a glass of juice). Language develops as a new means of achieving goals, which become more complex as the infant matures. For these theorists, the acquisition of language marks a fundamental change in the infant's ability to communicate; indeed, it is only at this point that they believe the infant can genuinely be said to be communicating. Other theorists who support a theory of innate communicative ability (e.g. Trevarthen; Tronick) view language as an extension of the shared interactions that the infant has participated in throughout his or her lifetime. The development of cognitive capacities makes it possible for language to emerge and therefore more complex methods of interaction to be exercised, but the structure of communicative interactions lies within earlier parent–infant exchanges. For these theorists, there is no qualitative shift in the infant's ability to communicate; although their skills are now much more elaborate, babies have been communicating since birth.

How do parents themselves explain the process of interpreting infants' actions?

The previous section examined the theoretical accounts offered by researchers to explain parental interpretation of infant actions. But how do parents themselves explain this process? Little research has approached the subject of parent–infant interaction from the perspective of the parent. This oversight reflects the traditional view of developmental psychologists that parents are biased and therefore the study of infants is better left in the hands of 'objective experts'. Auspiciously, parental report is increasingly being viewed as a valuable means of gathering data about children and is now used in a variety of areas, including language acquisition (Dale, Bates, Resnick and Morisset, 1989), infant temperament (Hubert and Wachs, 1985; Thomas, Chess and Korn, 1982), and identifying risk for developmental delay (Bricker and Squires, 1989; Diamond, 1993). This shift is encouraging, for parents are most knowledgeable about and have the most insight into the meaning of their children's behaviour. They can therefore bring important considerations to the study of child development. Admittedly, there are pitfalls in the use of parental report, but this is not a reason to exclude parental input altogether. (See Bates, 1994, for a more complete discussion of these issues.) We need, rather, to become aware of problems and guard against them, as is necessary with any method of data collection. Moreover, if we are to understand why parents behave in particular ways toward their children, it is crucial that we understand how parents themselves view their role.

In regard to understanding the meaning of infant behaviour, some recent research has approached the topic from the perspective of parents. Miller

(1988) asked parents of three- to twelve-month-olds to complete question-naires that assessed their beliefs about the meaning of infants' vocal beha-viour. Among her findings were those showing that parents were more likely to view vocalizations as meaningful if they were knowledgeable about infant development and that mothers were more likely than fathers to assign mean-ing to vocalizations. It is interesting to note that the findings also revealed that most parents did not endorse the idea of using 'babytalk', although observations of parent–infant interaction clearly show that most adults do engage in such behaviour. Miller (1988, p. 139) stresses that 'what parents think they are doing and what professionals think parents are doing may be quite different things'.

Kamel (1993) used a very different methodology to access parents' interpretations of infant behaviour. She filmed mothers and their infants interacting and then asked them to watch the tapes and to note all instances in which the infant's actions were meaningful to them. The number of instances they identified were compared to the number identified by non-parents. Results indicated, not surprisingly, that mothers selected more acts than did the non-parents and that they did so with more confidence. Kamel argued that in order to identify 'meaningful acts', one must first construct a set of criteria for what constitutes such an act. Mothers' greater experience with infants allows them to have a more diverse set of such criteria. It appears that parents' skills in identifying meaningful acts are not confined to use with their own children; Adamson, Bakeman, Smith and Walters (1987), using a method similar to Kamel's, found that even when parents observed the actions of infants who were not their own, they identified more meaningful acts than did non-parents.

Kamel's (1993) findings revealed particularly strong differences in mothers' and non-parents' interpretations about infants' intentions (as opposed to the meaning of infants' emotional expressions). Zeedyk (1994) attempted to identify the specific criteria that mothers use to decide when infant behaviour is intentional. After filming mothers and their infants inter-acting, she asked mothers to view the tape, stopping it each time they observed their child do something that 'they thought the infant *meant* to do'. They were then asked to articulate their reasons for coming to that conclusion. From their comments, Zeedyk was able to compile a list of maternal criteria for determining whether or not an infant meant to behave in a particular manner. The list included factors such as visual gaze, vocalizing, smiling, facial expressions, persistence, and intensity of the behaviour. It appears, then, that mothers can identify behaviours that they *believe* they are using in making decisions about infant behaviour. But how consistently do they actually apply such criteria? Zeedyk (1997) selected clips of infant activities (e.g. playing with mother, sneezing, reaching for toys) which, unknown to the mothers, contained a variety of the criteria. She asked the mothers to rate whether or not they thought the infant meant to perform the actions in the clips. The results revealed a very strong corre-lation between the number of behavioural criteria included in the clip and mothers' willingness to assign meaning to the actions. Therefore, it appears that mothers not only *say* they are using criteria to judge infant actions but that they are indeed *applying* such criteria, and in a fairly consistent manner.

Many of the criteria that mothers listed in Zeedyk's study are similar to those suggested by researchers for judging intention in infant behaviour (for reviews, see Willatts, 1989; Zeedyk, 1996). This suggests that mothers' and researchers' views may not be as discrepant as generally supposed. However, one criterion to which mothers have sole access is past experience with the infant. The participants interviewed in Zeedyk's (1994) study sometimes commented that they believed an action was intentional because they had previously observed the baby acting in a particular manner (e.g. 'he always reaches for his bottle like that') or that they knew the skill had been acquired over a period of time (e.g. 'she didn't always make that sound'). Researchers, of course, do not have access to such historical information in a laboratory setting, and its informative value is therefore too often overlooked in theoretical explanations of infant behaviour. However, it may be an important component to consider when constructing accounts of infant development, and one which parents can offer to professionals.

The results of studies such as these make it clear that parents can make important contributions to this area of study. This may not seem surprising, given their familiarity with infant behaviour, but as was pointed out earlier, their knowledge has traditionally been excluded from empirical work because of concerns about inherent bias. However, parents have much more opportunity than researchers to observe infant behaviour, and the nature of their relationship will give them privileged ways of understanding the behaviour. By making appropriate use of parents' expertise, we can expand the sources from which we are able to gather useful data. It is encouraging that an increasing number of developmental psychologists have begun to bring this awareness to their research.

What are the implications of early parent–infant interactions for later development?

Parents' interpretations of and responses to their infant can have important implications for the long-term development of the child. In this section, I will examine two topics that illustrate this process: cultural expectations and maternal depression. Both of these factors can influence parents' interpretations of children's actions. Interpretations give rise to parental actions, which in turn shape children's development in fundamental ways.

Cultural expectations

Cultural differences in parental expectations are often not immediately obvious, but they exert a strong influence on parental ideas about children's behaviour. For example, parents from westernized cultures tend to believe that infants develop more quickly than do parents from non-western cultures (e.g. Goodnow, Crashmore, Cotton and Knight, 1984; Hess, Kashigawi, Azuma et al., 1980; Hopkins and Westra, 1989). Ninio (1979; 1988), doing research in Israel, found that mothers of European descent believe that infants acquire basic cognitive skills at an earlier age than do mothers from Asian or African origins. Similarly, mothers from European backgrounds also believe that a number of parental actions should begin at an earlier age, including talking to babies, buying books for them, and reading them stories. Such differences in actions toward infants result in differential rates and patterns of development. In Asian and North African countries, where infant cognitive skills are considered to develop later, young infants are seldom talked to, played with, or supplied with toys (Goshen-Gottstein, 1980; Weintraub and Shapiro, 1968). These infants then have less opportunity to engage in social interaction, and this will naturally result in a different timetable of development.

Even within any particular culture, it is possible to find group differences. Tulkin and Kagan (1972), for instance, studying families who live in the Appalachian mountains of the USA, found that these mothers believed that their ten-month-old infants were not capable of communicating with others and that it was silly to talk to them because the babies could not understand what was being said. These expectations were correlated with differences in parental behaviour, such as a decreased proportion of recipro-cal vocalizations, less time spent in face-to-face interactions, and less use of objects with children. That is, parents in these groups spent less time talking to and playing with their young infants, and this appeared to be a result of their general expectations about babies. Given the importance of early inter-action for infant development, as discussed earlier, this style of parental interaction may be of concern.

Overall, these findings make it clear that parental ideas about the meaning of infants' actions and appropriate ways of communicating with them are heavily influenced by cultural factors. Parents' actions result from such beliefs, and the development of infants is then shaped by those actions. This process has obvious long-term implications, for the particular skills and capabilities that are shaped contribute to the overall qualities that make up each individual person. And, when infants have grown into adults with those particular qualities that have been reinforced by their culture, they will continue to encourage the same types of qualities in their own children.

Maternal depression

Depression has repeatedly been shown to affect mothers' interpretations of their children's behaviour. As with cultural expectations, when interpreta-tions differ, they give rise to divergent responses, and then the long-term development of the child is likely to be affected.

Depressed mothers have often been reported to make more negative inter-pretations of their children's behaviour than do non-depressed mothers (e.g. Breslau, Davis and Prabucki, 1988; Friedlander, Weiss and Traylor, 1986; Panaccione and Wahler, 1986). However, it is hard to draw firm conclusions from these findings, because mothers are evaluating their own children. Is the child's behaviour actually difficult, or is it merely the mother's perception that it is? Some investigators have suggested that depressed mothers' percep-tions are distorted, causing them to misinterpret the meaning of their child's actions (e.g. Griest, Wells and Forehand, 1979). Others argue that depressed mothers are accurate in their views and that their children do behave more negatively (e.g. Radke-Yarrow, Cummings, Kuczynski and Chapman, 1985). Indeed, studies using teachers' ratings (Richters and Pellegrini, 1989), peer ratings (Weintraub, Prinz and Neale, 1978), and children's own self-ratings (Weissman, Wickramarante, Warner et al., 1987) have also indicated that children of depressed parents are more maladjusted than are children of non-depressed parents. Whatever the nature of this relation, it appears that there is an association between the negative behaviour of children and depression in their mothers. However, most of these studies have focused on older children.

It is only recently that researchers investigating maternal depression have begun to extend their investigations downward in age to infants. The results available, nonetheless, support previous findings that depressed mothers interpret behaviours negatively. They exhibit more negative affect and facial expressions toward their infants (Cohn, Campbell, Matias and Hopkins, 1990; Field, Healy, Goldstein and Guthertz, 1990), and their sensitivity and responsivity to infants' cues are decreased (Bettes, 1988; Campbell, Cohn, Flanagan et al., 1992; Cohn, Campbell, Matias and Hopkins, 1990; Field, 1984). The verbal communication of depressed mothers is also more negative and less focused on infant experiences (Murray, Kempton, Woolgar and Hooper, 1993). Such differences may occur because the depression results in a general dampening of emotional responses on the part of the mother; alternatively, it may be that depressed mothers are interpreting infant actions as less meaningful (Zeedyk, 1994), and the decreased responsivity is therefore appropriate to their interpretation. Further exploration of these hypotheses is certainly in order.

One point of concern is the fact that not only are mother–infant interactions affected by such maternal responses, but the infants themselves are affected. They exhibit fewer positive expressions and more negative expressions than do infants of non-depressed mothers (Field, 1984). Dramatically, by the age of three months, infants of depressed mothers consistently engage in more negative behaviours (Field, Morrow and Adlestein, 1993). At older ages, differences can be seen in infants' cognitive development and in their attachment to mothers (Murray, 1992). Even physiological responses have been shown to be affected; Field's (1984) study revealed that infants of depressed mothers exhibit a lower activity level and heart rate. This suggests that infants may have adopted a passive coping style (Obrist, 1981), perhaps because they cannot control the stressful aspects of interactions with their mothers.

It is difficult to identify how, precisely, depression in mothers comes to affect the behaviour of infants. Therefore, a procedure labelled the 'still-face paradigm' has been developed to study this process (Cohn and Tronick, 1983). Using this methodology, infants are placed in a seat that is eye-level with the mother. The mother and baby interact normally for a few minutes, and then the mother is asked to hold her face still and to refrain from responding to any of the baby's actions. This is intended to simulate the facial expression and interactive style of depressed mothers. Results have repeatedly demonstrated that when mothers adopt a non-expressive face and are non-interactive, infants show a decrease in their own emotional expression and they look less frequently at the mother (e.g. Cohn and

Tronick, 1983; Field, 1984; Mayes and Carter, 1990). In effect, they make fewer attempts to interact with their mothers, and when they do so, it is with less emotion.

These startling changes in infant behaviour occur after only a minute or two of mothers' restrained responses. Imagine the effect if this style of interaction is the norm throughout a longer period of the infant's development. Recall that up until about five months of age, infants are attuned to social interactions. Therefore, they will be particularly sensitive during this period to any problems that occur within interactions. Unfortunately, this period is also the time during which post-natal depression is most likely to occur. Post-natal depression occurs in approximately 10–15 per cent of women after they give birth (O'Hara and Zekoski, 1988). For the majority of them, it fades within four to six months. Given the overlap between the needs of the infant and the decreased ability of the mother to meet them during this crucial period, it is easy to see why maternal depression is of concern to developmental psychologists.

This discussion is not meant to imply that post-natal depression makes a 'bad mother'. Instead, it highlights the degree to which a mother's emotional state has the capacity to affect her child's development, both during infancy and later on. Feminist theorists have argued that depression can be viewed as a natural response to a child's birth (e.g. Nicolson, 1986), given the social changes that surround it, including more demands on the mother's time and energy, loss of independence, a less fulfilling relationship with her partner, and isolation from other adults which was previously obtained during work or leisure activities. Therefore, greater societal acceptance of these changes to a woman's lifestyle is desirable. Rather than a wondrous, fulfilling experience, many women find motherhood, particularly in its early period, to be lonely and arduous. If women have a strong support system, they are better able to cope with the changes that accompany motherhood and may be less vulnerable to depressive symptoms. Additionally, if a variety of people interact with the baby, then he or she will have the opportunity to experience diverse interactive styles, many of which are likely to contain the kind of responsivity that is most beneficial for the infant's development and which can compensate for the effect of the decreased responsivity of a mother who is experiencing depression.

Nor is this discussion meant to suggest that the negative consequences of maternal depression are unalterable. Certainly providing increased or alternative types of input to the child at any point in development is desirable. However, the earliest months of infants' lives are those in which they are the most sensitized to social interaction. Indeed, theorists such as Trevarthen and Tronick would argue that the primary purpose of this early phase is to teach the child about the nature of social interactions. Never again will their attention be as singularly focused on social interaction as during this period. That is why the first few months after birth represent such a crucial period in the issue of maternal depression. We require much more research on the long-term implications of depression and a better understanding of how best to supplement infants' and mothers' experiences when depression does occur. It is only with this kind of information that we will be able to develop effective intervention programmes, directed toward both short- and long-term outcomes.

Under what circumstances can the interpretation of infants' actions be particularly problematic?

The topics already discussed present obvious circumstances under which parent–infant interactions can become problematic. Cultural beliefs can sometimes lead to styles of interaction that curb the child's development. Maternal depression can result in substantial difficulties in the ability of mother and infant to communicate smoothly and effectively. There are additional circumstances under which parent–infant interaction can become problematic and which highlight the importance of a parent's ability to interpret the meaning of his or her child's behaviour. In the remainder of this chapter, I will concentrate on two of these areas: non-typical patterns of development and child abuse.

Non-typical development

Many conditions occur that can cause children to experience and exhibit non-typical patterns of development. These include mental handicaps such as Down's syndrome and autism, or sensory impairments such as deafness and blindness. Each of these conditions results, not surprisingly, in changes within the parent–infant relationship and in a parent's ability to interpret the meaning of their child's behaviour.

In the case of infants with Down's syndrome, many social behaviours develop slowly. For example, the onset of eye contact, vocalizing, and smiling is usually delayed by several weeks, and emergence continues at a slower pace, accompanied by decreased intensity (Berger and Cunningham, 1981; 1985). Behaviours such as these are regarded as key components of successful social interactions. When they are absent, parents are forced to look for other ways of relating to their child and interpreting the meaning of his or her actions. How does a parent become aware of such alternatives, though? We have little exposure to developmentally delayed children in our culture. Training programmes could be offered by knowledgeable experts, but these are rarely available. Consequently, parents may be at a loss as to how to have fulfilling interactions with their baby. Indeed, parents of developmentally delayed infants often report difficulties in 'reading' their child's signals (Jones, 1980). This has an impact on their developing relationship with the child and on their confidence in their own parenting skills. While parents of 'typical' infants are free to concentrate on getting to know their newborn babies and to recognize their individual characteristics, parents of developmentally delayed infants are often distracted because they are mourning the loss of the healthy infant that they had envisioned (Emde and Brown, 1978).

Hearing impairment presents another circumstance under which the interaction of parent and infant can become problematic. Children who are deaf are denied one of the most fundamental modes of communication. In order to interact successfully, parents must adopt a communication style that is accessible to their child. However, research suggests that parents find it extraordinarily difficult to do this (Jamieson and Pedersen, 1993). For example, periods of joint attention (Moore and Dunham, 1995) are common when a child is learning to talk. The attention of both participants is directed toward the toy, and parents quite naturally comment on the object. For example, they might say, while pointing to the object, 'See the red ball? Can you roll it to me?' The hearing child and his or her parents can be communicating while neither of them are looking at the other, because they are both focused on the ball. In the case of the deaf child, though, it is impossible to have this kind of interaction with a parent, as the intake of information is limited to a single channel – vision. Because the child cannot look at the ball and the mother at the same time, he or she has to choose which of the two to attend to, and the information about the other is sacrificed.

Of course, it is possible that parents may communicate with their child via sign language. Parents who use sign language with infants modify it in much the same way vocal speech is altered when directed toward infants (Erting, Prezioso and Hynes, 1990). However, sign language is most likely to be used in families where another member of the family is deaf, and this occurs for only 10 per cent of hearing impaired children. Approximately nine out of ten deaf children come from families where no other members are deaf (Center for Assessment and Demographic Studies, 1989). This is of particular concern because the worst developmental outcomes for hearing impaired children occur for those who have hearing mothers (Jamieson and Pedersen, 1994). These children show less responsiveness and attentiveness to parents than do hearing children, and they initiate fewer conversations with their parents. This leads to continuing communication problems within the relationship (Koester, 1994).

A third example of non-typical development that presents particular difficulties for parent–infant interaction is visual impairment. Problems similar to those with deafness exist here. Because a blind infant and his or her parents cannot use visual gaze to communicate, fundamental components of normal social interaction are missing. As has been described, in the early months parents and infants interact most often by exchanges of visual gaze. A mother smiles at her baby; he smiles back; the mother makes a funny face; the baby smiles more intensely; perhaps the mother begins to play peek-a-boo. As infants get older, a parent will follow the baby's eye gaze to see what aspects of the environment he or she is interested in – the bottle on the table? the bird outside the window? the ball in the corner? It is episodes such as these that form the basis of relationships between parents and infants. Without visual gaze, the parent is denied intuitive ways of interacting with a baby and in interpreting his or her reactions to the world. Again, parents are often bewildered as to how to compensate for such a fundamental loss.

Unfortunately, little research has considered the early relationship of blind infants and their parents. Instead, much of the research on visual impairment has concentrated on the delay in language acquisition that blind infants exhibit (e.g. McConachie and Moore, 1994). Their acquisition of first words is delayed by several months, and they exhibit other atypical patterns of language use (Andersen, Dunlea and Kekelis, 1984). This is obviously due, in part, to the inability of blind children to see the objects around them and enquire about the name for the object. Indeed, there is a high proportion of repetitive labelling, rather than requesting, in the early stages of language acquisition in visually impaired children (Dunlea, 1989). However, it may be that the changed nature of the early relationship between blind infants and parents also contributes to the delay in language acquisition. As discussed, many theorists see early interactions as the basis for the development of later communication (e.g. Trevarthen, 1977; 1993; Tronick, 1981). Rattray (Rattray and Zeedyk, 1995) has recently begun work examining the early interactions of blind infants and their mothers and has found preliminary evidence to indicate that mothers of blind infants may talk less to their infants than do mothers of sighted infants. This is surprising, in that mothers of visually impaired infants might have been expected to talk *more* to their infants, in order to compensate for the loss of the visual channel. The decrease may reflect mothers' difficulties in adjusting to the needs of the infants. Other modes of communication may feel awkward, unfamiliar, or unfulfilling, and this is likely to lead to distress on the mother's part. Alternatively, the decrease in maternal speech may be encouraging. It may be that mothers use alternative modes of communication, such as touch, in communicating with their visually impaired infants.

Conflicting with Rattray's findings are those of Moore and McConachie (1994), who compared parental input to infants who were completely blind and those who were severely visually impaired (i.e. had a limited degree of visual perception). Their results indicated that even a very small amount of vision influenced the types of interaction that occurred in the two groups. Parents initiated more conversation if their infants were blind, in contrast to Rattray's findings. More importantly, their findings revealed qualitative differences in the style of interaction. For example, parents of totally blind infants more often requested verbal information from a child (e.g. 'What's that?', 'What do you want?'), while parents of severely visually impaired children, who had at least some vision, described objects for their children or requested that they perform an action with the object. Parents of blind children may use a requesting strategy to check that they have read the intentions of their child accurately, but this is problematic in connecting the child's experience to a particular object, which is achieved more successfully with a strategy of describing objects. Such differences, and others identified by Moore and McConachie (1994; see also Rowland, 1983; Urwin, 1984) highlight the difficulties faced by parents who are unable to read confidently the meaning of their child's actions and emphasize the fact that the interaction of parent and child is altered in critical ways. Much more research needs to be undertaken so that we can adequately understand the nature and impact of such differences.

Conditions such as Down's syndrome, deafness, and blindness provide examples of only a few of the conditions that may result from impairments in children's development. In all such circumstances, a common feature is that parents usually find it difficult to adjust to these changes, particularly in the earliest periods, and few programmes are available to help them cope or to adapt their styles of communication. When such programmes are available, relationships of parents and children can improve immensely. For example, Fraiberg (1974) designed a programme for parents of blind infants, in which she taught them to monitor the hand movements of their infants. It is possible to tell much about the excitement, tension, and general emotional state of an infant by being aware of their hands. Fraiberg reported that the mothers were better able to 'read' their babies, leading to much greater satisfaction in their relationships. Programmes such as this are rare, and additional research and resources are required in order to assist health professionals in developing such programmes.

Abuse

Another area in which parent–infant interactions may become problematic as a result of parents misinterpreting the meaning of infant behaviour is child abuse. Numerous researchers have examined the reasons that parents abuse their children, and certainly factors such as poverty, parental stress and the absence of support systems are major contributors (e.g. Sussman, Trickett, Iannotti et al., 1985). Another related factor may be the parent's interpretation of a child's particular behaviour.

As has already been stressed, a parent's response toward an infant is based, in large part, on his or her interpretation of the child's actions. For example, when a child cries for hours during the night, does the parent believe that that is due to discomfort, such as a tooth that is cutting, or does the parent believe that the child is just being stubborn and refusing to go to sleep? If a glass of milk is knocked over, is that viewed as a result of the child's undeveloped motor skills or an intention to create a mess? The parent's belief about which of these (or other) explanations is true will influence the response that he or she sees as appropriate. If the parent believes the child is misbehaving, then punishment may be viewed as warranted. On the other hand, if a parent believes the child is not responsible for the actions, then a different type of response is likely.

Research in this area indicates that some abuse may result from unreasonable expectations that parents hold in regard to the capabilities of their children (e.g. Rickel, 1989). For example, it is not uncommon for parents to expect toilet training to occur quickly or at an early age, although such expectations exceed children's physical ability to control their bladder. Parental education programmes have often been founded on the basis that knowledge about developmental timetables has an effect on parents' interpretations of infant behaviour. Their aim is to increase parental awareness of child development timetables and to increase their coping skills. Herrerias (1988) describes a programme for mothers who were at risk of abusing their children. While the programme addressed a variety of issues, including the self-esteem, depression, nutrition, and problem-solving skills of participants, one major component was dissemination of basic child development information. Encouragingly, after 20 weeks in the programme, mothers were found to engage children in play more often and they were using less physical disciplinary methods. Field and her colleagues (Field, Widmayer, Greenberg and Stoller, 1982) also developed a training programme for teenage mothers. Again, a variety of relevant issues were addressed, including education and job opportunities for the participants, but child-rearing attitudes constituted an important segment of the programme. For the two years of the evaluation period, infants in the experimental group consistently showed, among other differences, superior mental and motor skills and they weighed more. More relevant to the issue of parental interpretation, teenagers in the training programme rated their children as less difficult than did teenage parents in a control group, and their interactions with their infants were of a higher quality. They talked more to their infants, and their infants averted eye gaze less often.

These two programmes have been described to provide some sense of the breadth of parental education programmes that have now been developed to assist at-risk parents with parenting. There is a predominant attitude, at least with western cultures, that parenting skills are intuitive and are 'acquired with the birth of baby'. However, any parent can tell you this is not the case. Parenting skills are the result of hard won experience and trial-and-error testing. It appears that increased knowledge about child development alters, or at least broadens, the interpretations which parents make of their child's behaviour. This can only be beneficial for the interactions of parents and infants, as well as for the development of individual children.

What conclusions can be drawn from the consolidation of these research areas?

Because the behaviours of infants are so subtle and appear to be simplistic, the importance of the early relationship between parent and infant is often discounted. However, this relationship provides a critical foundation for parent–infant attachment, as discussed in more depth in Chapter 9, and it has a powerful impact on the longer term development of a child.

Understanding the more detailed aspects of this relation is possible because of the formidable amount of infancy research that has been carried out over the past 20 years. Unfortunately, most of this research has focused on typical parent–infant interactions. We are only beginning to investigate those circumstances under which interaction and communication are more problematic. It is vital that more research is directed toward such areas, because it is through such work that we learn how to combat difficulties. We become able to develop more effective intervention programmes and to target available resources more efficiently. Indeed, there is an increasing need for intervention programmes, given recent changes across a breadth of domains, including improvements in medical technology and shifting societal structures. For example, a high proportion of prematurely-born infants can now be saved, but their development is often subject to complications that result in physiological problems such as those described in this chapter. Likewise, families increasingly find themselves living under conditions in which traditional support structures, such as the extended family or social work services, are less accessible or even completely unavailable. The stress produced by these circumstances can push the relationship of parent and child into difficulties such as those discussed earlier. Of course adverse familial conditions may be temporary or physiological conditions sometimes corrected, but we require a greater understanding of the long-term effects of such conditions on a child's development. Are repercussions unavoidable; what factors increase or decrease their impact; can we mitigate later consequences with earlier attention? In other words, if problematic circumstances occur at any point in the child's development, how can parents and professionals respond most effectively?

Research directed toward these kinds of questions is typically classified as 'applied'. However, such work is also invaluable for more 'basic' research investigation of parent–infant communication. When we are able to observe situations in which particular aspects of interaction have gone awry or are absent or are even over-abundant, then we gain a better understanding of the degree to which specific factors are important in parent–infant interaction in general. Studying non-typical interactions also allows us to test theoretical assumptions, such as the views of the 'as-if' and 'innate' theorists previously summarized. We cannot fully address theoretical questions without working with both typical and non-typical samples.

Given our growing understanding of the significance of early parent–infant interactions for the long-term development of children, we can be optimistic that research in this area will expand. Researchers, professionals, and parents each have a contribution to make, and such diversity should be encouraged. Input from multiple sources can only serve to increase our awareness and strengthen our conclusions.

Applications

1. Become familiar with the normal pattern of infant development
Infants' abilities and preferences change rapidly, and in specific developmentally-driven ways, during the first year. Such differences will alter the kinds of activities that are appealing to infants and therefore the kinds of games that their parents will play with them. It is particularly important to be aware of this when giving advice to parents.

2. Be respectful of parents
It is not only 'experts' who are knowledgeable about infants. Parents can also make valuable contributions to our understanding of infant development, if given the opportunity.

3. Parents and infants benefit considerably when provided with support
Often difficulties between parents and infants result from the fact that parents are having trouble 'understanding' their infant. Supporting parents by providing them with information about their child's development can be extremely helpful (for example, how blindness is likely to affect children's facial expressions or why physical development restricts bladder control). Additionally, suggesting alternative meanings for a behaviour or other types of activities for parents to try out can significantly improve relationships (for example, pointing out that intense bouts of crying may not be intentional or encouraging the use of more touch for communicating with deaf children). Most parents report that they receive very little of this type of support.

Further reading

Messer, D. J. (1994). *The Development of Communication: From Social Interaction to Language.* Chichester: John Wiley and Sons.
Pope, C. (1994). *Baby Monthly.* London: BBC Books.

References

Adamson, L. B., Bakeman, R., Smith, C. B. and Walters, A. S. (1987). Adults' interpretation of infants' acts. *Developmental Psychology*, **23**, 383–7.
Andersen, E., Dunlea, A. and Kekelis, L. (1984). Blind children's language: resolving some differences. *Journal of Child Language*, **11**, 645–64.
Bates, E. (1979). *The Emergence of Symbols: Cognition and Communication in Infancy.* New York: Academic Press.
Bates, J. E. (1994). Parents as scientific observers of their children's development. In *Developmental Follow-up: Concepts, Domains, and Methods* (S. L. Friedman and H. C. Haywood, eds). New York: Academic Press.
Beebe, B., Jaffe, J., Feldstein, S., Mays, K. and Alson, D. (1985). Inter-personal timing: the application of an adult dialogue model to mother–infant vocal and kinesic interactions. In *Social Perception in Infants* (T. M. Field and N. Fox, eds). Norwood, NJ: Ablex.
Berger, J. and Cunningham, C. C. (1981). The development of eye contact between mothers and normal versus Down syndrome infants. *Developmental Psychology*, **17**, 678–89.
Berger, J. and Cunningham, C. C. (1985). Aspects of the development of smiling in young infants with Down syndrome. *Child: Care, Health and Development*, **12**, 13–24.
Bettes, B. A. (1988). Maternal depression and motherese: temporal and intonational features. *Child Development*, **59**, 1089–96.
Brazelton, T. B. (1982). Joint regulation of neonate-parent behavior. In *Social Interchange in Infancy: Affect, Cognition, and Communication* (E. Z. Gronick, ed.). Baltimore: University Park Press.
Breslau, N., Davis, G. and Prabucki, K. (1988). Depressed mothers as informants in family history research: are they accurate? *Psychiatry Research*, **24**, 345–59.
Bricker, D. and Squires, J. (1989). The effectiveness of parental screening of at-risk infants: the infant monitoring questionnaires. *Topics in Early Childhood Special Education*, **9**, 67–85.
Bushnell, I. W. R., Sai, F. and Mullin, J. T. (1989). Neonatal recognition of the mother's face. *British Journal of Developmental Psychology*, **7**, 3–15.
Camaioni, L. (1993). The development of intentional communication: a re-analysis. In *New Perspectives in Early Communicative Development* (J. Nadel and L. Camaioni, eds). London: Routledge.
Campbell, S. B., Cohn, J. F., Flanagan, C., Popper, S. and Meyers, T. (1992). Course and correlates of postpartum depression during the transition to parenthood. *Development and Psychopathology*, **4**, 29–47.
Center for Assessment and Demographic Studies (1989). *Annual Survey of Hearing Impaired Children and Youth, 1988–1989.* Washington, DC: Gallaudet University.
Cernoch, J. M. and Porter, R. H. (1985). Recognition of maternal axillary odors by infants. *Child Development*, **56**, 1593–8.
Cohn, J. R., Campbell, S. B., Matias, R. and Hopkins, J. (1990). Face-to-face interactions of postpartum depressed and nondepressed mother–infant pairs at two months. *Developmental Psychology*, **26**, 15–23.
Cohn, J. R. and Tronick, E. Z. (1983). Three-month-old infants' reaction to simulated maternal depression. *Child Development*, **54**, 185–93.
Cohn, J. F. and Tronick, E. Z. (1988). Mother–infant face-to-face interaction: influence is bidirectional and unrelated to periodic cycles in either partner's behaviour. *Developmental Psychology*, **24**, 386–92.

Dale, P. S., Bates, E., Reznick, J. S. and Morisset, C. (1989). The validity of a parent report instrument of child language at twenty months. *Journal of Child Language*, **16**, 239–49.

DeCasper, A. J. and Fifer, W. P. (1980). Of human bonding: newborns prefer their mother's voices. *Science*, **208**, 1174–6.

DeCasper, A. J., Lecanuet, J. P., Busnel, M. C., Granier-Deferre, C. and Maugeais, R. (1994). Fetal reactions to recurrent maternal speech. *Infant Behavior and Development*, **17**, 159–64.

Diamond, K. E. (1993). The role of parents' observations and concerns in screening for developmental delays in young children. *Topics in Early Childhood Special Education*, **13**, 68–81.

Dunlea, A. (1989). *Vision and the Emergence of Meaning: Blind and Sighted Children's Early Language*. Cambridge: Cambridge University Press.

Eisenberg, R. B. (1975). *Auditory Competence in Early Life: The Roots of Communicative Behavior*. Baltimore: University Park Press.

Emde, R. N. and Brown, C. (1978). Adaptation to the birth of Down syndrome infants. *Journal of American Academy for Child Psychiatry*, **17**, 299–323.

Erting, C. J., Prezioso, C. and Hynes, M. O. (1990). The interactional context of deaf mother–infant communication. In *From Gesture to Language in Hearing and Deaf Children* (V. Volterra and C. Erting, eds). Berlin: Springer-Verlag.

Field, T., Healy, B., Goldstein, S. and Guthertz, M. (1990). Behavior-state matching and synchrony in mother–infant interactions of nondepressed versus depressed dyads. *Developmental Psychology*, **26**, 7–14.

Field, T., Morrow, C. and Adlestein, C. (1993). Depressed mothers' perceptions of infant behavior. *Infant Behavior and Development*, **16**, 99–108.

Field, T., Widmayer, S., Greenberg, R. and Stoller, S. (1982). Effects of parent training on teenage mothers and their infants. *Paediatrics*, **69**, 703–7.

Field, T. (1984). Early interactions between infants and their postpartum depressed mothers. *Infant Behavior and Development*, **7**, 527–32.

Field, T. M., Woodson, R., Greenberg, R. and Cohen, D. (1982). Discrimination and imitation of facial expressions by neonates. *Science*, **218**, 179–81.

Fraiberg, S. (1974). Blind infants and their mothers: an examination of the sign system. In *The Effect of the Infant on its Caregiver* (M. Lewis and L. A. Rosenblum, eds). New York: Wiley.

Friedlander, S., Weiss, D. S. and Traylor, J. (1986). Assessing the influence of maternal depression on the validity of the Child Behaviour Checklist. *Journal of Abnormal Child Psychology*, **14**, 123–33.

Goodnow, J. J., Cashmore, J., Cotton, S. and Knight, R. (1984). Mothers' developmental timetables in two cultural groups. *International Journal of Psychology*, **19**, 193–205.

Goshen-Gottstein, E. R. (1980). Treatment of young children among nonwestern Jewish mothers in Israel: sociocultural variables. *American Journal of Orthopsychiatry*, **50**, 323–40.

Griest, D. L., Wells, K. C. and Forehand, R. (1979). An examination of predictors of maternal perceptions of maladjustment in clinic-referred children. *Journal of Abnormal Psychology*, **88**, 277–81.

Harding, C. G. (1984). Acting with intention: a framework for examining the development of the intention to communicate. In *The Origins and Growth of Communication* (L. Feagans, C. Garvey and R. Golinkoff, eds). Norwood, NJ: Ablex.

Herrerias, C. (1988). Prevention of child abuse and neglect in the Hispanic community: the MADRE parent education program. *Journal of Primary Prevention*, **9**, 104–19.

Hess, R. D., Kashigawi, K., Azuma, H., Price, G. G. and Dickson, W. P. (1980). Maternal expectations for the mastery of developmental tasks in Japan and the United States. *International Journal of Psychology*, **15**, 259–71.

Hobson, R. P. (1993). Perceiving attitudes, conceiving minds. In *Origins of an Understanding of Mind* (C. Lewis and P. Mitchell, eds). Hillsdale, NJ: Erlbaum.

Hopkins, B. and Westra, T. (1989). Maternal expectations of their infants' development: some cultural differences. *Developmental Medicine and Child Neurology*, **31**, 384–90.

Hubert, N. C. and Wachs, T. C. (1985). Parental perceptions of the behavioral components of infant easiness/difficultness. *Child Development*, **56**, 1525–37.

Jamieson, J. R. and Pedersen, E. D. (1993). Deafness and mother–child interaction: scaffolded instruction and the learning of problem-solving skills. *Early Development and Parenting*, **2**, 229–42.

Jones, O. M. H. (1980). Mother–child communication with prelinguistic Down's syndrome and normal infants. In *Studies in Mother–Infant Interaction* (H. R. Schaffer, ed.). London: Academic Press.

Kamel, H. (1993). Maternal intepretation of infant facial expressions: divergent perspectives, multiple meanings. Paper presented at Annual Meeting of British Psychological Society, Developmental Section. Birmingham, UK.

Kaye, K. (1982). *The Mental and Social Life of Babies: How Parents Create Persons*. London: Harvester Press Limited.

Koester, L. S. (1994). Early interactions and the socioemotional development of deaf infants. *Early Development and Parenting*, **3**, 51–60.

Kugiumutzakis, J. (1985). The origin, development, and function of the early infant imitation. PhD Thesis, University of Uppsala.

Kugiumutzakis, G. (1993). Intersubjective vocal imitation in early mother–infant interaction. In *New Perspectives in Early Communication Development* (J. Nadel and L. Camaioni, eds). London: Routledge.

McConachie, H. and Moore, V. (1994). Early expressive language of severely visually impaired children. *Developmental Medicine and Child Neurology*, **36**, 230–40.

Mayes, L. C. and Carter, A. S. (1990). Emerging social regulatory capacities as seen in the still-face situation. *Child Development*, **61**, 754–63.

Meltzoff, A. N. and Moore, M. K. (1983). Newborn infants imitate adult facial gestures. *Child Development*, **54**, 702–9.

Miller, C. L. (1988). Parents' perceptions and attributions of infant vocal behaviour and development. *First Language*, **8**, 125–42.

Moore, C. and Dunham, P. (1995). *Joint Attention: Its Origins and Role in Development*. Hillsdale, NJ: Erlbaum.

Moore, V. and McConachie, H. (1994). Communication between blind and severely visually impaired children and their parents. *British Journal of Developmental Psychology*, **12**, 491–502.

Murray, L. (1992). The impact of postnatal depression on infant development. *Journal of Child Psychology and Psychiatry and Allied Disciplines*, **33**, 543–61.

Murray, L., Kempton, C., Woolgar, M. and Hooper, R. (1993). Depressed mothers' speech to their infants and its relation to infant gender and cognitive development. *Journal of Child Psychology and Psychiatry and Allied Disciplines*, **34**, 1083–101.

Newson, J. (1978). An intersubjective approach to the systematic description of mother–infant interaction. In *Studies in Mother–Infant Interaction* (H. R. Schaffer, ed.). London: Academic Press.

Newson, J. (1979). Intentional behaviour in the young infant. In *The First Year of Life: Psychological and Medical Implications of Early Experience* (D. Shaffer and J. Dunn, eds). Chichester: John Wiley.

Nicolson, P. (1986). Developing a feminist approach to depression following childbirth. In *Feminist Social Psychology: Developing Theory and Practice* (S. Wilkinson, ed.). Milton Keynes: Open University Press.

Ninio, A. (1979). The naive theory of the infant and other maternal attitudes in two subgroups of Israel. *Child Development*, **50**, 976–80.

Ninio, A. (1988). The effects of cultural background, sex, and parenthood on beliefs about the timetable of cognitive development in infancy. *Merrill-Palmer Quarterly*, **34**, 369–88.

Obrist, P. A. (1981). *Cardiovascular Psychophysiology*. New York: Plenum.

O'Hara, M. W. and Zekoski, E. M. (1988). Postpartum depression: a comprehensive review. In *Motherhood and Mental Illness: Vol. 2. Causes and Consequences* (R. Kumar and I. F. Brockington, eds). London: Wright.

Panaccione, V. F. and Wahler, R. G. (1986). Child behavior, maternal depression, and social coercion as factors in the quality of child care. *Journal of Abnormal Child Psychology*, **14**, 263–78.

Radke-Yarrow, M., Cummings, E. M., Kuczynski, L. and Chapman, M. (1985). Patterns of attachment in two- and three-year-olds in normal families and families with parental depression. *Child Development*, **56**, 884–93.

Rattray, J. and Zeedyk, M. S. (1995). Early interactions of visually impaired infants and their mothers. Paper presented at the Annual Meeting of the British Psychological Society, Developmental Section. September, Glasgow.

Richters, J. and Pellegrini, D. (1989). Depressed mothers' judgments about their children: an examination of the depression-distortion hypothesis. *Child Development*, **60**, 1068–75.

Rickel, A. U. (1989). *Teen Pregnancy and Parenting*. New York: Hemisphere/Taylor and Francis.

Rowland, C. (1983). Patterns of interaction between three blind infants and their mothers. In *Language Acquisition in the Blind Child* (A. E. Mills, ed.). London: Croom Helm.

Schaffer, H. R. (1984). *The Child's Entry into a Social World*. London: Academic Press.

Schaffer, H. R. (1989). Early social development. In *Infant Development* (A. Slater and G. Bremner, eds). Hillsdale, NJ: Erlbaum.

Snow, C. E. and Ferguson, C. A. (eds) (1977). *Talking to Children*. Cambridge: Cambridge University Press.

Sussman, E. J., Trickett, P. K., Iannotti, R. J., Hollenbeck, B. E. and Zahn-Waxler, C. (1985). Child-rearing patterns in depressed, abusive, and normal mothers. *American Journal of Orthopsychiatry*, **55**, 237–51.

Templin, M. C. (1957). Certain language skills in children: their development and interrelationships. *University of Minnesota Institute of Child Welfare Monograph*, *26*.

Thomas, A., Chess, S. and Korn, S. J. (1982). The reality of difficult temperament. *Merrill-Palmer Quarterly*, **28**, 1–20.

Trevarthen, C. (1977). Descriptive analyses of infant communicative behaviour. In *Studies in Mother–Infant Interaction* (H. R. Schaffer, ed.). London: Academic Press.

Trevarthen, C. (1979). Communication and cooperation in early infancy: a description of primary intersubjectivity. In *Before Speech: The Beginning of Interpersonal Communication* (M. Bullowa, ed.). USA: Cambridge University Press.

Trevarthen, C. (1993). The function of motives in early infant communication and development. In *New Perspectives in Early Communication Development* (J. Nadel and L. Camaioni, eds). London: Routledge.

Tronick, E. (1981). Infant communication intent: the infant's reference to social interaction. In *Language Behavior in Infancy and Early Childhood* (Stark, ed.). New York: Elsevier.

Tronick, E., Als, H., Adamson, L., Wise, S. and Brazelton, T. B. (1978). The infant's response to entrapment between contradictory message in face-to-face interaction. *Journal of American Academy of Child Psychiatry*, **17**, 1–13.

Tulkin, S. R. and Kagan, J. (1972). Mother–infant interaction in the first year of life. *Child Development*, **43**, 31–41.

Urwin, C. (1984). Communication in infancy and the emergence of language in blind children. In *The Acquisition of Communicative Competence* (R. L. Schiefelbusch and J. Pickar, eds). Baltimore: University Park Press.

Vedeler, D. (1994). Infant intentionality as object directedness: a method for observation. *Scandinavian Journal of Psychology*, **35**, 343–66.

Vinter, A. (1986). The role of movement in eliciting early imitation. *Child Development*, **57**, 66–71.

Weintraub, D., Prinz, R. J. and Neale, J. M. (1978). Peer evaluations of the competence of children vulnerable to psychopathology. *Journal of Abnormal Child Psychology*, **6**, 461–73.

Weintraub, D. and Shapiro, M. (1968). The traditional family in Israel in the process of change: crisis and continuity. *British Journal of Sociology*, **19**, 284–99.

Weissman, M., Wickramarante, P., Warner, V., John, K., Prusoff, B. A., Merikangas, K. R. and Gammon, D. (1987). Assessing psychiatric disorders in children: discrepancies between mothers' and children's reports. *Archives of General Psychiatry*, **44**, 747–853.

Willatts, P. (1989). Development of problem-solving in infancy. In *Infant Development* (A. Slater and G. Bremner, eds). Hillsdale, NJ: Erlbaum.

Zeedyk, M. S. (1994). Maternal interpretations of infant intentionality. Unpublished doctoral dissertation. Yale University, USA.

Zeedyk, M. S. (1996). Developmental accounts of intentionality: toward integration. *Developmental Review*, **16**, 416–61.

Zeedyk, M. S. (1997) Maternal interpretations of infant intentionality: Changes over the course of infant development. *British Journal of Development Psychology*, **14**, 477–93.

9

The quality of care and attachment

Edward C. Melhuish

The vast majority of parents and infants have close emotional relationships. In everyday terms, they love each other. The best known psychological explanation of this experience is attachment theory, and this theory has been very influential both in stimulating research and in the formulation of guidelines for childcare. In this chapter Ed Melhuish reviews the current state of attachment theory research and considers the relationship between attachment and infant care. Are infants who receive day care from an early age less securely attached to their parents than those cared for at home? Does it matter who is caring – or is what they do more important? What is good quality parental care – or good quality day care? What consequences does childcare have for later development?

One of the most striking developments in the first year of life is the development of the infant's attachment to its primary caregiver, usually the mother. This development occurs almost universally, and where it does not deleterious consequences for future life may occur. The universality of early attachments by infants to caregiver applies to all cultures and all patterns of family life for which there is evidence. There are cultural variations but the central theme of the development of an emotional bond between infant and caregiver applies throughout the world. The functional significance of this attachment and the reverse attachment by caregiver toward infant is clear. Humans are an altricial species, i.e. are not capable of self-mobility or self-care in infancy and without this two-way bond between infant and caregiver, the care essential for the infant's survival would not happen. The infant's emotional bond toward the mother is the first love relationship and accumulating evidence suggests that it is the prototype or foundation for love relationships that develop in later life. It provides a 'working model' upon which later relationships are developed, perpetuating earlier forms of relationships.

Love relationships have long been a topic of interest to psychological theoreticians. Psychoanalytic theory (e.g. Freud, 1926) spent considerable effort in exploring their genesis, and a branch of psychoanalytic theory, object relations theory (e.g. Mahler, Pine and Bergman, 1975) makes such emotional bonds the main focus of study. However, the impact of this work on psychology as a whole *has* been limited. This situation began to change with the emergence of attachment theory. Bowlby (1958, 1969, 1973, 1980) produced a theoretical framework for the study of attachments through an integration of ideas from psychodynamic, ethological and systems theories. Within the theory the origin of the capacity for attachment derives from the child's initial attachment to the primary caregiver, usually the mother, and the theory goes on to consider how the development of attachments may proceed across the lifespan. However, the initial focus was on the infant–mother attachment.

The development of the relationship between a mother and her infant can be viewed from the perspective of the mother's bond to her infant and the perspective of the infant's attachment to the mother. The 'bonding' that occurs between mother and infant was addressed by Klaus and Kennel in a series of studies (Klaus and Kennel, 1976). They were influenced by ethological ideas and thought there may be a particularly sensitive period after birth when a special bond from mother to infant might be formed. They found that where infants received more hours of skin-to-skin contact with the mother during the first three days of life, the mothers cuddled, soothed and had more eye-contact with the babies. They found similar effects persisting two years later! As a result many hospitals changed procedures to facilitate such bonding. Subsequent research has been unable to substantiate Klaus and Kennel's findings (Eyer, 1993; Myers, 1984). The idea that there is a particular sensitive period is now viewed with scepticism. However the research did result in humanitarian reforms to many hospital procedures.

The other side of the mother–infant relationship is the infant's attachment to the mother. Attachment theory is predominantly concerned with this side of the relationship, although inevitably the two sides of the relationship are continually interacting. Sometimes the terms bonding and attachment are used interchangeably, as when insecure attachments are referred to as 'bonding disorders'. This is more common in the medical field. This chapter will focus on infant attachments to caregivers.

Earlier this century, stress was laid on the mother's role as a provider of food and comfort in explaining the development of the infant's attachment to the mother. Essentially the view was of infants' social responsiveness to the mother as motivated by a secondary drive. This view can be seen in early psychoanalytic thinking where the mother is seen as satisfying the orality needs of the child, when the child is in the oral stage of psycho-sexual development. It can also be seen in learning theory accounts (e.g. Sears, Maccoby and Levin, 1957) where secondary reinforcement value is seen as attached to the mother by virtue of her association with the satisfaction of the primary biological drives (e.g. feeding) of the infant.

Increasingly this view of the development of early social and emotional relationships came under attack. There was a variety of types of evidence which just did not fit this model. From animal ethology it was clear that certain species (e.g. geese, sheep) would form attachments purely on the basis of perceptual contact. Whether such imprinting occurs in other species has been a matter of debate, but it is clear that the simple association model of attachments did not hold for many animals. Also Harlow's (1958) work with monkeys showed that contact comfort was more important than satisfying biological drives in the choice of attachment object.

Research with human infants found evidence to suggest that the development of attachments was rooted in processes other than the provision of warmth and comfort. Schaffer and Emerson (1964) found that feeding schedules were unrelated to attachments and that infants commonly formed attachments to people who did not take part in the satisfaction of biological needs but only interacted with the infants through play and communication. In addition, Fantz's (1961) work showed very early, possibly innate preferences for face-like visual stimuli. In the auditory dimension infants also appeared to attend to the human voice and would orient their gaze to sounds

(Aronson and Rosenbloom, 1971). Hence they would turn to look at who was talking. Also evidence was accumulating for the special sensitivity of the infant's auditory apparatus for discriminating auditory linguistic distinctions (Eimas, Siqueland, Jusczgk and Vigorito, 1971). Mills and Melhuish (1974) showed that three-week-old infants had learnt to recognize their mother's voice, and later DeCasper and Fifer (1980) found even earlier voice recognition. In the smell/taste dimension MacFarlane (1975) reported that newborn infants quickly learnt to discriminate their own mother's breast milk from that of other mothers. Other work suggested that visual recognition of the mother was also occurring early in life. Such research as this provided evidence to suggest that infants' attachments develop out of their perceptual and cognitive interaction with people rather than from the satisfaction of primary biological drives. The work on infant perception and cognition suggests that infants are particularly adapted to receive communication from human sources. Other receptive channels for communication are touch, movement perception and proprioception (sense of bodily position), all of which are fully functional in infancy.

Besides this apparent preadaptation of receptive communication abilities, infants have a range of preadapted productive communication abilities. The cry is a powerful form of communication and can be differentiated into pain, hunger and irritable cries, which caregivers can learn to distinguish (Zeskind and Marshall, 1988). Other vocalizations quickly develop and almost invariably elicit responses from caregivers. Facial expressions are also present early on and easily convey mood. The smile is usually present by six weeks of age and is one of the infant's most powerful communications. Also there are a range of reflexes – the moro, sucking, rooting and grasping reflexes – which all play a role in the adaptation of the infant to communicating its needs, and maintaining contact with the caregiver. Recently evidence has accumulated for newborn imitation of others' facial movements, notably tongue protrusion (Maratos, 1971; Meltzoff and Moore, 1977). The precise age and precursors of imitation are still controversial but imitation by the infant of others' sounds, smiles and movements can be a very powerful form of communication. It is worth emphasizing how powerful these early communications are. It is difficult for adults to ignore the infant's cry, smile, coo or to ignore the appeal of the infant's very appearance.

There appears to be a congruence between the infant's perceptual capacities and human forms of communication, and between the infant's productive communicative abilities and adult susceptibility. It is as if there has been mutual adaptation in the evolutionary process, between the receptive and productive communicative apparatus of infant and adult. Such mutual adaptation of receptive and productive communication abilities means that the infant comes into the world with a ready-made communication system, which then undergoes rapid development and refinement.

When these aspects of the infant's communicative development are considered it would appear appropriate to consider their role in the development of parent–infant interaction (Chapter 8, this volume). This would suggest that the role of parent–infant interaction would be crucial to the development of attachments. Initial interaction would form the basis for recognition of specific individuals. Once such recognition had taken place then the child's attachment to individuals can proceed. Possibly different patterns of mother–infant interaction may result in different types of attachment. Certainly within Bowlby's theory such predictions might be made.

Initially Bowlby's theory had limited impact and if the theory had remained without empirical support it is likely that it would have had little effect on the development of psychology. However, Ainsworth took Bowlby's ideas and set about operationalizing them in ways conducive to empirical research, and this has brought the study of love relationships in from the cold and made attachment theory one of the most influential theories currently in psychology. The work by Ainsworth and her disciples produced the most widely used method for assessing the infant's attachment to a caregiver, the 'strange situation' (Ainsworth and Wittig, 1969).

The 'strange situation'

The strange situation consists of eight three-minute episodes involving two separations and reunions in an unfamilar setting, after the following format

- Episode one: infant and mother are shown to a comfortable unfamiliar room containing toys.
- Episode two: infant and mother together.
- Episode three: a stranger enters.
- Episode four: the mother leaves infant with stranger.
- Episode five: the mother returns and the stranger leaves.
- Episode six: the mother leaves infant alone.
- Episode seven: the stranger returns.
- Episode eight: the mother returns.

The procedure is designed to place the infant in increasingly stressful situations in order to produce an increased arousal of the attachment system and the elicitation of attachment-related behaviours. The infant's responses during the two reunions are particularly salient for the assessment of attachment. It is assumed that:

1. These experiences constitute a particular order of stressful events for infants;
2. Stress will change behaviour with a reduction of exploration and affiliation to unfamiliar people and increased attachment behaviours to familiar people.

Using this procedure a classification of infant attachments to mothers was developed. Securely attached infants (type B) show signs of missing mother upon separation and warmly greet her upon reunion. Insecurely attached infants might be insecure-avoidant (type A) and show little distress upon separation and avoid or ignore the mother at reunion, or insecure-ambivalent/resistant (type C) and show distress upon separation and while seeking contact upon reunion may show some resistance. These three major categories reflect earlier descriptions of types of attachment by Bowlby et al. (1956). There are several subcategories and for a full description of the procedure and classification the best source is Ainsworth, Blehar, Waters and Wall (1978). In much research, around 65–70 per cent of North American infants show secure attachment (type B) and 30–35 per cent show one of the insecure patterns (type A 20–25 per cent; type C 10–15 per cent).

One of the most interesting research findings is that the type of attachment is predictable from the characteristics of previous mother–infant interaction. In their research Ainsworth, Blehar, Waters and Wall (1978) followed children through the infancy period. At regular intervals they observed the child and mother together in the home and made assessments of mother–infant interaction. Later they were able to do the strange situation and produce classifications of attachment. They found that the mothers of children who had insecure attachment (A and C) classifications differed from mothers of children who had a secure attachment (B) classification. Securely attached infants had mothers who were more sensitive, responsive, accessible and cooperative in their care of their infants. They also showed more affection, tender holding of the infant and more adaptation to the baby's daily rhythm of activity. The four dimensions of sensitivity, responsivity, accessibility and cooperativeness were highly associated and appeared to form a dimension of sensitive mothering. Other studies have also documented the relationship between sensitive responsiveness in the care of infants and secure attachments (Goldsmith and Alansky, 1987; Isabella, Belsky and von Eye, 1989). Ainsworth, Blehar, Waters and Wall (1978) found that mothers of insecure avoidant infants were more rejecting with less affection, bodily contact, and less emotional expression. Mothers of insecure ambivalent infants showed less responsiveness to the infant's signals, but were otherwise like the mothers of securely attached infants.

The development of mutual dialogue in mother–infant interaction as a process in which both partners learn to time their communications to fit in with their partner, and hence have synchrony within the interaction, has been studied by numerous researchers (e.g. Schaffer, 1977; Stern, 1977). This work fills in the details of how sensitive responsiveness, which is the core of good quality care for infants, is established.

Such a notion of 'sensitive' mothering has been criticized as showing a lack of concern for the experiences of mothers. Woollett and Phoenix (1991) suggest that such sensitivity to the infant may require sacrifices by the mother, in terms of, possibly, the mother's self-esteem, career and adult relationships. Greater support for stressed mothers such as increased sharing of the parental load, with fathers playing a much greater role, may offset this somewhat.

Thus it is seen that earlier studies of parenting and attachment indicate that the quality of infant attachment was influenced by the quality of parental care, and hence factors which facilitate sensitive mothering are likely to facilitate secure attachment. Parenting requires behaving to fulfil the needs of another, i.e. altruistic behaviour. This contrasts with most behaviour which is oriented to fulfilling the needs of the self. If basic needs of the parent are unsatisfied, i.e. there is some form of stress, then personal needs will tend to predominate and this is likely to inhibit altruistic behaviour and sensitive parenting. In such circumstances insecure attachments become more likely. Supporting this view, Isabella (1994) found that maternal satisfaction was associated with more sensitive interactive behaviours with the child and also secure attachment.

In later studies researchers reported difficulties in categorizing some children into the A, B and C classifications. In particular researchers working with children from abusing families and high risk samples, where the quality of care is likely to be deficient, found this a frequent problem (e.g. Egeland and Sroufe, 1981; Crittenden, 1988). Main and Solomon (1986, 1990) proposed an additional classification of attachment, the D category, which is characterized by insecure and disorganized/disorientated behaviour. Children from such D dyads show a lack of consistency in behaviour, a lack of obvious goals, contradictory behaviour patterns and signs of confusion, apprehension and indecision toward the parent. Main and Solomon (1990) make the following points about the D classification.

1. The classification applies to the relationship and not the child, and children may display different attachment behaviours to other caregivers.
2. The parents in D relationships are likely to have unresolved attachment traumas.
3. The majority of infants of abusing parents have been judged as D classification (Lyons-Ruth, Connell, Zoll, and Stahl, 1987; Carlson, Cicchetti, Barnet and Braunwald, 1989).
4. The majority of children classified as D at one year are classified as controlling at six years (Main and Cassidy, 1988).

Some researchers (e.g. Kagan, 1982) have attributed attachment differences to temperamental differences rather than differences in the infant–child relationship per se. However, Sroufe (1988) points out that as infants may have a secure attachment with one caregiver and an insecure attachment with another; that security of attachment may vary with life circumstances; and that attachment classification can also be predictive of aspects of maternal behaviour, any explanation in terms of temperament differences is inadequate. Research indicates (e.g. Belsky and Rovine, 1987; Volling and Belsky, 1992) that attachment behaviour may be mediated by temperamental differences but not reduced to temperament alone, and Vaughn, Egeland, Sroufe and Walters (1979) found that while temperament and attachment were associated, the degree of association was not strong.

Most research has been conducted in the USA. Does the strange situation have cross-cultural validity? Research in several countries indicates that overall it does, but that there need to be qualifications in the interpretations of results reflecting cross-cultural variations. First, the distribution of infants across the attachment classifications varies from the white, middle-class patterns in the United States of 70 per cent B, 20 per cent A and 10 per cent C type infants. In Germany (Grossman, Grossman, Spangler et al., 1985) there is a higher percentage of type A infants. While in Japan (Miyake, Chen and Campos, 1985) and in Israeli Kibbutzim (Sagi, Lamb, Lewkowicz et al., 1985) the percentage of type C infants is higher. Van IJzendoorn and Kroonenberg (1988) analysed data from 32 studies in eight different countries. They concluded that while considerable variation in distributions between cultures do emerge, that the secure classification (B) is modal for all cultures and that the method appears valid for all cultures currently studied. However, there are distinct difficulties in transferring the procedure to very different cultures. Grossman, Fremmer-Bombik and Grossman (1990) report on the difficulties in classifying a substantial proportion of Japanese infants and that there appeared to be a range of responses, e.g. particularly intense and persistent crying to separation, that did not conform to the descriptions of behaviour produced by research in western cultures.

Other assessment methods for infants/toddlers

Other methods have been used to assess aspects of infant attachment to a caregiver. Amongst the most well-known is the interview procedure of Schaffer and Emerson (1964). This interview focused on seven common separation situations. For each situation, the presence, consistency, intensity and direction of infant distress was covered. Maternal bias was minimized by enquiring only about overt, easily observable behaviour. From the interview, the age of onset, intensity and breadth of attachments was estimated.

Observational methods include a structured observation in the home setting described by Melhuish (1987). The procedure involves a set sequence of approach behaviours by a stranger, followed by a separation and reunion episode. Behaviour signifying emotional reactions were coded at each stage. This procedure differentiated between 18-month-old children with differing day care histories. Another observation procedure is an adaptation of Ainsworth's methods used by Aber and Baker (1990) with toddlers in a clinical setting to enable aspects of attachment behaviour to be measured. This approach is particularly designed for clinical use and takes account of the different meanings behaviour may have with 19–24 month olds.

Infant attachment and day care

Early interest in the possible developmental effects of day care was motivated by emphasis within attachment theory that the child needs a close emotional bond with a stable caregiver who is responsive and loving. The regular separations that occur when a child uses non-parental day care were thought to threaten the stability of the infant–mother attachment. This might lead to an increased likelihood of insecure attachment and possible longer term consequences on social development, self concept, and emotional development.

Caldwell, Wright, Honig and Tannenbaum (1970) followed a group of children from infancy. Some had received full-time day care since one year of age, and others were home reared. Mothers' reports revealed no differences in attachment behaviours. However, possibly direct measurement of attachment might reveal differences. A study by Blehar (1974) was the first to test this proposition using the strange situation procedure to measure attachment. Blehar found that a group of two to three year olds who had experienced day care showed higher levels of insecure attachment than a comparable group of home-reared children. It is dubious whether the strange situation should be used to measure attachment with infants older than two and, as this early finding was not replicated (e.g. Moskowitz, Schwarz and Corsini, 1977; Ragozin, 1980), reviews of the day care literature of that period concluded that there was no strong evidence that day care experiences might influence the quality of the infant–mother attachment (Belsky and Steinberg, 1978; Clarke-Stewart and Fein, 1983; Rutter, 1981). However, in the 1980s several studies appeared in which the reunion behaviour and attachment security of infants with and without day care in the first year of life were compared. These studies found evidence that extensive non-parental care in the first year of life was associated with increased avoidance and insecurity in the infant–mother attachment (Jacobsen and Wille, 1984; Owen and Cox, 1988; Schwarz, 1983; Vaughn, Gove and Egeland, 1980).

The evidence was still equivocal in that some studies failed to find an association between non-parental care in the first year and insecure attachment (Burchinal and Bryant, 1986; Chase-Lansdale and Owen 1987; Owen, Easterbrooks, Chase-Lansdale and Goldberg, 1984). However the increasing accumulation of evidence suggesting a link between extensive non-parental day care in the first year of life and infant–mother attachment led some reviewers to conclude that there was cause for concern (Gamble and Zigler, 1986; Belsky, 1986). The major proponent of this viewpoint was Belsky (1988a,b). This represented an about-turn from his previous position that there was no good evidence of such a relationship (Belsky and Steinberg, 1978; Belsky, Steinberg and Walker, 1982).

Belsky pointed out that the methodologies of the studies were varied and this diversity produced confusing results. He argued that if you took studies with a certain commonality of methodology (i.e. they only used the proper 'strange situation' procedure (Ainsworth, Blehar, Waters and Wall, 1978)) as the measure of attachment and only considered day care children having at least 20 hours of day care per week for a large part of the first year of life, then the evidence was very consistent. Belsky (1988a) presented a meta-analysis of four studies (Barglow, Vaughn and Molitar, 1987; Belsky and Rovine, 1988; Chase-Lansdale and Owen, 1987; Jacobsen and Wille, 1984) with a total sample of 491 children and which could allow for any social class effects. The conclusion reached was that insecure avoidant attachment patterns were over-represented within the day care group as compared with the home-reared group (41 per cent versus 26 per cent). This report was immediately extremely controversial at least partly because of its ideological/political overtones. There were several papers which attacked Belsky's interpretation of the evidence. Thompson (1988) argued that the distribution of insecure attachments within the samples Belsky was using as evidence was not sufficiently different from distributions seen in normative data (e.g. Ainsworth, Blehar, Waters and Wall, 1978) to justify a conclusion that early day care is associated with attachment insecurity.

Another critic was Clarke-Stewart (1988) who argued that the 'strange situation' did not have equivalent ecological validity for day care and home-reared groups in that the procedure and attachment classifications were primarily developed for children reared at home. The meaning and functional significance of a separation and reunion would be different for a child with extensive day care experience and greatly more experience of separations and reunions. Hence day care infants would be expected to behave differently. Clarke-Stewart further argued that possibly greater independence on the part of day care infants was being interpreted as avoidance. These criticisms were followed up by a meta-analysis (Clarke-Stewart, 1989) of the four studies used by Belsky (1988) along with data from 12 other investigations (several unpublished). The 1200 cases represented were separated into those with more and less than 20 hours per week exposure to day care for a substantial period of the first year. The analysis revealed that 36 per cent of infants with 20+ hours per week of non-parental care were classified as insecurely attached as compared with 29 per cent of infants with reduced or no day care experience. This 7 per cent difference was statistically significant with the large sample, but was less than the difference found in Belsky's meta-analysis, and Clarke-Stewart argued that this level of difference was not sufficiently profound to warrant Belsky's conclusions, and could be explained by day care children being more used to separations and hence less stressed in the strange situation so that attachment behaviours would be less likely to be shown.

Clarke-Stewart's argument that day care children would be less stressed by separation and hence be less likely to show attachment-orientated behaviour in the strange situation was tested by Belsky and Braungart (1991). They observed 20 infants classified as insecurely avoidant (11 day care and 9 home care infants) in the 'strange situation'. The day care infants were rated by observers, blind to day care history, as being more distressed on separation than home care infants. While this study has a small sample, and generalization must be cautious, the data appear to contradict Clarke-Stewart's proposition that day care infants would be less stressed by separation. However the study included only insecure-avoidant children, and to be a complete test of Clarke-Stewart's proposition would need to include all attachment classifications. This was done in the NICHD (1996) study which did find that the strange situation was equally valid for home care and day care infants, while not finding any overall increase in stress for day care infants.

Yet another meta-analysis of 13 studies of attachment in the 'strange situation' and day care was conducted by Lamb, Sternberg and Ketterlinus (1992). These investigators found 37 per cent insecurely attached infants in the day care group and 29 per cent insecurely attached infants in the home care group. These figures almost exactly replicate those found by Clarke-Stewart's (1989) meta-analysis, which is not surprising given the large overlap in the studies included in both meta-analyses. Lamb, Sternberg and Ketterlinus (1992) argued that the greater proximity-seeking of home-reared children is open to a variety of interpretations. They also drew attention to methodological limitations of the studies, including the absence of assessments of the quality of day care, the often unrepresentative nature of the samples, and the reliance upon the 'strange situation' as a measure of infant–mother attachment.

In Lamb, Sternberg and Ketterlinus (1992) analyses the rate of insecure attachment was greater for infants starting day care between 7 and 12 months, than for infants starting day care earlier than 7 months. This suggests the possibility of a sensitive period for separation and day care effects, which is also suggested by a naturalistic observational study of reunions with 129 infants by Varin, Crugnola, Ripamonti and Molina (1996), where more difficult reunions were associated with starting day care either in the period 7–12 months or 18–24 months. Infants starting day care at other ages showed easier reunions and were less easily frustrated.

The fact that three separate meta-analyses all indicate a small but significant increase in insecure-avoidant attachment where children have substantial non-parental care in the first year does imply that there is a phenomenon to be explained. However, in all cases the size of the effect appears to be small, indicating that such an increase in risk is only a small part of the range of factors influencing attachment. Also these meta-analyses may be affected by the 'file drawer problem' as suggested by Roggman, Langlois, Hubbs-Tait and Rieser-Danner (1994). This refers to the likelihood that studies with non-significant results tend to be put in the file drawer rather than published. This, of course, is a problem of all research. Another limitation of these approaches to attachment is their reliance on one dominant measure, the strange situation, which is a limited sampling of the range of attachment behaviours.

When the samples in the studies showing slightly increased risk for insecure attachment are considered, it often appears that they are samples likely to be experiencing a high level of poor quality non-parental care. Studies where the day care is known to be of at least moderate quality (e.g. Pierrehumbert, Ramstein, Karmaniola and Halfon, 1996) fail to find a difference in attachment associated with non-parental care in the first year. Studies using measures of socio-emotional development other than the 'strange situation' find that quality of non-parental care may be influential (Melhuish, 1987; Howes, 1990). Using an observational measure of attachment behaviours in the home, Melhuish (1987) found that separation anxiety differed markedly for children who had experienced different types of child care. From the same study, Melhuish, Mooney, Martin and Lloyd (1990a) reported that these types of childcare varied markedly in terms of the quality of adult–child interactions occurring.

Taken together these reports indicate that attachment behaviour may well be mediated by the quality of interactions in the child's care environment. A study of infant day care in Greece also found evidence that variations in infant attachment behaviours were related to quality of day care environments (Petrogiannis, 1995). Hence the discrepancies reported in the literature with regard to the possible effects of day care on attachment are likely to reflect differences in the quality of day care. Taking this pattern of findings together it is possible that poor quality non-parental care may be a risk factor for attachment. This is the same principle that underlies Ainsworth, Blehar, Waters and Wall's (1978) finding with regard to the quality of home care, where insensitive mothering is associated with insecure attachment, and sensitive responsive care is associated with secure attachment.

A child from a home with poor quality care who experiences poor quality non-parental care is never in an environment which consistently provides sensitive responsive interaction. Such a situation would occur, for example, if the parents are stressed by the dual roles of worker and parent and the stress inhibits the altruistic attitude essential to good parenting. Such a child would be expected to be at particular risk for insecure attachment. Possibly the small risk effects revealed in the meta-analyses by Belsky (1988), Clarke-Stewart (1989) and Lamb, Sternberg and Ketterlinus (1992) may be due to children who experience this double dose of poor quality care. The influence of one aspect of stress – work-family interference – which is common amongst employed parents, on measures of attachment and behaviour problems has been documented by McCartney, Scarr, Rochelieu et al. (1997). These effects persisted after allowing for family and child care background factors.

The interpretation given here of increased risk for insecure attachment if there is poor quality care at home and in day care is supported by a recent study. The NICHD (1997) ten-site study of early childcare was able to assess attachment with the strange situation with 1200 infants at 15 months of age. This study found that non-parental care by itself was not related to attachment security. However, dual risks were associated with an increase in insecure attachment. If the mother was relatively insensitive and either the quality of day care was poor, or there was a lot of non-parental care, or there was unstable non-parental care; then there was more insecure attachment. Another dual risk was if the child was a boy and there was a high level of non-parental care, which was also associated with increased insecure attachment. Where dual risks existed, e.g. insensitive mothering and insensitive day care, then the degree of insecure attachment was 49–56 per cent; whereas if there was insensitive care in only one of the settings, home or day care, the degree of insecure attachment was 38 per cent. This study's results are very much consistent with the proposition that what matters is the overall quality of care, regardless of whether that care is at home or out of home.

Other studies also support the general proposition that the effects of non-parental care experience will be mediated by parental care experience. Benn (1986) found that where employed mothers provided sensitive responsive care, their infants were securely attached; by contrast, employed mothers showing less sensitive care had infants showing insecure attachments. Another example is a study of four year olds by Howes (1990) where early entry into day care was associated with less social competence only if children had previously established an insecure attachment to the mother.

Infants in day care form attachments to their caregivers. Such attachments are not determined by attachments with parents and security of attachment appears to be a function of sensitive care by caregivers (Goossens and van IJzendoorn, 1990; Howes and Hamilton, 1992a,b). The security of infant–caregiver attachment may also be increased by training (Galinsky, Howes and Kontos, 1995), presumably because caregivers become more sensitive to infant needs with training. Cummings (1980) and Barnas and Cummings (1994) found that toddlers showed stronger attachment behaviours to stable or regular caregivers rather than less familiar caregivers. The importance of stability of care is also supported by Howes and Hamilton (1993) who found that changes of caregiver were associated with increased aggression. With secure caregivers there is more advanced play (Howes, Matheson and Hamilton, 1994) and better peer relationships (Howes and Hamilton, 1993). It is likely that the effect of stability of care and sensitivity of care are linked. Infants communicate idiosyncratically, and caregivers unfamiliar with the child will not interpret communications appropriately and not respond appropriately. Stable caregivers come to understand a child's idiosyncratic communications and can respond sensitively and appropriately so fostering secure attachment.

The consequences of infant attachment for later development

The pioneering research by Ainsworth and colleagues has spawned a whole field of research. Ainsworth's method of assessment of attachment has become the standard for infants in the age range one to two years. If infant attachment had no longer term developmental consequences then interest in this aspect of development would not be very great. However several studies, notably by Sroufe and colleagues (Sroufe, 1983; Sroufe, Fox and Pancake, 1983; Sroufe, Egeland and Kreutzer, 1990; Suess, Grossmann and Sroufe, 1992; Elicker and Sroufe, 1992) have documented its predictive validity with regard to later socio-emotional development. Children who show insecure patterns of attachment in infancy have been found to have more problematic social and emotional development later in childhood, e.g. showing higher levels of behaviour problems, finding it harder to make friends.

The major criticism of attachment research revolves around the issue of whether infant attachment really does predict later development. Lamb, Thompson, Gardner et al. (1984) point out that while there are associations between prior caregiving experience, behaviour in the strange situation, and later socio-emotional development, such associations may well be attributable to stable aspects of infant and parental characteristics across development. For example, attachment at time 1 may be related to parenting at time 1; attachment at time 2 may be related to parenting at time 2. As parenting characteristics tend to be stable, attachment at times 1 and 2 may be linked because of their association with contemporaneous parenting. Hence reliable associations over time may reflect stability in these factors rather than the developmental consequences of early experience. Probably both types of factors are contributing to the predictability of developmental pathways.

The stability of attachment classification using the strange situation is an important consideration in that instability would suggest that the procedure is assessing transient characteristics likely to be of little consequence. Most studies of stability have focused on the 12–18 month age range and a number have found reasonably high levels of stability of 73 per cent to 85 per cent (e.g. Waters, 1978). However, lower stability has been found in some studies. Vaughn, Egeland, Sroufe and Waters (1979) and Egeland and Farber (1984) report stability of around 60 per cent over 12–18 months for disadvantaged families. Thompson, Lamb and Estes (1982) found stability of only 53 per cent between 12.5 and 19.5 months. There are indications in these studies that instability of attachment is associated with changes later in the care environments of children. The most striking evidence of stability comes from Main and Cassidy (1988) who found 84 per cent stability between one and six years. The high stability may well be a function of selection procedures which excluded birth complications, major life change, and separations from parents. Hence the study is dealing with a relatively homogenous sample with a reduced likelihood of disruptions to attachment patterns. It would appear that generally there is high stability in attachment if there is a stable environment with little major change.

The issue of predictive validity involves associations between infant attachment and later development. When the research on later development is considered, there are a number of differences which emerge between the developmental patterns of securely and insecurely attached infants. On average securely attached infants will later have higher sociability, self-esteem, obedience, empathy and attention span in play and problem solving. Insecurely attached infants, on average, will later show higher incidences of dependency, poor peer relationships, tantrums, aggression and behaviour problems (e.g. Sroufe, 1988). Overall the socio-emotional development of securely attached infants follows the more valued developmental trajectory. However, before jumping to conclusions about simple cause and effect relationships, there are some important aspects to be considered. The parent–child relationship and interactional style result from a particular set of family circumstances. It is probable that the family circumstances which give rise to a particular attachment in infancy will persist in later life. Hence the later characteristics of socio-emotional development may reflect the current effects of these family circumstances rather than the preceding infant attachment pattern. When developmental continuity is observed from infancy to later childhoood, there is also continuity in environmental circumstances.

The implication is that to change a developmental trajectory, the environment needs to be changed. This is not straightforward when dealing with relationships as an individual's attachment style, their way of relating to others, is based upon their own relationship history, which provides the 'working model' for current relationships. It is the power of past experience in determining current 'working models' and how that determines current interaction and attachments which can explain how a parent may transmit a relationship style to their own children and so produce inter-generational transmission of personality characteristics through environmental rather than genetic means. If the child who develops an insecure attachment in infancy is not to perpetuate such patterns, then the 'working model' of relationships must be altered. This may come about through the power of later love relationships in providing alternative 'working models' of how to relate to others. Such relationships may well alter trajectories of socio-emotional development. Such ideas are the focus of ongoing research.

Childcare, attachment and later development

The relationship between infant attachment and later socio-emotional development has led to expectations that, if infant attachment and day care are related, then later socio-emotional development will be affected. Evidence of longer term effects of day care experience on socio-emotional development studies indicate that children attending group day care interact more with their peers, both positively and negatively, and has usually led to conclusions that day care does not hinder socio-emotional development (e.g. Belsky, Steinberg and Walker, 1982; Clarke-Stewart, 1993) and may even promote some aspects of socio-emotional development (e.g. Hennessy and Melhuish, 1991; Clarke-Stewart, 1993). The research evidence contains examples of findings indicating negative, neutral and positive effects on aspects of social, emotional and behavioural development.

On the positive side group day care has often been associated with improved social competence with peers (Melhuish, 1991; McCartney, Scarr, Phillips et al., 1982; Field, Masi, Goldstein et al., 1988; Balleyguier and Melhuish, 1996) and also easier social interaction with adults (Cochran, 1977; McCartney, Scarr, Phillips et al., 1982; Clarke-Stewart, Gruber and Fitzgerald, 1994).

On the negative side, Moore (1975) found that children with preschool day care experience later appeared to be more aggressive and non-conformist and similar results were reported by Robertson (1982). Children with infant day care experiences have been found to be less compliant with adult requests and more aggressive with peers (Schwarz, Strickland and Krolick, 1974; Rubenstein, Howes and Boyle, 1981; Haskins, 1985; Field, Masi, Goldstein et al., 1988; Thornburg, Pearl, Crompton and Ispa, 1990). This aspect of children's social behaviour is sometimes represented negatively as greater aggression, uncooperativeness and non-compliance and sometimes, in a positive light, as increased assertiveness and independence.

To some extent the discrepancies between studies may reflect differences in ages of children studied. In Britain a longitudinal study found evidence of day care effects on socio-emotional development up to age three, but by age six all day care effects had disappeared, reflecting the increased equivalence in social experience of children in the study from three years onwards (Melhuish, Hennessy, Martin and Moss, 1990; Hennessy, Martin, Moss and Melhuish, 1992). Such age effects are likely to be closely tied to patterns of preschool and school provision and hence may differ for different countries or sections of society.

With regard to Haskins' finding of increased aggression in day care children in the Abecedarian project, when daily activities were altered to facilitate social skills and reduce aggression then the increased aggression was eliminated (Finkelstein, 1982). However most day care programmes do not have such characteristics. Recently Bates, Marvinney, Kelly, Dodge et al. (1994) in a study of 589 five-year-old children in two American states with poorly regulated child care, found that greater amounts of day care in the early years were associated with higher aggression, and lower social adjustment. These results held after controlling for family, child and background factors.

Two studies using a national US sample of four to six year olds (NLSY data set) reported similar findings for non-compliance (Belsky and Eggebeen, 1991) and behaviour problems (Baydar and Brooks-Gunn, 1991). Bearing in mind the often low quality of much American day care the results should be interpreted as applying to children who experience predominantly low quality day care. These results parallel earlier findings in a study in Texas. Vandell and Powers (1983) found that three to four year old children from high quality centres (good adult–child ratio, well-equipped, good staff training) showed more positive interactions with teachers than children from poorer quality centres (poor ratio, training and large groups). Four years later the children from lower quality centres seemed less socially competent (Vandell and Corasaniti, 1990). These last four American studies all attempted to differentiate early from later day care and controlled for background factors. They all found evidence of the effects of amount of day care and some evidence that day care in the first year might be more influential.

While American studies have often reported negative effects of day care, studies from countries where state support and regulations facilitate good quality day care have generally found rather different results. A longitudinal study in Sweden has found no evidence of day care effects (Cochran, 1977; Cochran and Gunnarson, 1985). Similarly another Swedish longitudinal study of children who experienced various types of early child care found no evidence of day care effects up to age three-and-a-half years (Hwang, Broberg and Lamb, 1991; Lamb, Hwang, Broberg et al., 1988; Sternberg, Lamb, Hwang et al., 1991). However at seven to nine years, while there was no overall home/day care difference, there was an indication that children who had been in individual day care were not as socially competent as children who had been in group day care (Wessels, Lamb and Hwang, 1996). In the same study there was also evidence that social competence and maturity of personality at seven years were partly predicted by quality of home care and quality of day care (Broberg, Hwang, Lamb and Ketterlinus, 1989; Lamb, Hwang, Broberg et al., 1988; Wessels, Lamb and Hwang, 1996). A study by Andersson (1986, 1989) of children from birth to 13 years of age reveals a positive effect on academic and social competence of early day care experience. Hence overall the Swedish studies reveal either neutral or positive effects of day care experience, with the possibility of some differences for different types of day care.

Norway has developed a system of child care provision with many similarities to Sweden, but has been slower in making provision generally available. A longitudinal study in Norway (Borge and Melhuish, 1995) found evidence of both positive and negative effects of day care experience. Firstly, good quality group day care from age four upwards was associated with less behaviour problems reported by parents. However, early day care in the first four years was associated with increased behaviour problems reported by teachers when the children were 10 years old. The day care in the first four years was informal, unregulated and of unknown quality. Hence the differential effects may reflect the differential quality of care available at different ages.

The importance of quality of care is indicated by a study of non-compliance and group day care by Howes and Olenick (1986). Non-compliance at 18, 24 and 36 months was studied at home, in day care, and in a structured observation. Non-compliance was not very consistent across situations indicating that this behaviour is likely to be strongly determined by the situation rather than the child. However in the structured observation, the best predictor of non-compliance was quality of care, with children from high quality centres showing more compliance and cooperativeness than children from low quality centres. Quality of care may be positively correlated with other aspects of social competence as reported by Howes (1990) in the USA and by Beller, Stahnke, Butz et al. (1996) in Germany. A change in Florida child care regulations enabled a study by Howes, Smith and Galinsky (1995) to find that improvements in care quality were associated with improvements in peer interactions. McCartney, Scarr, Rocheleau et al. (1997) used a measure of caregiver–child interaction derived from the overall quality ratings, and found that better caregiver–child interaction was associated with more social initiations by toddlers in childcare centres. Similarly, a multisite study in four American states found that quality of care was associated with better social competence after controlling for family background (Cost, Quality and Child Outcomes in Child Care Centers, 1995) and Phillips, Mekos, Scarr et al. (unpublished) found that centres with higher quality care had children who showed less aimless wandering, a higher level of peer play, and had higher perceptions of self-competence.

The importance of child–caregiver relationships as an aspect of quality of care is revealed in a longitudinal study reported by Howes, Hamilton and Matheson (1994). Children who showed secure attachments to caregivers were more competent in their social play, more sociable and less aggressive. Children without secure attachments to caregivers showed more social withdrawal and aggression. Volling and Feagans (1995) reported that socially withdrawn infants developed better peer relations in high quality day care centres yet their peer relations deteriorated if placed in centres with low quality care. In the Infant Health and Development Program intervention study with pre-term low birthweight infants, high quality day care, as part of the intervention was associated with a reduced incidence of behaviour problems for two to three year olds (Brooks-Gunn, Klebanov, Liaw and Spiker, 1993).

The quality of day care centres depends in part upon the characteristics of children who attend. The practice of segregating 'at risk' children into social service nurseries results in a clustering of children prone to behaviour problems. In such centres McGuire and Richman (1989) have reported high levels of aggressive behaviour and behaviour problems. It is likely that in such circumstances children are learning problematic behaviour patterns through peer interaction and observational learning, leading to an increase overall in such behaviours. Additionally, in such nurseries, McGuire (1991) found that socially withdrawn children did not benefit from the opportunities for social interaction. Vollings and Feagans (1995) found similar effects for socially withdrawn children in poor quality centres. They may well feel vulnerable and insecure in an environment where children show aggressive and disruptive behaviour. Peer interaction itself is an important component of quality of care.

A practical question often asked is does the type of childcare affect the quality of care or infant attachment or development. Infants may be cared for in a wide variety of contexts, with a relative (e.g. grandmother), childminder (family day care), day nursery (centre day care) or a mixture of these and other types of care. The results of research generally indicates that it is the quality of care rather than the type of care which is important. It is possible to find wide variations in the quality of care within all types. Melhuish, Mooney, Martin and Lloyd (1990) with 18 month olds and Melhuish, Martin and Mooney (1991) with three year olds found that relatives generally provided high quality care, and that there were instances of high and low quality care amongst childminders and day nurseries in their London-based study. The results of this study indicate that developmental effects were associated with quality rather than types of care. Generally the needs of infants are such that high quality care is more difficult and expensive to provide in the first year of life and becomes easier to provide as children grow older. Scandinavian countries acknowledge this in their parental leave policies which result in very few infants under 18 months of age being in nonparental care (Borge, Hartmann and Strom, 1996). The high level of provision of childcare in these countries is of such a high quality partly because the expense of childcare for young infants is largely avoided. One critical aspect of the quality of childcare is the stability of caregivers (Melhuish, 1994). Children will show different patterns of social interaction with stable than with less stable caregivers (Howes and Hamilton, 1992b). These differences were associated with some aspects of social development, such as dependency, social withdrawal and aggression with four year olds (Howes, Hamilton and Matheson, 1994). Instability of care has been found to be associated with effects on language development also (Melhuish, Lloyd, Martin and Mooney, 1990; Hennessey, Martin, Moss and Melhuish, 1992). Young children learning to communicate often use idiosyncratic speech and gestures. A regular, familiar caregiver learns such idiosyncrasies and can respond appropriately and sensitively, while an unfamiliar caregiver does not interpret the communication and does not respond appropriately. Hence stability of care is almost a prerequisite of sensitive responsiveness which is a central aspect of the quality of care and is associated with both attachment differences (Ainsworth, Blehar, Waters and Wall, 1978) and language development (Clarke-Stewart 1973; Melhuish, Hennessy, Martin and Moss, 1991). As with adult–child interaction, familiarity aids peer interaction. Good friends will show more prosocial behaviour and more sophisticated play (Young and Lewis, 1979). Hence stable peer groups in childcare will also foster the children's development and is another aspect of the quality of care.

However the quality of care either at home or out of home has to be considered in the context of the total ecology of the child. Egeland and Hiester (1995) have found with children from poor families that attachment in infancy was predictive of social adjustment for home-reared infants but not for children who received day care from infancy. Such a finding suggests that day care may be influential on development by altering the significance of other aspects of the child's ecology. As with the NICHD study cited earlier the effects of any pattern of experience in one niche of the child's environment is likely to be affected by what is happening in other niches of the child's ecology. In such circumstances interaction effects are likely to be most important in understanding developmental influence as Bronfenbrenner (1979) has pointed out.

Summary

The development of attachment is linked to the child's experience of relationships. Sensitive responsive interaction fosters the development of secure attachments. This association between interactive experience and type of attachment holds in both home and out-of-home environments. The environments conducive to particular types of attachment are likely to be consistent across time, and this will tend to lead to continuity of attachment. However, within attachment theory, the child's internal working model of attachment will tend to replicate itself in the child's newly developing attachments, which will again give rise to continuity. Therefore the child's socioemotional development can be set on a particular trajectory by the quality of the child's early interactive experience, or quality of care. Where the quality of care is consistently insensitive or unresponsive then insecure attachments are likely. However should the quality of care change, this offers the opportunity for a change in type of attachment. New attachments can themselves act as internal working models for subsequent attachments, setting the child on a different trajectory of socio-emotional development. Hence across development quality of care and attachment style are likely to be intimately linked.

Applications

1. Be sensitive to parenting variations. Parenting differs greatly across individuals, social class, ethnic groups and countries. Even within individuals, parenting practices may vary from time to time depending on factors such as stress, other commitments and the marital relationship. Attachment theory suggests that such variations matter.

2. Be aware of attachment differences in infants, children and adults. People's styles of relating to others differ. We could call such variations attachment differences. In infancy we have a way of categorizing these differences. Such differences show a tendency to be stable and to relate to other areas of development.

3. Be careful in considering the variety of childcare. Parenting differences are one aspect of childcare variations. However, who is caring for the child can vary as in the case of parental versus non-parental care; fathers rather than mothers taking a major role; and in the care offered by any one individual from day to day. Also the relative stability of care is a crucial component of quality. The evidence reviewed here suggests it is the quality of childcare rather than the who or where of childcare which is important.

4. Consider the total environment. Childcare and attachment relate to the total environment of the child and it is the relative stability of the quality of care from all sources which makes up the childcare experience of the child and may well influence attachment and development.

Further reading

Clarke-Stewart, K. A. (1993). *Day Care* (2nd edition). London: Fontana.
Eyer, D. E. (1993). *Mother–Infant Bonding: A Science Fiction.* New Haven, Conn: Yale University Press.
Hennessy, E., Martin, S., Moss, P. and Melhuish, E. C. (1992). *Childcare and Development: Lessons from Research.* London: Paul Chapman.
Melhuish, E. C. and Mass, P. (1991). *Day Care for Young Children: International Perspectives.* London: Routledge.

References

Aber, J. L. and Baker, A. J. L. (1990). Security of attachment in toddlerhood: modifying assessment procedures for joint clinical and research purposes. In *Attachment in the Preschool Years* (M. T. Greenberg, D. Cicchetti and E. M. Cummings, eds). Chicago: University of Chicago Press.
Ainsworth, M., Blehar, M. C., Waters, E. and Wall, S. (1978). *Patterns of Attachment.* Hillsdale, NJ: Lawrence Erlbaum.
Ainsworth, M. and Wittig, B. A. (1969). Attachment and exploratory behavior of 1-year-olds in a strange situation. In *Determinants of Infant Behaviour*, Vol. 4 (B. M. Foss, ed.). London: Methuen.
Andersson, B. E. (1986). *Home Care or External Care.* Report No. 2. Stockholm: Institute of Education.
Andersson, B. E. (1989). Effects of public day care: a longitudinal study. *Child Development*, **60**, 857–66.
Aronson, E. and Rosenbloom, S. (1971). Space perception in early infancy: perception within a common auditory-visual space. *Science*, **172**, 1161–3.
Balleyguier, G. and Melhuish, E. C. (1996). The relationship between infant day care and socio-emotional development with French children aged 3–4 years. *European Journal of Psychology of Education*, **11**, 193–200.
Barglow, P., Vaughn, B. E. and Molitar, N. (1987). Effects of maternal absence due to employment on the quality of infant–mother attachment in a low-risk sample. *Child Development*, **58**, 945–54.
Barnas, M. V. and Cummings, E. M. (1994). Caregiver stability and toddlers' attachment-related behavior towards caregivers in day care. *Infant Behavior and Development*, **17**, 141–7.
Bates, J. E., Marvinney, D., Kelly, T., Dodge, K. A., Bennett, D. S. and Pettit, G. S. (1994). Child-care history and kindergarten adjustment. *Developmental Psychology*, **30**, 690–700.
Baydar, N. and Brooks-Gunn, J. (1991). Effects of maternal employment and child care arrangements on preschoolers' cognitive and behavioral outcomes: evidence from the children of the National Longitudinal Study of Youth. *Developmental Psychology*, **27**, 932–45.
Beller, E. K., Stahnke, M., Butz, P., Stahl, W. and Wessels, H. (1996). Two measures of the quality of group care for infants and toddlers. *European Journal of Psychology of Education*, **11**, 151–68.
Belsky, J. (1986). Infant day care: a cause for concern? *Zero to Three*, **6**, 1–9.
Belsky, J. (1988a). The 'effects' of infant day care reconsidered. *Early Childhood Research Quarterly*, **3**, 235–72.
Belsky, J. (1988b). Infant day care and socioemotional development: the United States. *Journal of Child Psychology and Psychiatry*, **29**, 397–406.
Belsky, J. and Braungart, J. M. (1991). Are insecure-avoidant infants with extensive day-care experience less stressed by and more independent in the Strange Situation? *Child Development*, **62**, 567–71.
Belsky, J. and Eggebeen, D. (1991). Early and extensive maternal employment and young children's socioemotional development: children of the National Longitudinal Study of Youth. *Journal of Marriage and the Family*, **53**, 1083–98.

Belsky, J. and Rovine, M. N. (1987). Temperament and attachment security in the Strange Situation: an empirical rapprochment. *Child Development*, **58**, 787–95.

Belsky, J. and Rovine, M. N. (1988). Non-maternal care in the first year of life and the security of infant–parent attachment. *Child Development*, **59**, 157–67.

Belsky, J. and Steinberg, L. D. (1978). The effects of day care: a critical review. *Child Development*, **49**, 929–49.

Belsky, J., Steinberg, L. D. and Walker, A. (1982). The ecology of day care. In *Nontraditional Families: Parenting and Child Development* (M. E. Lamb, ed.). Hillsdale, NJ: Lawrence Erlbaum.

Benn, R. K. (1986). Factors promoting secure attachment relationships between employed mothers and their sons. *Child Development*, **57**, 1224–31.

Blehar, M. C. (1974). Anxious attachment and defensive reactions associated with day care. *Child Development*, **45**, 683–92.

Borge, A. I. H. and Melhuish, E. C. (1995). A longitudinal study of childhood behaviour problems, maternal employment and day care in a rural Norwegian community. *International Journal of Behavioral Development*, **18**, 23–42.

Borge, A. I. H., Hartmann, E. and Strom, S. (1996). The Norwegian perspective on issues of quality in day care. *European Journal of Psychology of Education*, **11**, 129–38.

Bowlby, J. (1958). The nature of the child's tie to his mother. *International Journal of Psycho-Analysis*, **39**.

Bowlby, J. (1969). *Attachment*, Vol. 1 of *Attachment and Loss*. London: Hogarth.

Bowlby, J. (1973). *Separation*, Vol. 2 of *Attachment and Loss*. London: Hogarth.

Bowlby, J. (1980). *Loss: Sadness and Depression*, Vol. 3 of *Attachment and Loss*. London: Hogarth.

Bowlby, J., Ainsworth, M. D. S., Boston, M. and Rosenbluth, D. (1956). The effects of mother-child separation: A follow-up study. *British Journal of Medical Psychology*, **29**, 211–47.

Broberg, A., Hwang, C. P., Lamb, M. E. and Ketterlinus, R. D. (1989). Child care effects on socioemotional and intellectual competence in Swedish preschoolers. In *Caring for Children: Challenge to America* (J. S. Lande, S. Scarr and N. Gunzenhauser, eds). Hillsdale, NJ: Lawrence Erlbaum.

Bronfenbrenner, U. (1979). *The Ecology of Human Development*. Cambridge, MA: Harvard University Press.

Brooks-Gunn, J., Klebanov, P. K., Liaw, F. and Spiker, D. (1993). Enhancing the development of low-birthweight, premature infants: changes in cognition and behavior over the first three years. *Child Development*, **64**, 736–53.

Burchinal, M. and Bryant, D. M. (1986). *Does Day Care Affect Infant–Mother Attachment Level?* Paper presented at the Annual Meeting of the American Psychological Association, Washington DC.

Caldwell, B. M., Wright, C. M., Honig, A. S. and Tannenbaum, J. (1970). Infant day care and attachment. *American Journal of Orthopsychiatry*, **40**, 397–412.

Carlson, V., Cicchetti, D., Barnett, D. and Braunwald, K. (1989). Finding order in disorganization: lessons from research on maltreated infants' attachments to their caregivers. In *Child Maltreatment: Theory and Research on the Causes and Consequences of Child Abuse and Neglect* (D. Cicchetti and V. Carlson, eds). New York: Cambridge University Press.

Chase-Lansdale, L. and Owen, M. T. (1987). Maternal employment in a family context: effects on infant–mother and infant–father attachments. *Child Development*, **58**, 1505–12.

Clarke-Stewart, K. A. (1973). Interactions between mothers and their young children: characteristics and consequences. *Monographs of the Society for Research in Child Development* (Serial No. 153), **38**.

Clarke-Stewart, K. A. (1993). *Day Care* (2nd edition). London: Fontana.

Clarke-Stewart, K. A. (1988). The 'effects' of infant day care reconsidered: risks for parents, children, and researchers. *Early Childhood Research Quarterly*, **3**, 293–318.

Clarke-Stewart, K. A. (1989). Infant day care: maligned or malignant? *American Psychologist*, **44**, 266–73.

Clarke-Stewart, K. A. and Fein, G. G. (1983). Early childhood programs. In *Handbook of Child Psychology*, Vol. 2: *Infancy and Developmental Psychobiology* (P. H. Mussen, series ed.; M. Haith and J. Campos, volume eds). New York: John Wiley.

Clarke-Stewart, K. A., Gruber, C. P. and Fitzgerald, L. M. (1994). *Children at Home and in Day Care*. Hillsdale, NJ: Lawrence Erlbaum.

Cochran, M. M. (1977). A comparison of group day care and family-based child rearing patterns in Sweden. *Child Development*, **50**, 601–16.

Cochran, M. M. and Gunnarson, L. (1985). A follow-up study of group day care and family-based childrearing patterns. *Journal of Marriage and the Family*, **47**, 297–309.

Cost, Quality and Child Outcomes in Child Care Centers (1995). Economics Department, University of Colorado at Denver, CO.

Crittenden, P. M. (1988). Relationships at risk. In *Clinical Implications of Attachment* (J. Belsky and T. Nezworksi, eds). Hillsdale, NJ: Lawrence Erlbaum.

Cummings, M. E. (1980). Caregiver stability and day care. *Developmental Psychology*, **16**, 31–7.

DeCasper, A. J. and Fifer, W. P. (1980). Of human bonding: newborns prefer their mothers' voices. *Science*, **208**, 1174–6.

Egeland, B. and Farber, E. (1984). Infant–mother attachment: factors related to its development and changes over time. *Child Development*, **55**, 753–71.

Egeland, B. and Hiester, M. (1995). The long-term consequences of infant daycare and mother–infant attachment. *Child Development*, **66**, 474–85.

Egeland, B. and Sroufe, L. A. (1981). Attachment and maltreatment. *Child Development*, **55**, 753–71.

Eimas, P. D., Siqueland, E., Jusczyk, P. and Vigorito, J. (1971). Speech perception in early infancy. *Science*, **171**, 303–6.

Elicker, J. and Sroufe, L. A. (1992). Predicting peer competence and peer relationships in childhood from early parent–child relationships. In *Family-peer Relationships: Modes of Linkage* (R. Parke and G. W. Ladd, eds). Hillsdale, NJ: Lawrence Erlbaum.

Eyer, D. E. (1993). *Mother–Infant Bonding: A Science Fiction*. New Haven, Conn: Yale University Press.

Fantz, R. L. (1961). The origins of form perception. *Scientific American*, **204**, 66–72.

Field, T., Masi, W., Goldstein, S., Perry, S. and Pearl, S. (1988). Infant day care facilitates preschool social behaviour. *Early Childhood Research Quarterly*, **3**, 341–59.

Finkelstein, N. W. (1982). Aggression: Is it stimulated by day care? *Young Children*, **37**, 3–9.

Freud, S. (1926). *Inhibitions, Symptoms and Anxiety*. The Complete Psychological Works of Sigmund Freud, Vol. 20. London: Hogarth.

Galinsky, E., Howes, C. and Kontos, S. (1995). *The Family Child Care Training Study*. New York: Families and Work Institute.

Gamble, T. J. and Zigler, E. (1986). Effects of infant day care: another look at the evidence. *American Journal of Orthopsychiatry*, **56**, 26–42.

Goldsmith, H. H. and Alansky, J. (1987). Maternal and infant temperamental predictors of attachment: a meta-analytic review. *Journal of Consulting and Clinical Psychology*, **55**, 805–16.

Goossens, F. A. and van IJzendoorn, M. H. (1990). Quality of infants' attachments to professional caregivers: relation to infant–parent attachment and day-care characteristics. *Child Development*, **61**, 832–7.

Grossmann, K., Grossmann, K. E., Spangler, G., Suess, G. and Unzer, L. (1985). In *Growing Points in Attachment Theory and Research* (I. Bretherton and E. Waters, eds). *Monographs of the Society for Research in Child Development*. Serial No. 209, Vol. 50, 3–35.

Grossmann, K., Fremmer-Bombik, E. and Grossmann, K. E. (1990). *Familiar and Unfamiliar Patterns of Attachment of Japanese Infants*. Research and Clinical Center for Child Development, Faculty of Education, Hokkaido University, Sapporo, Japan. Annual Report; Occasional Paper No. 2.

Harlow, H. (1958). The nature of love. *American Psychologist*, **13**, 673–85.

Haskins, R. (1985). Public school aggression among children with varying day-care experience. *Child Development*, **56**, 689–703.

Hennessy, E. and Melhuish, E. C. (1991). Early day care and the development of school-aged children: a review. *Journal of Reproductive and Infant Psychology*, **9**, 117–36.

Hennessy, E., Martin, S., Moss, P. and Melhuish, E. C. (1992). *Child Care and Development: Lessons from Research*. London: Paul Chapman.

Howes, C. (1990). Can the age of entry and the quality of infant child care predict behaviours in kindergarten? *Developmental Psychology*, **26**, 292–303.

Howes, C. and Hamilton, C. (1992a). Children's relationships with caregivers: Mothers and child care teachers. *Child Development*, **63**, 859–66.

Howes, C. and Hamilton, C. (1992b). Children's relationships with child care teachers: Stability and concordance with parental attachments. *Child Development*, **63**, 867–78.

Howes, C. and Hamilton, C. (1993). The changing experience of child care: changes in teachers and in teacher–child relationships and children's social competence with peers. *Child Development*, **63**, 867–78.

Howes, C., Hamilton, C. E. and Matheson, C. C. (1994). Children's relationships with peers: differential associations with aspects of the teacher–child relationship. *Child Development*, **65**, 253–63.

Howes, C., Matheson, C. C. and Hamilton, C. E. (1994). Maternal, teacher and child care history correlates of children's relationships with peers. *Child Development*, **65**, 264–73.

Howes, C. and Olenick, M. (1986). Family and child care influences on toddlers' compliance. *Child Development*, **57**, 202–16.

Howes, C., Smith, E. and Galinsky, E. (1995). *The Florida Child Care Improvement Study*. New York: Family and Work Institute.

Hwang, P. C., Broberg, A. and Lamb, M. E. (1991). Swedish childcare research. In *Day Care for Young Children* (E. C. Melhuish and P. Moss, eds). London: Routledge.

Isabella, R. A. (1994). Origins of maternal role satisfaction and its influences on maternal interactive behaviors and infant–mother attachment. *Infant Behavior and Development*, **17**, 381–8.

Isabella, R. A., Belsky, J. and von Eye, A. (1989). Origins of infant–mother attachment: an examination of interactional synchrony during the infant's first year. *Developmental Psychology*, **25**, 12–21.

Jacobsen, J. L. and Wille, D. E. (1984). Influence of attachment and separation experience on separation distress at 18 months. *Developmental Psychology*, **20**, 477–84.

Kagan, J. (1982). *Psychological Research on the Human Infant: An Evaluative Summary*. New York: W.T. Grant Foundation.

Klaus, M. H. and Kennel, J. H. (1976). *Mother–Infant Bonding*. St Louis, MO: Mosby.

Lamb, M. E., Hwang, C. P., Broberg, A. G. and Bookstein, F. L. et al. (1988). The determinants of parental involvement in primiparous Swedish families. *International Journal of Behavioural Development*, **11**, 351–79.

Lamb, M. E., Sternberg, K. J. and Ketterlinus, R. (1992). Child care in the United States. In *Child Care in Context* (M. E. Lamb, K. Sternberg, C. P. Hwang and A. G. Broberg, eds). Hillsdale, NJ: Lawrence Erlbaum.

Lamb, M. E., Thompson, R. A., Gardner, W. P., Charnov, E. L. and Estes, D. (1984). Security of infantile attachment as assessed in the 'strange situation': its study and biological interpretation. *Behavioral and Brain Sciences*, **7**, 121–71.

Lyons-Ruth, K., Connell, D., Zoll, D. and Stahl, J. (1987). Infants at social risk: relationships among infant maltreatment, maternal behavior, and infant attachment behavior. *Developmental Psychology*, **23**, 223–32.

MacFarlane, A. (1975). Olfaction in the development of social preferences in the human neonate. *Parent–Infant Interaction (CIBA Symposium 33)*. Amsterdam: Elsevier.

Mahler, M., Pine, F. and Bergman, A. (1975). *The Psychological Birth of the Human Infant*. London: Hutchinson.

Main, M. and Cassidy, J. (1988). Categories of response to reunion with the parent at age six: predicted from infant attachment classifications and stable over a one-month period. *Developmental Psychology*, **24**, 415–26.

Main, M. and Solomon, J. (1986). Discovery of a new, insecure disorganized/disoriented attachment pattern. In *Affective Development in Infancy* (M. Yogman and T. B. Brazelton, eds). Norwood, NJ: Ablex.

Main, M. and Solomon, J. (1990). Procedure for identifying insecure-disorganized/disoriented infants within the Ainsworth strange situation. In *Attachment During the Preschool Years* (M. T. Greenberg, D. Cicchetti and E. M. Cummings, eds). Chicago: University of Chicago Press.

Maratos, O. (1971). *Imitation in Infancy*. PhD dissertation, University of Geneva.

McCartney, K., Scarr, S., Phillips, D., Grajek, S. and Schwarz, J. C. (1982). Environmental differences among day care centers and their effects on children's development. In *Day Care: Scientific and Social Policy Issues* (E. Zigler and E. Gordon, eds). Boston: Auburn House.

McCartney, K., Scarr, S., Rocheleau, A., Phillips, D., et al. (1997). Teacher-child interaction and child care auspices as predictors of social development in infants. *Merrill-Palmer Quarterly*, **43**, 426–50.

McGuire, J. (1991). Social interactions of young, withdrawn children in day nurseries. *Journal of Reproductive and Infant Psychology*, **9**, 169–79.

McGuire, J. and Richman, N. (1986). The prevalence of behavior problems in three types of preschool group. *Journal of Child Psychology and Psychiatry*, **27**, 7–32.

Melhuish, E. C. (1987). Socio-emotional behaviour at 18 months as a function of day care experience, temperament, and gender. *Infant Mental Health Journal*, **8**, 364–73.

Melhuish, E. C. (1991). Research on day care for young children in the United Kingdom. In *Day Care for Young Children* (E. C. Melhuish and P. Moss, eds). London: Routledge.

Melhuish, E. C. (1994). Preschool care and education: lessons from the 20th for the 21st century. *International Journal of Early Years Education*, **1**, 19–32.

Melhuish, E. C., Hennessy, E., Martin, S. and Moss, P. (1990). A longitudinal study of day care and social development. Paper presented at the IVth European Conference in Developmental Psychology, Stirling, Scotland.

Melhuish, E. C., Mooney, A., Martin, S. and Lloyd, E. (1990). Type of childcare at 18 months–I: differences in interactional experience. *Journal of Child Psychology and Psychiatry*, **31**, 849–59.

Melhuish, E. C., Lloyd, E., Martin, S. and Mooney, A. (1990). Type of childcare at 18 months–II: relations with cognitive and language development. *Journal of Child Psychology and Psychiatry*, **31**, 861–70.

Melhuish, E. C., Hennessy, E., Martin, S. and Moss, P. (1991). Does day care affect development over the first six years? Paper presented at the Conference of the International Society for the Study of Behavioural Development, Minneapolis, July, 1991.

Melhuish, E. C., Martin, S. and Mooney, A. (1991). Differing experiences of three-year-olds within various types of care. *Journal of Reproductive and Infant Psychology*, **9**, 116–27.

Meltzoff, A. N. and Moore, M. K. (1977). Imitation of facial and manual gestures by human neonates. *Science*, **198**, 75–8.

Moore, T. W. (1975). Exclusive early mothering and its alternatives–the outcome to adolescence. *Scandinavian Journal of Psychology*, **16**, 255–72.

Mills, M. and Melhuish, E. C. (1974). Recognition of mother's voice in early infancy. *Nature*, **252**, 123–4.

Miyake, K., Chen, S. J. and Campos, J. J. (1985). Infant temperament, mother's mode of interaction, and attachment in Japan: an interim report. In *Growing Points in Attachment Theory and Research* (I. Bretherton and E. Waters, eds). *Monographs of the Society for Research and Child Development*, **50** (1–2, Serial No. 209).

Moskowitz, D. S., Schwarz, J. C. and Corsini, D. A. (1977). Initiating day care at three years of age: effects on attachment. *Child Development*, **48**, 1271–6.

Myers, B. J. (1984). Mother–infant bonding: the status of the critical period hypothesis. *Developmental Review*, **4**, 240–74.

NICHD Early Child Care Network (1996). *Infant Child Care and Attachment Security: Results of the NICHD Study of Early Child Care*. International Conference on Infant Studies, Providence, RI.

NICHD Early Child Care Research Network (1997). The effects of infant child care on infant–mother attachment security: Results of the NICHD Study of Early Child Care. *Child Development*, **68**, 860–79.

Owen, M. T. and Cox, M. (1988). Maternal employment and the transition to parenthood. In *Maternal Employment and Children's Development: Longitudinal Research* (A. E. Gottfried and A. W. Gottfried, eds). New York: Plenum.

Owen, M. T., Easterbrooks, M. A., Chase-Lansdale, P. L. and Goldberg, W. A. (1984). The relationship between maternal employment status and the stability of attachments to mother and father. *Child Development*, **55**, 1894–901.

Petrogiannis, K. G. (1995). Psychological development at 18 months of age as a function of child care experience in Greece. PhD Thesis, University of Wales.

Phillips, D., Mekos, D., Scarr, S., McCartney, K. and Abbott-Shim, M. (unpublished). Paths to quality in child care: structural and contextual influences on children's classroom environments. Unpublished manuscript, Department of Psychology, University of Virginia, Charlottesville, VA.

Pierrehumbert, B., Ramstein, T., Karmaniola, A. and Halfon, O. (1996). Child care in the pre-school years: attachment, behaviour problems and cognitive development. *European Journal of Psychology of Education*, **11**, 201–14.

Ragozin, A. S. (1980). Attachment behavior of day care children: naturalistic and laboratory observations. *Child Development*, **51**, 409–15.

Robertson, A. (1982). Day care and children's responsiveness to adults. In *Day Care: Scientific and Social Policy Issues* (E. Zigler and E. Gordon, eds). Boston, MA: Auburn House.

Roggman, L. A., Langlois, J. H., Hubbs-Tait, L. and Rieser-Danner, L. A. (1994). Infant day-care, attachment and the 'file-drawer problem'. *Child Development*, **65**, 1429–43.

Rubenstein, J. L., Howes, C. and Boyle, P. (1981). A two-year follow-up of infants in community-based day care. *Journal of Child Psychology and Psychiatry*, **22**, 209–18.

Rutter, M. L. (1981). Social-emotional consequences of day care for preschool children. *American Journal of Orthopsychiatry*, **51**, 4–28.

Sagi, A., Lamb, M. E., Lewkowicz, K. S., Shoham, R., Dvir, R. and Estes, D. (1985). Security of infant–mother, –father, and –metapelet among kibbutz reared Israeli children. In *Growing Points in Attachment Theory and Research* (I. Bretherton and E. Waters, eds). *Monographs of the Society for Research in Child Development*, **50** (1–2, Serial No. 209), 257–75.

Schaffer, H. R. (ed.) (1977). *Studies in Mother–Infant Interaction*. London: Academic.

Schaffer, H. R. and Emerson, P. E. (1964). The development of social attachments in infancy. *Monographs of the Society for Research in Child Development*, **29**, No. 3.

Sears, R., Maccoby, E. and Levin, H. (1957). *Patterns of Childrearing*. Evanston, Ill: Row, Peterson.

Schwartz, P. (1983). Length of day care attendance and attachment behaviour in eighteen-month-old infant. *Child Development*, **54**, 1073–8.

Schwarz, J. C., Strickland, R. G. and Krolick, G. (1974). Infant day care: behavioural effects at preschool age. *Developmental Psychology*, **10**, 501–6.

Sroufe, L. A., Fox, N. E. and van Pancake, R. (1983). Attachment and dependency in developmental perspective. *Child Development*, **54**, 1615–27.

Sroufe, L. A. (1983). Infant–caregiver attachment and patterns of adaptation in preschool: the roots of maladaptation and competence. In *Minnesota Symposium in Child Psychology* (M. Perlmutter, ed.). Hillsdale, NJ: Lawrence Erlbaum.

Sroufe, L. A. (1988). The role of infant–caregiver attachment in adult development. In *Clinical Implications of Attachment* (J. Belsky and T. Nezworski, eds). Hillsdale, NJ: Lawrence Erlbaum.

Sroufe, L. A., Egeland, B. and Kreutzer, T. (1990). The fate of early experience following developmental change: longitudinal approaches to individual adaptation in childhood. *Child Development*, **61**, 1363–73.

Stern, D. (1977). *The First Relationship: Infant and Mother*. London: Fontana.

Sternberg, K. J., Lamb, M. E., Hwang, C. P., Broberg, A., Ketterlinus, R. D. and Bookstein, F. L. (1991). Does out-of-home care affect compliance in preschoolers? *International Journal of Behavioural Development*, **14**, 45–66.

Suess, G. J., Grossmann, K. E. and Sroufe, L. A. (1992). Effects of infant attachment to mother and father on quality of adaptation in preschool: from dyadic to individual organisation of self. *International Journal of Behavioural Development*, **15**, 43–66.

Thompson, R. A. (1988). The effects of infant day care through the prism of attachment theory: a critical appraisal. *Early Childhood Research Quarterly*, **3**, 273–82.

Thompson, R. A., Lamb, M. E. and Estes, D. (1982). Stability of infant–mother attachment and its relationship to changing life circumstances in an unselected middle-class sample. *Child Development*, **53**, 144–8.

Thornburg, K. R., Pearl, P., Crompton, D. and Ispa, J. M. (1990). Development of kindergarten children based on child care arrangements. *Early Childhood Research Quarterly*, **5**, 27–42.

Vandell, D. L. and Corasaniti, M. A. (1990). Variations in early child care: do they predict subsequent social, emotional, and cognitive differences? *Early Childhood Research Quarterly*, **5**, 555–72.

Vandell, D. L. and Powers, C. P. (1983). Day care quality and children's free play activities. *American Journal of Orthopsychiatry*, **53**, 493–500.

van IJzendoorn, M. H. and Kroonenberg, P. M. (1988). Cross-cultural patterns of attachment: a meta-analysis of the Strange Situation. *Child Development*, **59**, 147–56.

Varin, D., Crugnola, C. R., Ripamonti, C. and Molina, P. (1996). Sensitive periods in the development of attachment and age of entry into day care. *European Journal of Psychology of Education*, **11**, 215–30.

Vaughn, B., Egeland, B., Sroufe, L. A. and Waters, E. (1979). Individual differences in infant–mother attachment at twelve and eighteen months: stability and change in families under stress. *Child Development*, **50**, 971–5.

Vaughn, B., Gove, F. L. and Egeland, B. (1980). The relationship between out-of-home care and the quality of infant–mother attachment in an economically disadvantaged population. *Child Development*, **51**, 1203–14.

Volling, B. L. and Belsky, J. (1992). Infant, father and mother antecedents of infant–father attachment security in dual-earner and single-earner families. *International Journal of Behavioural Development*, **15**, 83–100.

Volling, B. L. and Feagans, L. V. (1995). Infant day care and children's social competence. *Infant Behavior and Development*, **18**, 177–88.

Waters, E. (1978). The reliability and stability of individual differences in infant–mother attachment. *Child Development*, **49**, 483–94.

Waters, E. and Deane, K. D. (1985). Defining and assessing individual differences in attachment relationships: Q-methodology and the organization of behavior in infancy and early childhood. In *Growing Points in Attachment Theory and Research* (I. Bretherton and E. Waters, eds). *Monographs of the Society for Research in Child Development*, **50** (Serial No. 209).

Wessels, H., Lamb, M. E. and Hwang, C.-P. (1996). Cause and causality in day care research: an investigation of group differences in Swedish care. *European Journal of Psychology of Education*, **11**, 231–45.

Woollett, A. and Phoenix, A. (1991). Psychological views of mothering. In *Motherhood: Meanings, Practices and Ideologies* (A. Phoenix and A. Woollett, eds). London: Sage.

Young, G. and Lewis, M. (1979). Effects of familiarity and maternal attention on infant peer relations. *Merrill-Palmer Quarterly*, **25**, 105–19.

Zeskind, P. S. and Marshall, T. R. (1988). The relation between variations in pitch and maternal perceptions of infant crying. *Child Development*, **59**, 193–6.

10

From feeds to meals: the development of hunger and food intake in infants and young children

Robert Drewett, Peter Wright and Bridget Young

Should babies be breastfed or bottlefed? The political and health controversies over breast- and bottlefeeding have dominated research in this area for several decades. More recently, though, researchers have begun to move away from the (relatively) simple question of whether 'breast is best', for whom and in what circumstances, and towards a more developmental perspective on infant feeding. This chapter by Robert Drewett, Peter Wright and Bridget Young provides an excellent introduction to this approach. It considers not only the consequences of the mode of feeding for physical health and cognitive development, but also how infants feed and psychological aspects of weaning, the process by which solid foods gradually replace milk as the main source of nourishment.

Introduction

The evolution of lactation and the feeding of their young on milk has been of fundamental importance to the biology of mammals, as it freed mammalian species from the need to restrict themselves to environments where their newborn young can find their own food. It is a spectacularly successful adaptation. Even today in areas of the world where hunger is endemic the growth of infants is usually satisfactory while they are breastfed; it is during the weaning period that malnutrition generally begins (Waterlow, Ashworth and Griffiths, 1980).

Considered either in relation to other mammals, or cross-culturally, western Europeans are unusual in two ways. First, we have developed procedures for feeding infants cows' milk from bottles. Second, we maintain our capacity to digest the lactose in milk, breaking it down into glucose and galactose, into adult life, so extending into adulthood the period over which milk is drunk. These, however, are specific modifications to the general system for feeding infants which we share with most other human populations and most other mammals. In the general system milk is a food only for infants; the milk is provided by the mother, and then at some later stage the infant is weaned onto the solid foods taken by adults.

The general system is itself quite complex. A nursing infant does not simply take in milk, but stimulates physiological responses in the mother that have far-reaching effects. Weaning is also complex: half way through the first year of life the nursing infant has to learn a completely new method of feeding. In this chapter we shall deal with the general system, i.e. with nursing and weaning, and also consider two additional practical problems. These are the choice between breast- and bottlefeeding in the United Kingdom and its consequences; and the feeding of infants born pre-term, which is the source of much of the evidence that breast milk has specific components that are important to psychological development.

The terminology of lactation is confused, and has been for many years. An infant feeding at the breast is properly described as being suckled or nursed. Initially babies are nursed at intervals through the day and night; the details of nursing patterns vary across cultures. While babies are nursed they suck, and sucking patterns are species-typical and, as far as we know, essentially the same in different human populations. The human species-typical sucking pattern shows a burst-pause pattern, with each suck during a burst of sucking taking up to a second, and pauses of varying lengths between bursts of sucking (Chetwynd, Diggle, Drewett and Young, 1998). Sucking can be nutritive, or non-nutritive, as it is when an infant sucks on a dummy.

Nutritive sucking combines negative pressure with a stripping movement of the tongue. Its effect is not only to swallow the milk, but also to act as an afferent stimulus to neuroendocrine neurones in the mother's central nervous system. Neuroendocrine neurones act both as neurones and as endocrine glands. They conduct nerve impulses like other neurones, but also secrete hormones into the circulation. Sucking stimulates hypothalamic neurones, with axons which project from the base of the brain down into the posterior pituitary gland and secrete a polypeptide hormone, oxytocin, into the systemic circulation. The oxytocin contracts myoepithelial cells which surround the milk secreting alveoli in the breast, causing milk to flow. This is the milk-ejection reflex, upon which successful breastfeeding depends. Sucking also stimulates milk production in the mother, through the release of a second anterior pituitary hormone, prolactin.

These behavioural and physiological interactions between the mother and the child are only part of the system controlling milk intake in the infant. The other part is internal to the child, and involves its own homeostatic control.

Homeostasis is a term that has a core and an extended use. In the core use homeostasis is the preservation of the constancy of the 'internal environment'. It is achieved physiologically, for example by the release of insulin in response to rising blood glucose levels, and behaviourally, for example by drinking in response to water deprivation. Homeostasis is achieved partly by negative feedback, and in its extended sense the term is also applied to other biological or social systems that involve negative feedback.

Here we are using the term in its core sense, and a central and so far unanswered question concerns the nature of the homeostatic systems that control milk intake in infancy. We often talk as if milk intake in infants is controlled by the same hunger system that controls food intake in adults – essentially a system for regulating energy intake. There is, indeed, evidence that infants very early in life do regulate their energy intake, for example by changing the volume of milk they drink to compensate for changes in its energy yield (Fomon, Filer, Thomas et al., 1975). Yet in the rat, the only species on which we have reasonably good evidence both on the regulation of milk intake in suckling pups and on food intake in adults, the evidence seems to show that milk intake in the pup is controlled by an independent motivational system in its own right, and not by the hunger system that controls food intake in older animals (Drewett, 1978).

Suckling has other, non-homeostatic, effects. The most important of these is that it reduces the probability of the mother becoming pregnant. This effect is used in the lactation amenorrhea method of family planning (LAM), which has now been properly evaluated. The requirements of the method are that the infant is less than six months old; that the mother remains amenorrheic (i.e. that there is no return of menstrual cycles); and that the infant is fully or nearly fully breastfed (i.e. that there is no substantial use of supplements). Used in this way, the pregnancy rate with LAM was as low as 0.7 per hundred women over the first six months, in a summary of data from studies in eight different countries (Kennedy and Visness, 1993). This is a lower actual pregnancy rate than is found with most other contraceptive methods, with the exception of tubal ligation and vasectomy.

Infant feeding and infant health

In Great Britain we have good quality data on infant feeding practices from quinquennial surveys carried out by the Social Survey Division of OPCS. The first was in 1975, and the latest for which published data are available was in 1990 (White, Freeth and O'Brien, 1992). The sample comprised 11,105 infants born in the summer and autumn of 1990. Questionnaires were sent to the mothers when the infants were six to ten weeks old. If the mothers had not replied after two reminders an interviewer visited them personally. This is an important improvement over the usual postal sampling procedures, which tend to have rather poor response rates, giving rise to a risk of samples biased, for example, against respondents with poor literacy. The mothers were contacted again when the infants were four and nine months old.

The 'incidence' of breastfeeding is the proportion of infants breastfed at least once, and in 1990 it was 63 per cent in Great Britain. The incidence was 65 per cent in 1980 and 64 per cent in 1985, so there is no evidence that the efforts made to increase breastfeeding rates over the decade have had any appreciable effect on its incidence.

There are a number of stable associations with the choice of infant feeding method. First, it is associated with the social class of the family. In the infant feeding surveys the families were classified on the occupation of the mother's husband or partner. The percentage who breastfed their infant initially ranged from 86 per cent in social class I to 41 per cent in social class V. Second, the choice is associated with the mother's age, with a breastfeeding incidence (for first babies) of 39 per cent in mothers under 20 rising to 86 per cent in mothers over 30. This association is not simply due to social class differences in mother's ages: the trend is also seen within each social class. Third, infant feeding practices are associated with other health related behaviour within each social class. The most important of these is smoking. In social class I 80 per cent of smokers started breastfeeding, while 88 per cent of non-smokers did. In social class V the proportions were 36 per cent and 45 per cent respectively.

These results show clearly why examining the effects of infant feeding on health is not easy. A randomly selected group of breastfed infants compared with a randomly selected group of bottlefed infants will generally be born into a higher social class and have older and better educated mothers who are less likely to smoke. Each of these is likely to improve their health independently of how they are fed. Smoking by the infant's mother during pregnancy, for example, affects the infant prenatally and reduces average birthweight. Smoking after the birth increases the incidence of respiratory disorders in the infant.

To show effects of infant feeding itself, therefore, requires careful matching of the infants on these other variables, or the use of statistical procedures that have an equivalent effect. For example, Howie, Forsyth, Ogston et al. (1990) examined the effect of breastfeeding on the health of infants in the first year, in a prospective observational study of 674 mothers and infants. They divided them into bottlefeeders, early weaners (infants breastfed for less than 13 weeks) and breastfeeders; this group was itself subdivided into partial breastfeeders (who introduced supplements before 13 weeks) and full breast-feeders (who did not). As expected, the mothers of the bottlefed infants tended to be younger, of lower social class and more likely to smoke. Even after statistical adjustment for these confounding variables, however, it was clear that breastfeeding significantly reduced the incidence of gastro-intestinal illness in the infants. There was also some evidence that respiratory illnesses were reduced.

These beneficial effects of breastfeeding, which are present but relatively small in Great Britain, are of great importance in countries in which sanitation and water supplies are poor. In Malasia, for example, infants who live in households without piped water or a toilet are five times more likely to die after the first week if they are not breastfed (Habicht, DaVanzo and Butz, 1988). It is the combination of these health benefits of breastfeeding with its birth-spacing effect that makes it so important in health promotion in developing countries.

Mothers and infants

In the first few days of life, before lactation is fully established, breastfed infants consume less milk than bottlefed infants. This results in increased hunger in the breastfed baby, and more frequent and persistent crying. First time mothers who have elected to breastfeed but who are unaware of differences in the behaviour of breast- and bottlefed infants often attribute difficulties in feeding at this time to their own lack of milk, and unless provided with support may discontinue breastfeeding. For breastfeeding to become established and be successfully maintained, it is important that health professionals understand how bottle- and breastfed infants differ in their behaviour.

The process of feeding enables behaviour in the newborn to become more organized, with the mother calming and organizing the infant by responding to feeding cues and working to keep the infant in a quiet state. It is useful to think of such interactions as taking place in what Vygotsky called the zone of proximal development. This term is used in relation to a phase prior to independent performance in which the infant who has some skills needed for a task can complete it but only with the assistance of a more capable person. A mother may assess the infant's hunger and satiation cues, and tacitly operating in the zone of proximal development, arrange and support the feeding interactions so that their infants can manage components of the feeding on their own terms.

The most important variable to influence the behaviour associated with feeding in infants is whether they are fed from the breast or fed infant formula from a bottle. The choice of feeding method results in differences in the pacing of feeds which seem to be related to this establishment of control over actions by the infant. Milk feeds are not a continuous period of suckling but are interrupted by the removal of the bottle or breast for a variety of reasons such as choking, winding, possetting of milk or changing to another breast. When filmed feeds were analysed to see whether it was the baby or the mother who initiated these breaks in feeding, for bottlefed babies the interruptions were found to be almost entirely under the control of the mother, but for breastfed infants there was a predominantly baby-determined pattern. Whereas bottlefeeding mothers have immediate feedback available to them in the form of amount of milk consumed, breastfeeding mothers do not. When they were asked about the criteria they use to decide if their baby has had enough milk, falling asleep was recognized as a satiety cue more commonly by breastfeeding mothers, but bottlefeeding mothers were more likely to terminate feeds only when the baby spat out the teat (Wright, 1987). There are several stages in the process of terminating the feed: the baby slows down its sucking rate, becomes drowsy and, if the mother still continues the feed, refuses to open its mouth, or spits out the teat if it is forced into the mouth. In terms of this progression it would seem that some bottlefeeding mothers are more likely to override the early signals of satiety and are thus in greater danger of overfeeding their baby.

Bottlefed infants are offered and take a fixed amount of formula at regular intervals in the first few months of life, whereas breastfed infants develop a pronounced diurnal pattern of meal size by the age of 6–8 weeks, with the largest meals at the beginning of the day. These estimates are based on mothers' weighings of their infants immediately before and after each breastfeed. When mothers attending baby clinics were asked if they were aware of any differences in their baby's level of hunger across the day, breastfeeding mothers were more likely to report hunger variation than bottlefeeding mothers. The mothers identified a wide range of behaviours and attributions as evidence for increased hunger in their infants, which Wright (1987) classified into five categories:

1. *Avidity measures.* Comments concerning the intensity of the sucking or the speed or length of sucking: 'desperate, sucks everything'; 'sucks rapidly'; 'sucks slowly and rhythmically'.
2. *Distractibility.* The baby is said to be more hungry because it is less distractible and more single-minded about the feed: 'gets on with it'; 'sustained concentration'; 'no rests for looking about'.
3. *Cries and screams.* 'Screams until fed'.
4. *Very frequent feeding.* The baby demands feeds more frequently: 'fed in under three hours'; 'wants lots of little feeds'; 'has to be fed very often'.
5. *Maternal inference.* The mother makes an inference to support her claim for increased hunger at this stage of the day: 'has gone all night without food, and so must be more hungry'.

Inevitably the feeding method chosen focuses the mother on different cues for hunger. Bottlefeeding mothers identify the vigour of sucking as the most common reason for believing their infant to be particularly hungry.

In contrast, breastfeeding mothers cite the increased frequency or demand for feeds at particular times of the day. Feeding method also leads to changes in the patterns of night waking, with bottlefed babies beginning to sleep through the night at a significantly earlier age than breastfed babies. Such pronounced differences in the experience of mothers feeding their babies are often unacknowledged by health visitors; yet sleeping through the night is an important milestone in development which parents eagerly strive to attain, and it is something that breastfed infants can be trained to do (Pinella and Birch,1993).

Pre-term infants

Pre-term infants are those born before 37 weeks of gestation. Pre-term birth is a common reason for low birthweight (<2500 g) though a low birthweight can be found for other reasons. The survival of pre-term infants has improved dramatically in recent years. This has led to difficult problems of care, among which nutritional problems are of great importance. Growth rates of the fetus at the end of pregnancy are very high, and it is difficult to maintain satisfactory growth after a pre-term birth, when the infant is no longer fed via the placental circulation but is insufficiently developed to feed by mouth in the normal way.

A number of interesting issues arise in connection with pre-term infants. The first is the developmental issue. At what developmental age is an infant capable of breastfeeding? A traditional assumption is that bottlefeeding needs to be established first, but recent research does not suggest that this assumption is well founded.

Meier and Pugh (1985) carefully compared breast- and bottlefeeding in the same three pre-term infants over an extended period of time. The infants were 35–37 weeks old at their first feed, and weighed less than 1500 g. The infants needed to be taught to attach to the breast, but then sucked for extended periods (often longer than 45 minutes). This was considerably longer than the duration of bottlefeeds in the same infants (15 to 20 minutes). The difference appeared to be due to the breastfeeds being more infant-paced than the bottlefeeds, just as they are in term infants.

During feeding infants have to synchronize sucking, swallowing and breathing, and difficulty with this is one of the problems of pre-term infants. Meier (1988) examined the transcutaneous oxygen pressure and temperature of a group of five pre-term infants who were again both breast- and bottlefed. At the first feed the infants weighed less than 1500 g and were under 35 weeks old. The interesting finding was that it was during breastfeeds that the oxygen pressure was less likely to decline, apparently because sucking, swallowing and breathing were better co-ordinated during breastfeeds. The babies also kept warmer.

In small mammals and primates early nutrition has potentially important long-term effects on blood lipids, plasma insulin, obesity, atherosclerosis, as well as on behaviour and learning ability. Breastfed and bottlefed baboons have long-term differences in their lipid metabolism and in the degree of atherosclerosis. Lucas (1991) suggests that a similar form of 'nutritional programming' operates in humans, i.e. that when an early stimulus or insult occurs at a critical or sensitive period, it can result in a permanent or long-term change in structure or function.

That the mode of feeding in early infancy might have long-term influences on development is an idea that has been around for most of this century, but only recently has there been acceptable evidence that breast milk itself may have long-term beneficial effects on cognitive outcome. We have seen earlier in this chapter that the way an infant is fed in the United Kingdom is strongly associated with the social class of their family, and that the feeding inter-actions between mother and infant depend on whether the infant is breast- or bottlefed. The difficulty in investigating cognitive or other psychological effects of feeding has been in finding grounds for distinguishing between three possibilities. These are:

- First, that cognitive differences between breast- and bottlefed infants are derived from the associated social class characteristics of their families, and are not directly affected by how the infant is fed.
- Second, that they are derived from behavioural interactions between mothers and infants that differ in breast- and bottlefeeding. As noted above, the nature of the interactions between mother and infant lead to feeds being more paced by the infant when the infant is breastfed. This experience, which enables the infant to establish a degree of control over a crucial part of their environment, may generalize to other ways of exploring and manipulating the environment. Establishment of what he referred to as 'mastery' is a key element in Vygotsky's theory of cognitive development (a view in part shared by Piaget), so this could give breastfed infants some developmental advantage over infants that are bottlefed.
- The third possibility is that cognitive or other psychological differences between breast- and bottlefed infants derive directly from nutritional differences between breast milk and formula milks.

Substantial improvements in IQ tested at nine years have now been reported in recent research in the UK in premature babies provided with human breast milk via a nasogastric tube in the first month post partum (Lucas, 1991). The pre-term infant is suited to such research because it is possible to some extent to randomly assign the kind of early diet fed to the infants. The diets in this study included human milk, standard formula, and nutrient enriched pre-term formula, though in the part of the study that showed this outcome the breast milk was not assigned randomly but according to the choice of the mother. The authors of the study attribute the improved IQ measured at a later age solely to the breast milk, although it is clear from the data that the greatest gains are seen in the infants whose mothers established successful breastfeeding and continue breastfeeding following discharge from the hos-pital. That dietary variation over such a brief period has a lasting effect seems to imply that the neonatal period is important for nutrition after a pre-term birth.

One problem is that although this research strongly suggests that early feeding has implications for long-term development, this may be true only for the pre-term infant, and not for the majority of infants, who are born at term. However a substantial body of evidence now shows that breastfed infants do better both on developmental tests in the first two years (Morrow-Tlucak,

Haude and Ernhart,1988; Rogan and Gladen, 1993) and on tests of cognitive ability and educational attainment at school age (Rodgers, 1978; Taylor and Wadsworth, 1984). These studies controlled for obvious confounders such as social class. One study also controlled for the IQ of the mother, and still found a small residual difference of about 2 IQ points in favour of breastfed infants (Fergusson, Beautrais and Silva, 1982).

The pre-term baby work would imply that some component of human breast milk, perhaps long-chain fatty acids or nerve growth factors, are key components which promote brain development. More recent work indicates that children who are born with mild neurological damage as revealed in a neonatal assessment have better neurological status at the age of 9 years if they are breastfed rather than bottlefed (Lanting, Fidler, Huisman et al., 1994). There is also evidence from a controlled trial that the addition of a source of docosahexaenoic acid, one of the long-chain fatty acids in breast milk, to formula milk improves both early visual acuity and scores on the mental development index of the Bayley Scales of Infant Development (Carlson, Werkman, Peeples and Wilson, 1994). The extent to which these effects endure is not clear at the moment.

Weaning and feeding on solids

Starting on solids is an important new step for the infant, who is exposed for the first time to a wide range of tastes, flavours and textures. There are new motor skills to learn, beginning with removing food from a spoon and moving on to the mastery of complex skills involved in self-feeding. The introduction of solids also entails a switch to an externally controlled three to four meals per day, at least in western cultures. Starting on solids also introduces the infant to food and eating as important aspects of a wider social life. The change in terminology as 'feeds' come to be referred to as 'meals' signify that the infant has moved to a more generally social arena. No longer cradled in the enclosed and semi-prone position characteristic of milk feeding, the infant is now sat upright among other family members, and with a clear view of proceedings is able to participate more fully in meal times.

Weaning is the term used to describe the process by which other foods gradually replace milk as the primary source of nutrition. To refer to these other foods as 'solids' is something of a misnomer as the initial weaning foods are more likely to have the consistency of a puree; however 'solids' is the term most commonly used even to refer to the first foods. For infants in Britain weaning normally begins between two and four months and almost all infants will have been offered foods other than milk by six months of age (White, Freeth and O'Brien, 1992). Whether they accept the other foods is a different matter: a number of mothers reported their infants would not accept solids even at nine months. In contrast to the onset of weaning, it is difficult to clearly define when weaning ends in the United Kingdom because of the extended use of milk and milk products throughout childhood and into adulthood. Twenty-six per cent of calorie intake is based on milk and milk products in one to two year olds, and 16 per cent even in three to four year olds (Gregory, Collins, Davies et al., 1995).

There is very little basic descriptive research on feeding behaviour in infants over the weaning period, and there are still no conclusive answers to a range of elementary questions concerning the duration of meal times, the way infants express satiety and the way parents respond to infant satiety cues. The weaning period is a complex period in which milk feeding and solids feeding must be considered simultaneously, and weanlings are not usually readily accessible for research purposes in hospitals or schools in the way newborn infants and older children are. These practical problems have led to a lack of behavioural research in the weaning period, in spite of it being the period in which the most widespread and important nutritional problems in childhood arise.

Black, Cole, Wiles and White (1983) examined daily variation in food intake in infants from 2–18 months. Dietary intake was measured using four-day weighed intake records. Day-to-day variation for the whole group was relatively low while infants were fully breastfed, rose slightly as infants were weaned and increased markedly to a level comparable to that of adults when infants were aged 15–18 months. There were also individual differences between infants in their levels of variability with some having quite consistent levels of intake from day to day, while others fluctuated quite widely.

An exploratory study by Connolly and Dalgleish (1989) investigated the development of tool using skills in feeding behaviour in one to two year olds. The focus of the study was on the use of spoons. The children were videoed every month at meal times for a period of six months. A detailed analysis of the video tapes revealed an orderly progression in spoon using skill. This was divided into four broad stages by the authors. Firstly there is a stage of repetitive actions. The spoon is repeatedly pushed in and out of food or in and out of the mouth with little apparent understanding of its function. Secondly, the child moves to a more complex sequence of behaviour where the spoon is placed into the food and then into the mouth. Thirdly, specific attempts are made to fill the spoon with food. Thus instead of merely dipping the spoon into the bowl, it is brought across the food in a purposeful scooping movement. At this stage the authors suggest the child has understood the function of the spoon. Finally, in the fourth stage certain correction routines appear; for example the infant begins to check that there is sufficient food on the spoon and if necessary makes a second attempt at loading before it is brought to the mouth. On a more general level, actions are accomplished more rapidly and smoothly and there is greater consistency in the use of the preferred hand and style of grasping the spoon. The sequence is similar in different children, but with some variability in the timing of the different stages.

Taste sensitivity and taste preferences in infants have generally been measured by examining the intake of food with different taste properties, although other indicators such as facial expression and sucking behaviour have also been used. Beauchamp, Cowart and Moran (1986) studied developmental changes in the acceptance of salt solutions and water in two groups of infants aged 2–4 and 4–7 months. The younger infants consumed equal quantities of saline and water, but the older infants took significantly more saline than water. This suggests that prior to four months infants are unable to discriminate the taste of salt, and illustrates a maturational change in behaviour.

But does this increased consumption of salty water, a substance which adults find aversive, demonstrate that infants would actually prefer the taste of salt in food? Sullivan and Birch (1994) presented 4–6-month-old infants with either salted or unsalted versions of two different vegetables (peas and green beans) which they had never before tasted. Each infant was given the same vegetable for the duration of the study. In assessment meals at the beginning and end of the study measures of intake for both salted and unsalted versions of the vegetable were taken on separate days. In addition adults' ratings of the infants' preferences were made from video-tapes of the meals. Between assessments each infant was consistently offered only one version of one vegetable at lunch times for an exposure period of ten days. There was no evidence that the addition of salt increased consumption. Comparisons of intake of the salted and unsalted vegetable before and after exposure showed no evidence that infants develop a strong preference for the version of the vegetable fed over the ten-day period. Infants who were fed the salted peas increased their consumption of both unsalted and salted peas following the exposure period. The adult ratings of the infants' preferences for foods correlated with their intake of them.

These results on children in the first year contrast with results on a comparable study by Sullivan and Birch (1990) on children two to three years old. Older children, it seems, do not develop such generalized preferences. If they are exposed to one version of the vegetable, whether salt has been added or not, they appear to develop an actual aversion for the version of the vegetable to which they are not exposed.

A recurrent suggestion has been that there may be a sensitive period during the middle of the first year of life when infants are particularly open to the introduction of new foods. This phase purportedly lasts until about the first birthday when the infant becomes more discriminating and less flexible in patterns of food acceptance. This suggestion, though mostly based on anecdote, has a certain appeal in evolutionary terms. At about the time milk is ceasing to be adequate for their nutritional needs infants are relatively adaptable in accepting new foods which are generally offered by parents; then as they become increasingly mobile and in danger of ingesting toxic substances they also becomes neophobic towards unfamiliar foods. However, the only research to come close to addressing this question throws an element of doubt on these ideas. Rozin, Hammer, Oster et al. (1986) investigated preschool children's readiness to taste a variety of food and non-food items. Children at 16–29 months of age were still more ready to taste a variety of items than older children.

Whatever the evidence for developmental changes in food acceptance patterns, there is little doubt that repeated experience with foods is a powerful shaper of infant and young children's food acceptance patterns. This was investigated by Birch and Marlin (1982) in preschool children aged two to three years. Children were exposed to varying extents to unfamiliar fruits and cheeses over a period of 25 days. Their later preferences were found to be highly correlated with exposure frequency; 13 out of 14 children chose foods they were more familiar with.

Many psychologists have become interested in feeding because they saw this kind of interaction as the source of subsequent social communication. Some therapists have suggested that the root of eating disorders such as anorexia nervosa and bulimia may be due to inadequate learning experiences about hunger in early infancy, and recent evidence indicates that babies may themselves be vulnerable to their mothers' concerns about their own bodies and weight (see Cooper and Stein, 1994).

A longer established area of interest, though, is the way in which weight gain in infancy predisposes to obesity, and here early ideas of 'nutritional programming' have turned out to be ill-founded. Although they have a slightly increased risk of doing so, over-weight infants do not usually become over-weight adults. There are, in fact, two periods of increased adiposity in childhood. The median BMI (body mass index, i.e. weight divided by the square of height) in the United Kingdom (Cole, Freeman and Preece, 1995) increases from 10.6 at 35 weeks of gestation to a peak of 17.6 at eight months. It then drops to 15.5 at five years before increasing again during childhood. It is the later increase that is associated with childhood obesity, not adiposity in infancy. Correspondingly, avidity measures based on sucking in infants predict later adiposity in infancy, but do not predict adiposity beyond the age of six (Agras, Kraemer, Berkowitz et al., 1987, 1990).

It may well be, therefore, that behavioural studies after eight months will be more revealing in respect of later weight problems than studies in the lactation period, and several observational studies have been conducted concerning the possible role of parent modelled feeding behaviour and parental feeding strategies on the development of obesity in children. Agras, Berkowitz, Hammer and Kraemer (1988) examined the relationship between the eating behaviour of 18-month-old children and their parents. All the family members ate alone in a controlled laboratory environment but their mothers were present when observations were conducted on children. Children with higher levels of caloric intake at the test meal tended to have mothers who ate rapidly and fathers who spent more time eating. Klesges, Holzer, Woolfrey and Vollmer (1983) investigated the influence of parent–child interaction during meal times on children's feeding behaviour and relative weight. Families of children aged 12–30 months were observed at meal times in the home. High correlations were observed between the relative weight of children and the number of times parents intervened to encourage and prompt children to eat. A lower but still statistically significant correlation was observed for the number of times parents offered food to their children. There are, of course, genetic components to obesity; but the recent studies in this area do not suggest that more than about half the variance in the body mass index can be explained genetically in European populations, so these intra-familial influences may be important, and are open to change in a way that the genetic influences are not.

Linear growth and weight gain in the early years are related to an unexpectedly wide range of outcomes in childhood and adult life, including cognitive development (Dowdney, Skuse, Heptinstall et al., 1987), diabetes and hypertension (Barker, Winter, Osmond et al., 1989; Fall, Vijayakumar, Barker et al., 1995) and death from suicide (Barker, Osmond, Rodin et al., 1995). We are a long way from understanding the mechanisms underlying these associations. It would be wrong to start, however, from the assumption that infants are simply passive recipients of food: they are, on the contrary, active participants in the feeding process.

Their participation needs to be understood developmentally. Essentially there are two phases in food intake: an early infant, milk-based phase, in which sucking is the infant's principle behaviour, and a childhood phase based on a variety of solid and liquid foods. Correspondingly there are two phases in fat deposition. But additionally there is a prolonged transitional phase of weaning, in which extensive sensory, motor and motivational learning takes place, and initial childhood habits come to be formed. The transition is a complex one, and it should not be surprising that weaning is often accompanied by behavioural and nutritional problems (Douglas, 1995; Waterlow, Ashworth and Griffiths, 1980).

Applications

1. Infants are partners
From the moment of birth, infants are actively regulating their own intake, partly through their sucking and partly through signals to the mother. The feeding interaction between mothers and infants has rather different properties in breast- and bottlefeeding, especially in the relative autonomy of the infant.

2. Weaning is difficult
Over the weaning period an infant engages in a complex process of sensory and motor learning, and begins to acquire habits and preferences that endure into childhood. The weaning process is complex, and it is not surprising that it often causes difficulty.

3. Infant feeding may have long-term consequences
It is important to be aware of the long-term consequences of infant nutrition, and also important not to exaggerate them. In term infants, breastfeeding has clear physical advantages, the importance of which depends on the physical environment: in tropical countries they are very important. It appears also to have advantages to neural and psychological development, but these are less certain and their magnitude is probably not great.

Further reading

Birch, L. L. and Fisher, M. S. (1995). Appetite and eating behaviour in children. *Pediatric Clinics of North America*, **42**, 931–53.

Forsyth, J. S. (1995). The relationship between breast-feeding and infant health and development. *Proceedings of the Nutrition Society*, **54**, 407–18.

St. James-Roberts, I., Harris, G. and Messer, D. (1993). *Infant Crying, Feeding and Sleeping: Development Problems and Treatments*. New York: Harvester Wheatsheaf.

Wright, P. and Woollett, A. (1987). Breastfeeding. *Special Issue of Journal of Reproductive and Infant Psychology*, **5**, 125–90.

References

Agras, W. S., Berkowitz, R. I., Hammer, L. C. and Kraemer, H. C. (1988). Relationships between the eating behaviors of parents and their 18-month-old children: a laboratory study. *International Journal of Eating Disorders*, **7**, 641–8.

Agras, W. S., Kraemer, H. C., Berkowitz, R. I. and Hammer, L. D. (1990). Influence of early feeding style on adiposity at 6 years of age. *Journal of Pediatrics*, **116**, 805–9.

Agras, W. S., Kraemer, H. C., Berkowitz, R. I., Korner, A. F. and Hammer, L. D. (1987). Does a vigorous feeding style influence early development of adiposity? *Journal of Pediatrics*, **110**, 799–804.

Barker, D. J. P., Osmond, D., Rodin, I., Fall, C. H. D. and Winter, P. D. (1995). Low weight gain in infancy and suicide in adult life. *British Medical Journal*, **311**, 1203.

Barker, D. J. P., Winter, P. D., Osmond, C., Margetts, B. and Simmonds, S. J. (1989). Weight in infancy and death from ischaemic heart disease. *Lancet*, **ii**, 578–80.

Beauchamp, G. K., Cowart, B. J. and Moran, M. (1986). Developmental changes in salt acceptability in human infants. *Developmental Psychobiology*, **19**, 17–25.

Birch, L. L. and Marlin, D. (1982). I don't like it; I never tried it: effects of exposure on two-year-old children's food preferences. *Appetite*, **3**, 353–60.

Black, A. E., Cole, T. J., Wiles, S. J. and White, F. (1983). Daily variation in food intake of infants from 2 to 18 months. *Human Nutrition: Applied Nutrition*, **37A**, 448–58.

Carlson, S. E., Werkman, S. H., Peeples, J. M. and Wilson, W. M. (1994). Long-chain fatty acids and early visual and cognitive development of preterm infants. *European Journal of Clinical Nutrition*, **48** (Suppl. 2), S27–S30.

Chetwynd, A. G., Diggle, P. J., Drewett, R. F. and Young, B. (1998. A mixture model for sucking patterns of breast-fed infants. *Statistics in Medicine*, in press.

Cole, T. J., Freeman, J. V. and Preece, M. A. (1995). Body mass index references curves for the UK, 1990. *Archives of Disease in Childhood*, **73**, 25–9.

Connolly, K. and Dalgleish, M. (1989). The emergence of tool-using skill in infancy. *Developmental Psychology*, **25**, 894–912.

Cooper, P. and Stein, A. (eds) (1994). Monographs in child pediatrics 5, *Feeding Problems and Eating Disorders in Children and Adolescents*. Switzerland: Harwood Academic Publishers.

Douglas, J. E. (1995). Behavioural eating problems in young children. In *Nutrition and Child Health* (D. P. Davies, ed.). Royal College of Physicians of London.

Dowdney, L., Skuse, D., Heptinstall, E., Puckering, C. and Zur-Szpiro, S. (1987). Growth retardation and development delay amongst inner-city children. *Journal of Child Psychology and Psychiatry*, **28**, 529–41.

Drewett, R. F. (1978). The development of motivational systems. In: maturation of the nervous system. *Progress in Brain Research*, **48**, 407–17.

Fall, C. H. D., Vijayakumar, M., Barker, D. J. P., Osmond, C. and Duggleby, S. (1995). Weight in infancy and prevalence of coronary heart disease in adult life. *British Medical Journal*, **310**, 17–19.

Fergusson, D. M., Beautrais, A. L. and Silva, P. A. (1982). Breast-feeding and cognitive development in the first seven years of life. *Social Science and Medicine*, **16**, 1705–8.

Fomon, S. J., Filer, L. J., Thomas, L. N., Anderson, T. A. and Nelson, S. E. (1975). Influence of formula concentration on caloric intake and growth of normal infants. *Acta Paediatrica Scandinavica*, **64**, 172–81.

Gregory, J. R., Collins, D. L., Davies, P. S. W., Hughes, J. M. and Clarke, P. C. (1995). National diet and nutrition survey: children aged 1.5 to 4.5 years. *Volume I: Report of the Diet and Nutrition Survey*. London: HMSO.

Habicht, J.-P., DaVanzo, J. and Butz, W. P. (1988). Mother's milk and sewage: their interactive effects on infant mortality. *Pediatrics*, **81**, 456–61.

Howie, P. W., Forsyth, J. S., Ogston, S. A., Clark, A. and du V. Florey, C. (1990). Protective effect of breast feeding against infection. *British Medical Journal*, **300**, 11–16.

Kennedy, K. I. and Visness, C. M. (1993). Contraceptive efficiency of lactational amenorrhea. *Lancet*, **339**, 227–30.

Klesges, L. M., Holzer, B., Woolfrey, J. and Vollmer, J. (1983). Parental influences on children's eating behavior and relative weight. *Journal of Applied Behavior Analysis*, **14**, 371–8.

Lanting, C. I., Fidler, V., Huisman, M., Touwen, B. C. L. and Boersma, E. R. (1994). Neurological differences between 9-year old children fed breast-milk or formula milk as babies. *Lancet*, **344**, 1319–22.

Lucas, A. (1991). Programming by early nutrition in man. In *The Childhood Environment and Adult Disease* (Ciba Foundation Symposium 156). Chichester: Wiley.

Meier, P. (1988). Bottle- and breast-feeding: effects on transcutaneous oxygen pressure and temperature in preterm infants. *Nursing Research*, **37**, 36–41.

Meier, P. and Pugh, E. J. (1985). Breast-feeding behavior of small preterm infants. *Maternal and Child Nursing*, **10**, 396–401.

Morrow-Tlucak, M., Haude, R. H. and Ernhart, C. B. (1988). Breast-feeding and cognitive development in the first 2 years of life. *Social Science and Medicine*, **28** (6), 635–9.

Pinella, T. and Birth, L. L. (1993). Help me make it through the night: behavioral entrainment of breast-fed infants' sleep patterns. *Pediatrics*, **91**, 436–44.

Rodgers, B. (1978). Feeding in infancy and later ability and attainment: a longitudinal study. *Development Medicine and Child Neurology*, **20**, 421–6.

Rogan, W. J. and Gladen, B. C. (1993). Breast-feeding and cognitive development. *Early Human Development*, **31**, 181–93.

Rozin, P., Hammer, L., Oster, H., Horowitz, T. and Marmora, V. (1986). The child's conception of food: differentiation of categories of rejected substances in the 16 months to 5 year age range. *Appetite*, **7**, 141–51.

Sullivan, S. A. and Birch, L. L. (1990). Pass the sugar, pass the salt: experience dictates preference. *Developmental Psychology*, **26**, 546–51.

Sullivan, S. A. and Birch, L. L. (1994). Infant dietary experience and acceptance of solid foods. *Pediatrics*, **93**, 271–7.

Taylor, B. and Wadsworth, J. (1984). Breast-feeding and child development at five years. *Developmental Medicine and Child Neurology*, **26**, 73–80.

Waterlow, J. C., Ashworth, A. and Griffiths, M. (1980). Faltering in infant growth in less-developed countries. *Lancet*, **ii**, 1176–8.

White, A., Freeth, S. and O'Brien, M. (1992). Infant Feeding 1990. Office of Population Censuses and Survey. London: HMSO.

Wright, P. (1987). Mothers' assessment of hunger in relation to meal size in breastfed infants. *Journal of Reproductive and Infant Psychology*, **5**, 173–81.

Wright, P. (1993). Mothers' ideas about feeding in early infancy. In *Infant Crying, Feeding and Sleeping* (I. St. James-Roberts, G. Harris and D. Messer, eds). New York: Harvester Wheatsheaf.

11

Infants' sleep: patterns and problems

David Messer and Carol Parker

As most new parents will testify, infants' sleeping patterns are not the same as those of adults, and being woken during the night by a crying baby is a common experience of parenthood. In this chapter, David Messer and Carol Parker trace the development of sleeping patterns during infancy and consider the definition and treatment of sleeping difficulties. Are infants' sleeping difficulties really 'problems' for them – or simply part of a developmental pattern with which parents in western cultures are not able to cope? They raise questions such as whether some babies are more likely to experience sleeping difficulties than others or whether patterns of feeding or caregiving have greater effects. For example, does sleeping in the same bed as their parents reduce sleeping problems? They go on to consider whether health professionals can help with sleeping difficulties in infancy; for example, is behavioural management, currently the most popular approach, an effective intervention?

Introduction

Babies spend about two thirds of their days in sleep and adults spend about a third of their days in sleep. At first sight these figures would suggest that infants are relatively undemanding on adults' time. However, these simple biological facts fail to capture the complexity of the relationship between infant and adult sleep patterns, and the ways in which infants and adults affect one another's sleeping. In discussing these issues we will start with outlining the developmental course of sleeping and consider typical patterns together with individual differences. This leads on to a consideration of sleeping difficulties and the factors that are associated with such difficulties. Then the effects of sleeping difficulties on development and well-being are briefly considered. The last section addresses the issue of what advice and methods of treatment can be provided about sleeping difficulties. This is discussed from a cultural perspective where it is argued that sleeping processes need to be viewed within a cultural context.

Before moving on to this material it is worth explaining the impact that the sleeping patterns of infants can have on adults. In many ways the term infant or child sleeping difficulties is something of a misnomer. In most cases the biggest impact is on adults who suffer the consequences of disrupted night time sleeping and do not have the opportunity to take naps during the day. Maternal depression is associated with infant sleeping difficulties, and the literature on child abuse contains a number of reports about lack of sleep and persistent crying being precipitating factors in such violence (Messer and Richards, 1993). Furthermore, if one has experienced the disruption of sleep and the lack of sleep over months, and in some cases years, then one can readily appreciate the impact of these simple events on the functioning and mood of the caregivers.

The development of infant sleep patterns

An obvious feature of adult sleep is that it is linked to diurnal (daily) patterns of light and darkness. Typically our biological clocks are set in such a way that we sleep at night and are awake during the day, furthermore adults tend to sleep for 8 hours. However, the newborn baby does not come into the world with a biological clock attuned to the differences between day and night. Furthermore, the sleeping and waking is organized around a 3–4 hour cycle, so that new-borns will usually sleep for this time, wake and be fed, and then sleep for another similar period. Thus, at the beginning life infant and adult biological rhythms are not synchronized with one another, and this has important consequences for the caregivers. Such a pattern is normal and not unusual; however, many first time parents fail to appreciate the consequences such a regime imposes on their lives. It is one thing to be told about being repeatedly woken up, it is another to experience this.

One other characteristic of early infant sleep-wake functioning that deserves comment is that there has been a tendency to differentiate *infant state* into more phases than a simple awake-asleep contrast. For example, the following five states are often identified: deep sleep; light sleep with some movements and irregular breathing; awake but quiet and alert; active with vigorous movements, and crying. In adults a widespread distinction is made between REM (rapid eye movement) and NREM (non-rapid eye movement) sleep, with the former involving dreaming. REM are infrequent in pre-term infants, but are rapidly increased by the term date. However, they do not correspond to an adult pattern until about two to six months.

The classic study by Parmelee, Wenner and Schulz (1964) provided one of the first comprehensive descriptions of early sleep patterns. Mothers filled in a sleep chart about the pattern of their baby's sleeping every day over the first five months. This involved entering information accurate to about a quarter of an hour about when their baby had been asleep. These records showed that newborn babies were sleeping about 16 hours a day, and there was only a slight decline in the total amount so that by 16 weeks the babies were on average sleeping 15 hours a day. The study identified the early pattern of sleeping in 3–4 hour bouts which was outlined in the first paragraph of this section.

Parmelee, Wenner and Schulz's data also revealed that there were important changes during the first four months. The longest period awake increased from 2.4 to 3.6 hours over this period, and more significantly the longest period asleep increased from 4.1 to 8.5 hours. In addition, by four months infants were sleeping twice as much at night as during the day. Thus, during the first four months many infants adapt to a pattern of sleeping which is much more congenial for their parents. However, not all infants adapt to this pattern. Moore and Ucko (1957) report that by 3 months 70 per cent of babies are sleeping through the night, with 81 per cent of babies achieving this at 4 months. The remaining 20–30 per cent of infants who wake at night are likely to be seen as having sleeping difficulties and we will return to this topic later on in the chapter. There also are suggestions that later on in the first year infants who have been sleeping through the night might begin waking again (Anders and Keener, 1985; Ferber, 1987).

Sleeping in older infants has been described by Jacklin, Snow, Gahart and Maccoby (1980). Mothers filled in a sleep diary about a single day. This was done at 6, 12, 18, 26 and 33 months with a sample of between 65 and 145 reports. There was not much change in the total amount of time spent asleep, although there was a gradual decrease from 14 hours sleep at 6 months to 11 hours sleep at 33 months. The longest period asleep was about 9–10 hours throughout the age range. There was moderate stability in the number of wakings, but the correlations decreased in strength as the time gap between data points increased.

A longitudinal study of sleeping through the preschool years has been provided by Beltramini and Hertzig (1983). Their information was obtained from interviews with 109 mothers every year from one year of age to five years. Throughout this age range a substantial proportion of children were reported to wake every night; the highest proportion was 33 per cent at three years, and the lowest proportion was 19 per cent at five years. Furthermore, at every age, around 60 per cent of the children were reported to wake at least once a week. With increasing age, bedtimes became more problematic and took longer, more children took longer to fall asleep, there were more recalls of parents after the light had been switched out, and more nightmares were reported. Thus, difficulties with sleeping continue to be present during the preschool years and affected a reasonably high proportion of children. In addition, the nature of difficulties appears to change with there being more problems with settling children to sleep.

Is there continuity in infants' patterns of sleeping across age? Are there some consistently good sleepers and some consistently poor sleepers? The studies reviewed so far provide some evidence in support of continuity, so that having one type of sleeping pattern at one age means that the infant is likely to have a similar set of patterns at a later age. A longitudinal investigation of this issue was conducted by Jenkins, Owen, Box and Hart (1984) on infants who were aged 6, 12, 18 and 24 months. Sleep problems were rather liberally defined as waking once or more a night and associated problems of settling. Out of a sample of 150 infants, 63 per cent did not have sleeping difficulties at any age, and those infants who were sleeping through the night at six months were highly likely to continue to sleep through the night. Thus, there appears to be a reasonably high proportion of infants whose sleep is unproblematic for parents. The remaining infants showed an interesting pattern of development. At 12 and 18 months, and for any condition (i.e. having sleeping difficulties or not having them), about half of the infants changed from having sleeping difficulties to not having sleeping difficulties, and about half changed in the opposite direction. Thus, if the infant was not a consistently good sleeper, there was about a 50 per cent probability that there would be a change in his or her behaviour at 12 months and at 18 months. As a result of this there were very few infants who had sleeping difficulties at every age, only 5 per cent. Overall, these figures indicate that there is a reasonably high proportion of infants whose sleeping is unproblematic, but for the remainder there is considerable variability in sleeping patterns across age. Fortunately for parents, there seem to be relatively few infants with consistent sleep problems at all age points.

Summary

The organization of young children's sleep can have a profound effect on parents. Immediately after birth infants have a sleep-wake cycle of about 3–4 hours with sleeping patterns being relatively unaffected by whether it is day or night. The most dramatic developmental change in sleeping occurs at about four months. At this age the majority of infants start to sleep for longer periods at night. However, throughout the preschool years somewhere between a fifth to a third of infants continue to have patterns of sleep which are problematic for their parents.

Assessing infant sleeping and sleeping difficulties

Most of the studies reviewed so far have involved maternal reports of infant sleeping; often the mothers have filled in a diary in which they have to indicate whether their child is awake or asleep in every given period of time (often 15 minutes) throughout 24 hours. However, the limitations of this method of collecting data need to be recognized. Such reports provide a very good picture of the behaviour that the parents notice. This is very useful for examining the impact of children's sleeping on parents. However, it can be argued that this form of data collection suffers from a number of limitations if one is concerned with accurately describing the patterns of children's sleeping (Messer and Richards, 1993).

The most obvious problem is that mothers will only identify children as being awake at night if the child calls out and requires attention, or if the parents are in sufficiently close proximity to notice that the child is awake (e.g. if the child is in the same bed as the parents). Furthermore, there is some evidence from video recordings using an infra-red camera to suggest that at least at around 12 months some infants wake for brief periods and settle themselves back to sleep (Anders and Keener, 1985). Such occurrences are likely to be missed by many parents. However, it is also worth adding that checks between infra-red recordings and parental reports have typically shown a reasonably high degree of agreement (Anders and Sostek, 1976; Jacklin, Snow, Gahart and Maccoby, 1980).

EEG recordings have also been used to obtain information about sleep state, as it is possible to use these patterns to identify not only when a child is asleep or awake, but also to identify the different forms of sleeping. But again, one cannot assume that there is always a one-to-one mapping between EEG recordings and child behaviour, and there is the possibility that the very method of using electrodes may disrupt child behaviour. Similarly, infra-red video recordings can be useful, but because time lapse recordings are often made, these only provide an incomplete record of sleeping. Thus, it is important to be aware that there is no 'perfect' method of recording; all are likely to have some advantages as well as drawbacks and limitations.

A related issue to the description of children's sleeping is the issue of whether or not children have sleeping difficulties. There is no standard definition of what constitutes sleeping difficulties. A useful rule of thumb is that a child who is waking several times a night, and doing this several nights in a week can be considered to have sleeping difficulties. Other behaviours may also be problematic such as difficulties over bedtime or early waking, although these are often associated with night waking. This definition is based on the characteristics of infant behaviour. However, it is important to realize that similar infant behaviour can have different effects on parents. There are some parents who have a child waking every night of the week, but do not consider this to be a problem, while there are others who have a child waking once or twice a week and do consider this to be a problem. Thus, parental perceptions of what is normal and appropriate, and what impact it has on them, are both likely to influence their perception of whether or not their child has sleeping difficulties.

Effects of sleep on development and health

Surprisingly little information exists about the relation between sleeping patterns and other outcomes in children and parents. Furthermore, caution needs to be exercised when interpreting these correlational findings as the presence of a correlation does not necessarily indicate a causal relation.

Early sleeping difficulties in the first 18 months do not appear to be associated with other major behavioural problems (Zuckerman, Stevenson and Bailey, 1987; Pollock, 1992; Messer and Richards, 1993). Examination of the relationship between sleeping difficulties at eight months and problems at three-and-a-half years, failed to find many relations (Zuckerman, Stevenson and Bailey, 1987), although poor sleepers at the later age were more likely to have temper tantrums.

Pollock (1992) using a National Birth Cohort sample (of over 13,000 children) examined the relation between sleep patterns at five years and the parents' recall of earlier sleep in infancy. The sleep difficulties in infancy were related to various health problems at five years; these included admission to hospital, GP home visits and frequency of sore throats requiring medical attention. Children who had sleep difficulties were also found to score just *above* the mean on a vocabulary test. Furthermore, there was a small association between infant sleeping difficulties and reading ability at ten years. Pollock (1994) in a later and similar analysis on the same data, reports that parental perception of sleeping difficulties at five years was related to variables at ten years which indicate a sub-optimal outcome. These variables include: eczema, hay fever, abdominal pains, migraines, wheezing, seen GP and seen health visitor in last month, and temper tantrums. It should be borne in mind that at five years very few children were rated as having 'severe' sleeping problems (only 1.4 per cent), although 22.1 per cent were rated as having mild problems. As these were global ratings of parental perception rather than reports of wakings and other related behaviours, these relations may be coloured by parents already having general difficulties with the care of their children.

Thus, early sleeping difficulties have been found to be associated with later health problems. It is difficult to know whether this is a causal relation, whether children who are less healthy have both sleeping difficulties and more illness, or whether sub-optimal health is a cause of early sleep difficulties. An interesting feature of Pollock's findings is an association between sleeping difficulties and later vocabulary and reading. However, the effect was not a strong one and only may have been detected because of the large sample he was able to analyse.

Sleeping difficulties

Given the relatively high incidence of night wakings, what might be the cause? Answering this question is hampered by the fact that it is usually not possible to conduct experimental studies to identify causal relationships between variables and sleeping difficulties. Instead, researchers are usually limited to identifying those variables which are associated with sleeping difficulties (e.g. whether problems in labour are associated with later sleeping difficulties) and it should be remembered that an association does not establish causality. To complicate matters further, there may be an association because both variables are influenced by a common third factor (the infant's sleeping and maternal behaviour might be associated with difficulties in labour), or there may be an association because the sleeping difficulties give rise to an associated variable (e.g. sleeping difficulties might result in mothers using certain strategies).

A number of studies have identified variables associated with infant sleeping difficulties. In some of the reports the argument has been made that sleeping difficulties are the result of either infant or of maternal characteristics, and evidence can be marshalled in support of both positions. In one case the parents are absolved of any 'fault', in the other case 'fault' is attributed to them. Such arguments may be an oversimplification of a rather complex process by which infants influence and are influenced by maternal behaviour, and over time a system of behaviour in relation to sleeping evolves within a family (Messer and Richards, 1993). Bearing all this in mind we will review the variables that are related to sleeping difficulties under the following three headings: infant characteristics, caregiving and maternal characteristics and demographic variables.

Infant characteristics

Three forms of infant characteristic have received the most attention because of their potential causal relation with sleeping difficulties, they are: labour difficulties; birthweight and prematurity, and temperament.

Difficulties in delivery
Babies who experience more problematic deliveries seem to be at greater risk for later sleep difficulties. There are a range of characteristics which appear to increase this risk. Mild asphyxia at birth was found by Moore and Ucko (1957) to be related to a failure to sleep through the night at three months. Blurton-Jones, Rosetti Ferreira, Farquar Brown and McDonald (1978) and Richman (1985) both found that a sleep problem group contained more infants who had experienced problems in pregnancy, delivery and labour than control groups without sleeping difficulties. Pollock (1994) in an analysis of the national birth cohort reports that sleeping difficulties at five years

are more likely if there was an admission to hospital during pregnancy, and there had been forceps or vacuum extraction.

Birthweight and prematurity
In babies who are not considered to be of low birthweight, there does not seem to be a relation between their birthweight and later sleeping problems (Moore and Ucko, 1957; Grunwaldt, Bates and Guthrie, 1960). However, Pollock (1994) found a slight effect of having a birthweight between 2992 and 3445 grams which was associated with later sleeping difficulties. A comparison of sleep patterns between premature babies and those born at term by Anders and Keener (1985) failed to detect any major differences during the first year in a study that used infra-red cameras. Similarly, a large scale study by Wolke, Meyer, Ohrt and Riegel (1995) failed to detect any major differences between pre-term infants and full-term infants who were matched for birthweight, indeed the pre-term infants had slightly better sleeping at 5 months, and there was no difference at 20 and 56 months of age.

Temperament
There has been controversy about whether it is possible to identify different forms of temperament in infancy. In relation to sleeping difficulties there has been interest in the possibility that difficult temperament in infancy is associated with problems in going back to sleep and soothability. Carey (1974) found that a group with sleeping difficulties at 6 months had a lower threshold of sensitivity on the Thomas and Chess temperament questionnaire filled in by the mother. This suggests that the group of infants with sleeping difficulties were more easy to arouse and disturb. Weissbluth (1981) employed the Carey temperament questionnaire, which is based on maternal report. Analysis revealed that the infants' mood, rhythmicity, adaptability, and approach-withdrawal were related to the duration of sleeping, and that infants classified as having a difficult temperament slept less (i.e. these infants were regarded as more difficult to sooth and quieten, and to be more irritable, etc.). Other studies have also found similar relations. However, there is a problem in knowing whether the infants with a difficult temperament are more likely to have sleeping difficulties, or whether sleeping difficulties influence maternal perceptions so that these infants are perceived as being more difficult, more irritable, and more difficult to soothe.

Caregiving and maternal characteristics

Which caregiving and maternal characteristics are associated with sleeping difficulties? This section first examines birth order, then feeding, and lastly weaning and co-sleeping.

Birth order
It is often expected that first borns should be more likely to have sleeping difficulties than later borns. This is because parents of later borns will have greater experience of managing sleeping. Admittedly, there are some studies which report a higher rate of sleeping difficulties in first borns (Moore and Ucko, 1957; Richman, 1985). An analysis of the national cohort study of over 13,000 children by Pollock at five years revealed that there was a slightly

higher likelihood of first-time parents rating their children as having sleeping difficulties. However, there are also a number of studies which have failed to detect this effect (Grunwaldt, Bates and Guthrie, 1960; Zuckerman, Stevenson and Bailey, 1987; Bernal, 1973). It is also of interest that no effect of parity was detected in two studies using automatic recording devices (Thoman and Whitney, 1989; Anders and Keener 1985). This raises the possibility that parity differences that have been detected could be a product of parental concern and awareness of changes in sleeping rather than any difference in objective behaviour.

Feeding
Breastfeeding brings many benefits to infant and child, but it is associated with a slightly higher incidence of night waking (see also Chapter 8). Mothers who bottlefeed are able to stop feeding in the early hours of the morning at an earlier age than those who are breastfeeding (10 weeks compared to 16 weeks; Wright, Fawcett and Crow, 1980; Wright, Mcleod and Cooper, 1983). This may be due to there being shorter durations of sleep periods in breastfed infants. In addition, Wright (1993) comments that bottlefed infants are introduced to solids at an earlier age than breastfed infants. This he attributes to bottlefed infants starting to wake again at 3–4 months, after sleeping through the night, and the mothers perceiving hunger to be the cause of this waking. Interpreting these associations between feeding and sleeping is complicated by the association between breastfeeding and other caregiving characteristics.

These patterns appear to continue. At five months more breastfed than bottlefed babies are reported as waking at least four times a week (52 per cent compared to 20 per cent; Carey, 1975; see also Wailoo, Peterson and Whittaker, 1990). Even more extreme figures have been reported by Wolke et al. (in press) in their Bavarian sample. About 45 per cent of five month infants who were breastfed (full or partial) were waking five or more nights a week, while 18 per cent of the mothers who had changed to bottlefeeding reported this, whilst only 8 per cent of those who had bottlefed their infant from birth reported night waking. This was interpreted as being due to breastfed infants becoming used to a more responsive routine than bottlefed babies. Zuckerman, Stevenson and Bailey found a similar direction of effect at eight months, although the difference was not quite as large (32 per cent compared to 15 per cent). Even in nursery school children Wright, McLeod and Cooper (1983) found that breastfeeding during infancy was associated with sleeping difficulties at the older age. An exception to this general pattern of findings comes from a study conducted in the 1970s which examined sleeping in a small sample at 14 months and found no difference in the sleeping of infants who have been breast- or bottlefed (Bernal, 1973).

There is evidence that the content of milk might effect sleeping patterns. An experimental study by Yogman and Zeisel (1983) manipulated the amount of tryptophan and valine in bottlefed babies in their last feed of the day. If more tryptophan is available then this increases the levels of serotonin in the brain, and studies have shown both substances influence sleep patterns in adults. Furthermore, it is known that there are quite large naturally occurring variations in the levels of tryptophan in mothers' breast milk. The infants who were given tryptophan and glucose went to sleep more quickly than infants given formula milk, although there was no difference in the total amount of sleep. Infants given valine, which reduced the uptake of tryptophan, took longer to fall asleep than those given formula milk. Thus, the composition of milk can influence settling, but it is unclear whether levels of tryptophan influence night waking.

An investigation of allergies to cows' milk suggests that for some infants this is a factor in night disturbances. Kahn, Mazin, Rebuffet et al. (1989) eliminated dairy products from the diet of children who had failed to show any improvement after a behavioural management treatment programme (see below). The infants showed improvement and a later 'challenge' by the re-introduction of cows' milk led to a return to sleeping difficulties. Consequently, it may be that for a minority of children, dietary problems could be responsible for sleeping difficulties.

Weaning and co-sleeping

It is sometimes thought that the early introduction of solids might help with sleeping as infants would not be woken by nutritional needs (Reisman, 1958; Wright, McLeod and Cooper, 1983), this also seems to be a common perception among parents. Despite such suggestions several studies have failed to find support for this claim. No relationship was found between the age at which solids are introduced and the age of sleeping through the night by Moore and Ucko (1957), Grunwaldt, Bates and Guthrie (1960) and Parmelee, Wenner and Shulz (1964).

Elias, Nicolson, Bora and Johnston (1986) have questioned whether the findings from these studies can be applied to more recent feeding practices. They argue that infants who are weaned later are more likely to wake at night. The basis for this argument was a study of mothers who were members of La Leche League (LLL), and a comparison group of 'typical' mothers. The League promotes close physical contact between mother and infant and a delay in weaning. Data was collected until the infants were 24 months old. The mothers in the LLL (except one) continued breastfeeding until 24 months, while in the comparison group the average age of the termination of breastfeeding was 13 months. In addition, mothers in the LLL were significantly more likely to share their bed with their infant (co-sleep) than mothers in the comparison group. Were there differences in infant sleeping? Overall the infants in the comparison group appeared to sleep better. In the comparison group, the longest duration of sleep was 8 hours at four months of age; the infants whose mothers were in the LLL did not achieve this until 24 months and often were sleeping for less than 4 hours at a time. Further analysis indicated that weaned infants slept for longer that nursing infants, although it should be remembered this might have been confounded by co-sleeping and group status.

The issue of co-sleeping also has been examined by Lozoff, Wolf and Davis (1984). They note that while most advice to North American parents counsels against co-sleeping, in practice an appreciable number of parents and infants sleep in this way. They found that nearly a third of white mothers and nearly three-quarters of black mothers routinely shared their bed with their infants. Co-sleeping in both groups was associated with a caregiving style that involved the infant falling asleep when they were not in their bed, when an adult was present, and when there was bodily contact with a caregiver.

In the white families, co-sleeping was linked to more bedtime struggles (these were defined as at least three a week; 47 per cent of the co-sleeping sample had these, 14 per cent of the no co-sleeping group had these), and a higher percentage waking three or more nights per week occurred in the co-sleeping group (55 per cent and 23 per cent respectively). Interestingly, 29 per cent of all co-sleeping parents rated their children's wakings as disruptive, while 10 per cent of all non-sleeping parents rated their children as being disruptive. Thus, a significant number of white parents who engaged in co-sleeping found this had negative consequences for their own sleep.

A different pattern was present in black families. Here there was no significant difference in bedtime struggles (19 per cent and 22 per cent respectively), but there were more children who woke three or more times a week in the co-sleeping group (48 per cent) than in the non-co-sleeping group (11 per cent). In relation to these figures of waking three or more times a week, it is interesting that few of the black co-sleeping mothers described their child's wakings as disruptive (10 per cent of the whole co-sleeping sample used this description), while all of the non-co-sleeping mothers described these wakings as disruptive. Thus, more co-sleeping occurred in black families, but only a relatively small proportion of mothers reported that this produced what they regarded as disruptive behaviour. In contrast, the black mothers who did not co-sleep found night wakings more disruptive.

These are complicated findings. They suggest that although co-sleeping appears to be associated with more night wakings, this is not always regarded as being disruptive by the mother. The most problematic group in Lozoff, Wolf and Davis's sample were the white co-sleeping mothers; 29 per cent of them found their child's behaviour disruptive. An explanation for this is that co-sleeping has different meanings and associations in the two groups. For whites, co-sleeping was only practised by a minority who tend to be less well educated and of lower SES; these may be a more vulnerable group. In contrast, co-sleeping was the majority activity in the black sample and is likely to be a more accepted practice. It may also be that the black families have strategies which minimize the disruptions of co-sleeping, and that these strategies are absent in white families.

In relation to this, our own research suggests that co-sleeping is not simply a response to having to deal with sleep problems. In a sample of English mothers those who said they were likely to co-sleep before the birth of their baby were more likely to co-sleep with their infant. Furthermore, plans about co-sleeping and the actual practice of co-sleeping were related to more night waking at 17 months. In addition, it is interesting that Wolke, Meyer, Ohrt and Riegel (1995) in a study of Bavarian families found that at 56 months about a quarter reported that the child slept in their bed at some point during the night, and overall about 7 per cent of families reported problems with their child's sleeping. These latter figures suggest that for some families co-sleeping may be an acceptable strategy in dealing with child waking.

In other cultures co-sleeping is an accepted practice. In the Kipsigis of Kenya, infants sleep with their mother and suckle when they wake in the night (Super and Harkness, 1982). Interestingly, in comparison to North American babies studied by Parmelee, Wenner and Shulz (1964), the

Kipsigis infants, at 16 weeks, slept significantly less and had a shorter maximum sleep length (4 hours versus 8 hours). In Japan the traditional practice is for the whole family to sleep together and the incidence of sleeping problems is reportedly low (Nugent, 1994).

The issues of feeding, weaning and co-sleeping appear to be closely intertwined and it is notable that advice about co-sleeping often arouses strong feelings in mothers and professionals. It can be argued that breastfeeding and co-sleeping are often related because the process of breastfeeding is long, so that sharing a bed allows the mother to rest in comfort, and it may also be the case that mothers who breastfeed desire a more intimate and physical relation with their child which predisposes them to co-sleep. Furthermore, Carey may be correct in suggesting that breastfeeding sets up expectations in babies which make them more likely to demand a response when waking at night, and breastfeeding may simply be more rewarding than bottlefeeding. It is also possible that these factors make weaning more difficult, especially if breastfeeding is a quick and reliable way settle infants back to sleep.

As has just been mentioned, arguments against co-sleeping often generate strong feelings. Arguments for co-sleeping are often made on the basis that it is a more natural arrangement as well as providing greater responsiveness and security for infants. However, it is also important to place the issue of co-sleeping in relation to the wishes of parents and the culture in which we live. If the lives of parents are so demanding that they have difficulty functioning with frequent night wakings and disturbances then clearly something has to give somewhere in the organization of their lives. It might be argued that in western culture what has 'give' are childcare practices such as co-sleeping which can disturb parental sleep. This in turn can affect day time functioning with the consequences being clearly apparent when both parents are employed. Consequently, there may have grown a tendency for parents in western cultures to want children to sleep alone in their own rooms, and for night time disturbances to be seen as a 'problem' rather than a natural occurrence. Those that argue for co-sleeping are identifying what they see as a valuable part of parenting and attempting to reverse a trend present in our cultural practice. Thus, what is important is to recognize that there is no right or wrong way to make sleeping arrangements, but rather parents should be given the information to make decisions for themselves, and to recognize that issues about childrearing are not ones of right and wrong, but of what we value and what we are prepared to accept in the way of consequences.

Demographic variables

Many child characteristics are related to SES, parity and gender. None of these three variables show a consistent and powerful relation to sleeping difficulties, as can be seen from the following material.

Socio-economic status

A number of investigations have failed to detect a relation between SES and sleeping difficulties in prospective samples (e.g. Moore and Ucko, 1957; Bernal, 1973). Nor was this association found in the national childbirth cohorts where the large sample should enable even small effects to be detected (Butler and Golding, 1986; Pollock, 1994). Neither is there strong evidence, from a comparison of children with sleeping difficulties and those without difficulties, that there are differences according to SES, home ownership, age of the mother or overcrowding (Zuckerman, Stevenson and Bailey, 1987).

However, Scott and Richards (1989) have reported that dissatisfaction with housing and overcrowding (the number of bedrooms divided by the number of children and adults in a dwelling) were both related to sleeping difficulties. Pollock (1994) in the national birth cohort sample finds a similar effect of crowding (person per room in home). Analysis of our own data has also provided similar findings (Messer and Parker, 1995). Furthermore, we found that overcrowding was related to certain plans the mothers had about the way to deal with sleeping. Before the birth mothers who had a higher level of overcrowding reported that they were more prepared to take the future baby into their bed, and were more prepared to do this to help them go to sleep at night. These patterns may not be a simple effect of overcrowding leading mothers to use strategies to avoid waking other individuals, but of overcrowding leading to changes in the mothers' pre-natal perceptions, which also contribute to both plans and later behaviour.

A related issue to SES is that there appear to be differences between cultures in the incidence of sleeping difficulties. Zuckerman, Stevenson and Bailey (1987) in a study of different ethnic groups in Britain found equivalent percentages of sleeping difficulties in white mothers and mothers originating from Asia (16 per cent and 17 per cent respectively), while mothers of Afro-Caribbean origin reported a much higher rate (46 per cent). Pollock (1994) also reports similar findings with there being an elevated rate for mothers born in the West Indies and Africa.

Sex of infant
For many disorders in early childhood boys are more vunerable than girls. Therefore it is surprising that this does not seem to be the case for sleeping difficulties. The lack of differences according to the sex of the infant has been reported in a number of investigations (Moore and Ucko, 1957; Bernal, 1973; Jacklin, Snow, Gahart and Maccoby, 1980; Zuckerman, Stevenson and Bailey, 1987). Nor have studies using automatic recording devices detected any differences (Thoman and Whitney, 1989; Anders, Keener and Kraemer, 1985).

Summary

It can be seen that there are a range of variables associated with sleeping difficulties. Somewhat surprisingly birth order does not appear to be strongly related to sleeping difficulties. In contrast, it is clear that breastfeeding carries a higher risk for sleeping problems. The issues related to weaning and co-sleeping are complex, but there are suggestions that later weaning and co-sleeping are both related to a higher frequency of night waking. Furthermore, the evidence points to the causes of sleeping difficulties not being the 'fault' of the mother or of the infant. Instead the evidence suggests that both may contribute to this pattern. If maternal experience was an important factor one would expect later borns to sleep much better than first borns; the lack of this effect suggests that infant characteristics have an important role in determining the pattern of sleeping. Similarly, the associations between birth experiences and sleeping difficulties suggest a role for infant characteristics. However, it is also true that pre-natal plans and features of caregiving like breastfeeding are also related to sleeping difficulties. As Messer and Richards (1993) have argued, sleeping difficulties are likely to be due to a complex interplay between infant and maternal characteristics, and these are in turn influenced by environmental and demographic factors.

Advice and intervention

An implication of the material that already has been presented is that if infant sleeping was an easy matter to deal with, then there would not be a need for this chapter or such an interest in the topic. Thus, it is important to bear in mind that sleeping difficulties are probably the result of complex processes which are not usually solved in a single short intervention. If they were then one would expect a much lower incidence of sleeping difficulties.

Sedatives can be used to influence the sleeping of infants. In the past these have sometimes been thought of as a useful form of treatment. The logic is that if one can change the pattern of sleeping then infants may continue with the improved pattern when the drugs are no longer administered. Ousted and Hendrick in 1977 reported that by 18 months a quarter of the first borns in their sample had been given sedatives because of sleeping difficulties. Three years later, Chavin and Tinson (1980) reported that nearly three-quarters of infants who had sleeping difficulties in their sample had been given drugs at some time. Although drugs were widely used, controlled investigations have generally revealed that although sleeping improves while the drug is being administered, sleeping difficulties re-emerge when the drug is no longer administered. This pattern was shown in a study by Richman (1985). A double blind procedure was used to study the effects over two weeks of administering trimeprazine tartrate in comparison to a placebo. The infants who were administered the drug fell asleep more quickly and were less likely to wake at night, and there was a lower rate of night waking during treatment than during a baseline period (3.7 against 5.2 times a week). However, Richman noted that although improvements were made, night waking had not been eliminated. Furthermore, a six-month follow-up showed no difference in sleeping in comparison to the pre-treatment baseline. Similar findings have been presented by Simonoff and Stores (1987).

Thus, sedatives and other drugs do not appear to have long term impact on sleeping difficulties. This is now recognized and consequently the use of such drugs is much lower. There are, however, arguments that sedatives may be useful in cases where there is a short term crisis where the parents need respite in the form of better sleep (Douglas and Richman, 1982), but without other procedures there are unlikely to be any long term benefits from the use of sedatives.

The behavioural management approach

As the limitations of drug based approaches became apparent the application of behavioural management techniques became increasingly popular. The behavioural management approach uses the principles of learning theory to attempt to modify behaviour. The approach involves a careful analysis of the cause of the problem and then realistic advice, using learning principles, to remove the reinforcing consequences of the problem behaviour or set up new associations which will mean that parental intervention is less likely to be required.

One core assumption of the behavioural management approach is that sleeping difficulties usually stem from the inability of children to settle themselves to sleep (Douglas and Richman, 1982). This basic difficulty is the reason why some children need help both to go to sleep at bedtime and when they wake in the night. Furthermore, it is assumed that the sleeping difficulties are maintained if not caused by the actions of the parent. Consequently, the therapy requires a full and accurate description of the sleeping patterns of the infant and the behaviour of the parents in relation to this behaviour. This is designed to identify the consequences of the child's sleeping difficulties. Often the parents are asked to fill out a sleep diary so that there is a precise written record of what is happening.

There are several techniques which are used in behavioural management programmes; the main ones are fading, extinction and the use of association. Fading involves promoting a gradual change in the target behaviour by gradually removing a stimulus which is associated with the behaviour. This may involve processes such as a parent gradually physically distancing themselves from the child so that they are no longer required to be present for the child to fall asleep. Thus, an adult may first sit with the child, then move a chair gradually away from the child, until eventually they are sitting outside the bedroom. Another technique is to start bedtime routines at a late time in the evening when the infant may be more responsive to settling themselves to sleep, and then gradually move the bedtime forward. The advantage of these types of strategies is that confrontations with the infant are minimized; however, such strategies can take several months in which the adults have to be both patient and motivated to complete the programme.

In contrast with fading the use of extinction can be relatively rapid. Extinction is a technical term which refers to circumstances when rewards are no longer given when a target behaviour is produced; in such circumstances there is a reduction and eventually cessation of the target behaviour. For infants it is supposed that the effects of primary reinforcements such as feeding are due to their physiological properties in satisfying primary drives (e.g. hunger). There are also secondary reinforcements, such as attention and social responses, which are supposed to be acquired by their association with primary reinforcements (although some might now dispute this claim).

The use of extinction in relation to sleeping difficulties involves parents no longer responding when their child cries out at night, the rewarding effects of parental attention thereby being removed. In such circumstances children can become very upset with long periods of crying and distress. Sometimes it is recommended that parents go to see their child every 5 minutes to reassure themselves about the child; however, such visits should not involve social interaction as this will only serve as a reinforcement. Parents and professionals are divided about the use of extinction techniques. Some parents feel that they are not able to listen to the distress of their infants for long periods, while others who find the procedure difficult are never the less glad to achieve an improvement in sleeping by the use of the technique over a few days or weeks. When using this technique it is essential that parents appreciate that if they decide to abandon it, then their behaviour will only have served to reinforce the child's behaviour. An infant who has found that if he or she cries for long enough will eventually receive a reinforcing response, is likely to be more motivated to continue crying.

Other group of techniques commonly employed by therapists using the behavioural management approach involves the strengthening or altering of the cues which are associated with going to sleep. When sleeping difficulties occur the parents usually provide a cue which helps the infant fall asleep. By introducing other cues it is possible to help the child to fall asleep without the assistance from adults. One obvious way to achieve this is to try to help the child associate sleeping with the place they sleep at night. To do this it is sometimes recommended that children should be put in their bed when they are about to go to sleep for their day time nap. In cases where there are difficulties at bedtime it is usually recommended that a consistent routine be adopted so that this provides a set of cues which prime an infant about sleeping.

Reinforcement by the use of external rewards is usually only effective in children who have a language age of about three years or above. This is because of the need to verbally explain the process to the children. Reinforcement often involves star charts or similar devices to reward positive behaviour. The scheme should be organized so that the child is rewarded for doing something (i.e. staying in bed) rather than not doing something (i.e. not getting up). Such schemes can often be effective especially if this is accompanied by explanations of the parents' needs.

The effectiveness of the behavioural management approach

Sometimes the behavioural management approach appears to be merely common sense. However, as we will see these techniques are not always effective and it is possible to underestimate the skills needed to identify the causes of the sleeping difficulties, the appropriate remedies, and the support that is needed to sustain the parents' motivation. Further, it should be appreciated that the behavioural management approach does not involve a set of mechanical instructions which are automatically given in relation to the infant's and parent's behaviour.

What do investigations of these treatment techniques show? Two of the more successful studies have been conducted by Richman (1985) and by Seymour and his colleagues (Seymour, Bayfield, Brock and During, 1983; Seymour, Brock, During and Poole, 1989). Richman reports a high rate of success (90 per cent) in one to four year olds who entered a six-month intervention programme. However, there was a high drop-out rate from the study, which if taken into account reduces the overall success rate. The programme consisted of six sessions where there was a diagnosis of the cause of the problem on the basis of the content of sleep diaries and then an agreed programme designed to modify the child's behaviour. Success was considered to involve a marked improvement or a complete improvement as judged by two of the therapists from the sleep diaries and parental reports.

An analysis of the effects of therapy on 208 families seen over 12 years was carried out by Seymour, Bayfield, Brock and During (1983). The children were under six years of age with most being under three years. The programme began with an analysis of the sleep patterns of the child. In the intervention condition the role of the parents in being able to effect a change was emphasized, as was the reinforcing nature of some parental behaviours, and the need for routines. It was recommended that parents only stayed briefly with their child after settling them down for the night, to ignore night time crying, and if it was necessary to return the child to his or her bed with the minimum of interaction. The parents were given written instruction and initially daily telephone calls were made to offer support and advice. The use of extinction was defended by Seymour, Bayfield, Brock and During (1983) as providing greater overall psychological gains to the families than losses. A decline of night wakings from four nights a week before treatment had begun, to one night a week one month after the beginning of treatment was achieved. Seven per cent of families did not continue with the programme.

A later study by Seymour, Brock, During and Poole (1989) found that a group given written instructions improved to a similar extent to a group who had intervention sessions with a therapist, whilst a waiting-list control group failed to show significant improvement. The group given written instructions were given details about the way to implement a behavioural management programme. The therapist used a behavioural management programme to advise the parents with follow-up telephone calls. The written instruction group improved from 12 wakings per week to 5, and the comparable figures for the therapist programme were 16 and 7. The implications from the study is that some improvements can be made by parents with very little assistance; however, it should be noted that all groups were still showing some sleeping difficulties. Furthermore, another study, in which non-directive written information was provided to mothers of infants under a year old was not found to be effective in reducing sleeping difficulties (Scott and Richards, 1989).

In contrast, other investigations of behavioural management techniques indicate that such interventions are not always effective. In studies which have used control groups there has not always been a difference between the intervention and comparison group (Weir and Dinnick, 1988; Messer and Richards, 1993; but see Seymour, Bayfield, Brock and During, 1989). Furthermore, many studies have reported a success rate of about 50 per cent (Weir and Dinnick, 1988; Chavin and Tinson, 1980; Jones and Verduyn, 1983; Messer and Richards, 1993; but see Seymour, Brock, During and Poole, 1983 and Richman, 1985; the studies are described above). Although 50 per cent improvement may appear like a reasonable rate of success, it would appear on closer scrutiny that one can expect about half of the children in a sample to improve, without any intervention. Such a rate has been reported in longitudinal studies which have been interested in examining the rates of sleeping problems over various age ranges (e.g. Jenkins, Owen, Bax and Hart, 1984; Zuckerman, Stevenson and Bailey, 1987; Wolke, Meyer, Ohrt and Riegel, 1995) and this rate has been found in control groups (Weir and Dinnick, 1988; Messer and Richards, 1983). What seems to be happening in the longitudinal studies without any intervention, is that there is a reasonable rate of improvement, which is balanced by a similar or slightly fewer number of children developing sleeping problems. This explains why the incidence of sleeping difficulties remains fairly static over the first few years.

Because of these issues it is worth examining studies which fail to find a positive effect in more detail. Sanger, Weir and Churchill (1981) involved health visitors in an intervention programme, where the precise therapy was discussed with a child psychiatrist before it was implemented. The therapy involved collecting information about the sleeping difficulties and then using the techniques of extinction, reinforcement, shaping, cueing and fading. After four months it was found that 9 out of 16 children had shown 'much improvement', with 5 children showing little or no improvement. Another study involving health visitors was conducted by Weir and Dinnock (1988). After the collection of details about the sleep patterns, these were discussed by a group of professionals and an intervention programme was identified. A comparison group was identified who received no treatment but 'normal' advice from their health visitor. Both treatment and comparison groups showed improvement over a six-month period, with 62 per cent of the treatment group having a mild or no problem at the end of 6 months; the comparable figure for the comparison group was 42 per cent. Despite the difference in percentages there was no significant difference between the two groups. A similar finding was resorted in a study of group treatment of sleeping difficulties (Messer and Richards, 1993).

Both the treatment and a waiting list control group showed a significant improvement with about half of the children in each group sleeping better at the end of a 4–6 week period. Jones and Verduyn (1983) assessed an intervention programme which involved a careful analysis of the difficulties, identification of joint goals, and the gradual movement towards these goals. There were usually about five or six sessions every two weeks. At the end of treatment 53 per cent of the 19 children in their programme showed complete success and 37 per cent showed a partial resolution.

Summary

There is some uncertainty about the success of intervention programmes using behavioural management techniques. Although some studies report significant gains (e.g. Richman, 1985; Seymour et al., 1989), other do not. Such differences can be attributed to the skill and experience of therapists, but such possibilities are difficult to investigate.

Psychoanalytic interventions

Interestingly Daws (1985a, b) using a psychoanalytic perspective has employed similar techniques to those described in the behavioural management approach. The difference between the approaches is the way the problem is viewed. The behavioural management approach assumes that it is the responses of the parents which maintain the sleeping difficulties. In contrast, the psychoanalytic perspectives tend to assume that the difficulties are the result of a failure to resolve issues about the relationship between the infant and parents. Daws regards the main problematic issue for infant and mother as one of separation. Therapy is designed to make both individuals better able to deal with separation and so the infant is able to fall asleep by themselves. The intervention is designed to help the mother understand why the issue of separation is important for them, and gives advice about ways to distance herself from her infant. Here techniques such as fading and the development of routines are suggested.

Conclusions

Children who wake at night or exhibit other difficulties related to sleeping routines can have a profound impact on their parents. Furthermore, between a fifth and a third of parents of preschool children report such difficulties. All babies wake frequently at night during the first three months, but between four and five months the majority of babies change their sleep pattern and sleep for most of the night. The infants who fail to achieve this are likely to continue to have problems with sleeping during the preschool years. The causes of sleeping difficulties are still not yet well understood, but it seems likely that they are caused by an interplay between infant, parental and environmental characteristics, all of which are associated with sleeping difficulties. The behavioural management approach is the most popular form of treatment; however, evaluations of this method have not been uniformly successful. Thus, although children's sleeping is very important for many parents, the limited nature of the research that has been conducted means that there are still many more uncertainties about the causes and the best methods of treatment than is desirable.

Applications

1. Use of sedatives
These only seem to be effective in the short term in helping children get to sleep more quickly and reducing the amount of night waking. Research indicates that there are little or no long term benefits in terms of changed sleeping patterns.

2. Behavioural management approach
This is the most popular current approach. For this approach to be successful there needs to be a careful collection of information, usually obtained through the use of a sleep diary. The therapist then needs to use a problem solving approach to the difficulty, using the techniques of extinction, shaping, cueing and reinforcement. It is easy to obtain the impression that this technique is effective; however, there are a number of studies which have reported that control groups make as good progress as treatment groups.

3. Alternative methods
The psychoanalytic approach offers a different perspective about sleeping difficulties, but many of the techniques are similar to those employed in behavioural management. There do not appear to have been any formal evaluations of this approach. Other techniques are sometimes suggested such as relaxation, aromatherapy and altering the diet of the child. As with the psychoanalytic technique there do not appear to be any research evaluations of these approaches.

Acknowledgement

Funding from Wellbeing and the NHS Research and Development Directorate assisted the writing of this chapter.

References

Anders, T. F. and Keener, M. A. (1985). Developmental course of nighttime sleep-wake patterns in full-term and premature infants during the first year of life. I. *Sleep*, **8** (3), 173–92.

Anders, T. F., Keener, M. A. and Kraemer, H. (1985). Sleep-wake state organisation neonatal assessment and development in premature infants during the first year of life. II. *Sleep*, **8** (3), 193–206.

Anders, T. F. and Sostek, A. (1976). The use of time-lapse videorecording of sleep-wake behaviors in human infants. *Psychophysiology*, **13**, 155–8.

Beltramini, A. U. and Hertzig, M. E. (1983). Sleep and bedtime behavior in preschool-aged children. *Pediatrics*, **71** (2), 153–8.

Bernal, J. (1973). Night waking in infants during the first 14 months. *Developmental Medicine and Child Neurology*, **14**, 362–72.

Blurton-Jones, N., Rosetti Ferreira, M. C., Farquar Brown, M. and McDonald, L. (1978). The association between perinatal factors and later night waking. *Developmental Medicine and Child Neurology*, **20**, 427–34.

Butler, N. R. and Golding, J. (eds) (1986). *From Birth to Five*. Oxford: Pergamon.

Carey, W. B. (1974). Night waking and temperament in infancy. *Behavioral Pediatrics*, **84**, 756–8.

Carey, W. B. (1985). Temperament and increased weight gain. *Developmental and Behavioral Pediatrics*, **6**, 128–31.

Chavin, W. and Tinson, S. (1980). Children with sleep difficulties. *Health Visitor*, **53**, 477–80.

Daws, D. (1985a). Sleep problems in babies and young children. *Journal of Child Psychotherapy*, **11**, 87–95.

Daws, D. (1985b). *Through the Night: Helping Parents and Sleepless Infants*. London: Free Association Books.

Douglas, J. and Richman, N. (1982). *Sleep Management Manual*. Institute of Child Health, revised 1985.

Elias, M. F., Nicolson, N. A., Bora, C. and Johnston, J. (1986). Sleep/wake patterns of breast-fed infants in the first 2 years of life. *Pediatrics*, **77**, 322–9.

Ferber, R.(1987). Sleeplessness, night awakening, and night crying in the infant and toddler. *Pediatrics in Review*, **9**, 69–82.

Grunwaldt, M. D., Bates, T. and Guthrie, D. (1960). The onset of sleeping through the night in infancy. *Pediatrics*, **26**, 667–8.

Jacklin, C. N., Snow, M. E., Gahart, M. and Maccoby, E. E. (1980). Sleep pattern development from 6 through 33 months. *Journal of Pediatric Psychology*, **5**, 295–303.

Jenkins, S., Owen, C., Bax, M. and Hart, H. (1984). Continuities of common behaviour problems in preschool children. *Journal of Child Psychology and Psychiatry*, **25**, 75–89.

Jones, D. P. H. and Verduyn, C. M. (1983). Behavioural management of sleep problems. *Archives of Disease in Childhood*, **58**, 442–4.

Kahn, A., Mazin, M. J., Rebuffet, E., Sottiaux, M. and Muller, M. F. (1989). Milk intolerance in children with persistent sleeplessness. *Pediatrics*, **84**, 595–603.

Lozoff, B., Wolf, A. W. and Davis, N. S. (1984). Cosleeping in urban families with young children in the United States. *Pediatrics*, **72**, 171–82.

Messer, D. J. (1993). The treatment of sleeping difficulties. In *Infant Crying, Feeding and Sleeping* (I. St-James-Roberts, G. Harris and D. Messer, eds). Hemel Hempstead: Harvester Wheatsheaf.

Messer, D. J. and Richards, M. P. M. (1993). The development of sleeping difficulties. In *Infant Crying, Feeding and Sleeping* (I. St-James-Roberts, G. Harris and D. Messer, eds). Hemel Hempstead: Harvester Wheatsheaf.

Messer, D. J., Lauder, L. and Humphrey, S. (1994). The effectiveness of group therapy in treating children's sleeping problems. *Child: Care, Health and Development*, **20**, 267–77.

Messer, D. J. and Parker, C. (1995). Infant sleep patterns and maternal responses. Paper presented at the Society for Reproductive and Infant Psychology, Leicester.

Moore, T. and Ucko, L. E. (1957). Night waking in early infancy. *Archives of Disease in Childhood*, **32**, 333–42.

Nugent, K. (1994). The sleep environment of Japanese and US infants. Paper presented at the Society for Reproductive and Infant Psychology, Dublin.

Ousted, M. K. and Hendrick, A. M. (1977). The first-born child: patterns of development. *Developmental Medicine and Child Neurology*, **19**, 446–53.

Parmelee, A. H. (Jr), Wenner, W. A. and Schulz, H. R. (1964). Infant sleep patterns: from birth to 16 weeks of age. *Journal of Pediatrics*, **65**, 576–82.

Pollock, J. I. (1992). Predictors and longterm associations of reported sleeping difficulties in infancy. *Journal of Reproductive and Infant Psychology*, **10**, 151–68.

Pollock, J. (1994). Night waking at 5 years of age: predictors and prognosis. *Journal of Child Psychology and Psychiatry*, **35**, 699–708.

Reisman, M. C. (1958). Feeding of solid foods to infants. *Pediatrics*, **22**, 604–5.

Richman, N. (1985). A double-blind drug trial of treatment in young children with waking problems. *Journal of Child Psychology and Psychiatry*, **26**, 591–8.

Sanger, S., Weir, K. and Churchill, E. (1981). Treatment of sleep problems: the use of behavioural modification techniques by health visitors. *Health Visitor*, **54**, 421–2.

Scott, G. and Richards, M. P. M. (1989). Night waking in infants: effects of providing advice and supports for parents. *Journal of Child Psychology and Psychiatry*, **31**, 551–69.

Seymour, F. W., Bayfield, G., Brock, P. and During, M. (1983). Management of night-waking in young children. *Australian Journal of Family Therapy*, **4**, 217–23.

Seymour, F. W., Brock, P., During, M. and Poole, G. (1989). Reducing sleep disruptions in young children: evaluation of therapist-guided and written information approaches: a brief report. *Journal of Child Psychology and Psychiatry*, **30**, 913–18.

Simonoff, E. A. and Stores, G. (1987). Controlled trial of trimeprazine tartrate for night waking. *Archives of Disease in Childhood*, **62**, 253–7.

Super, C. M. and Harkness, S. (1982). The infant's niche in rural Kenya and Metropolitan America. In *Cross-cultural Research at Issue* (L. C. Adler, ed.). New York: Academic.

Thoman, E. B. and Whitney, M. P. (1989). Sleep states of infants monitored in the home: individual differences, developmental trends, and origins of diurnal cyclicity. *Infant Behaviour and Development*, **12**, 59–75.

Wailoo, M. P., Peterson, S. A. and Whittaker, H. (1990). Disturbed nights and 3–4 month old infants: the effects of feeding and thermal environment. *Archives of Disease in Childhood*, **65**, 499–501.

Weir, X. and Dinnick, I. K. (1988). Behavioural modification in the treatment of sleep problems occurring in young children: a controlled trial using health visitors as therapists. *Child: Care, Health and Development*, **14**, 355–67.

Weissbluth, M. (1981), Brief clinical and laboratory observations. Sleep duration and infant temperament. *Journal of Pediatrics*, **99**, 817–19.

Wolke, D., Meyer, R., Ohrt, B. and Riegel, K. (1995). The incidence of sleeping problems in preterm and fullterm infants discharged from neonatal special care units: an epidemiological longitudinal study. *Journal of Child Psychology and Psychiatry*, **36**, 203–23.

Wright, P., Fawcett, J. and Crow, R. (1980). The development of differences in the feeding behaviour of bottle and breast fed human infants from birth to two months. *Behaviour Processes*, **5**, 1–20.

Wright, P., McLeod, H. A. and Cooper, M. J. (1983). Waking at night: the effect of early feeding experiences. *Child: Care, Health and Development*, **9**, 309–19.

Yogman, M. and Zeisel, S. H. (1983). Diet and sleep patterns in newborn infants. *New England Journal of Medicine*, **309**, 1147–9.

Zuckerman, B., Stevenson, J. and Bailey, V. (1987). Sleep problems in early childhood: continuities, predictive factors, and behavioral correlates. *Pediatrics*, **80**, 664–71.

12

Pain in neonates

Sheila Glenn, Rhoda Martin and Maureen F. Horgan

Can newborn babies feel pain? In this chapter, Sheila Glenn, Rhoda Martin and Maureen Horgan review the evidence which suggests that, although babies can't tell us that they are in pain, they can and do experience it. They consider the physiological mechanisms which might allow pain sensations to occur in infants and go on to ask how we can tell when an infant is in pain. How can we measure the degree of pain they feel if they can't verbalize their experience? If pain can be felt and measured in infancy, then the implication is that it can be controlled or limited by analgesia or other techniques, and the chapter concludes with a consideration of this.

The issue of whether or not neonates feel pain has been debated for centuries, as has the question of whether analgesics should be routinely used with this age group. Anand and McGrath (1993b) provide a detailed historical account of the debate over the existence of pain and its management in infancy; for example, Hippocrates (460–357BC) believed that infants are less tolerant of pain than adults, and Susutra (a Hindu physician, 550BC) did prescribe drugs and analgesics for children. On the other hand Celsus (25BC–50AD), described analgesics as powerful drugs which would be bad for infants and Bigelow (1848) stated that anaesthesia was unnecessary for infants as they lacked 'the remembrance of suffering'. Yet another element was introduced by Wolff and Wolff (1958) who argued that there are specific receptors and pathways for pain perception, and these are not sufficiently well developed in neonates for them to be able to perceive pain.

Thus in the 1970s and '80s anaesthesia during surgery was often not given to premature and full-term neonates on the grounds that:

1. Lack of CNS maturity and absence of myelination meant that pain was, probably not perceived.
2. Even if it was, lack of memory for the experience meant it did not matter; there would be no long term effects.
3. The use of drugs might have a deleterious effect on the infant because of their poor clinical condition and unstable vital signs. Therefore the requirement to save life took precedence over the requirement to reduce suffering.

Others, including the authors of this chapter, argue that neonates can feel pain; that there are long term effects of this experience; and that safe analgesics and anaesthetics can be produced. These arguments are presented in Sections 1, 2 and 3 of this chapter.

Also relevant to this debate is the fact that outside a medical context, i.e. in the home situation, caregivers would be severely criticized if they did not respond to the pain signals of their infants. It seems that it is only within a medical setting that the general belief that we should not hurt babies, or allow them to be in pain if we can do something to prevent it, is suspended. In recent years however, increased consumer involvement in health services has influenced both public opinion and clinical management. There is some evidence that attitudes are changing and that protocols for the prevention and management of pain in neonates are increasingly being used. Even so we can read Lawson's account of the clinical management of her son born at 25–26 weeks gestation; he had patent ductus arteriosus surgery using a paralysing agent but no general anaesthetic. She comments '. . . Somehow it was possible for professionals who perceived a baby as too fragile to tolerate general anaesthesia to perceive that same infant as able to withstand open-chest surgery without pain relief' (Lawson, 1988, p. 1).

The debate that she articulates is still going on and this chapter will attempt to elucidate some of the issues surrounding it and draw together the relevant empirical evidence. It concentrates first on the controversy surrounding the existance of pain in neonates, drawing on evidence from premature babies and the fetus, on the grounds that if they demonstrate the capacity to feel pain, then it must be present in all infants in the first year of life. Second, it considers whether there are long term effects of pain in infants; and, third, it discusses whether the use of analgesia and anaesthesia are more harmful to the baby than any experience of unrelieved pain.

Before addressing these issues, we might sensibly ask why such debate exists. After all, we virtually all experience pain as adults, and many infants are exposed to experiences which older children and adults would describe as painful; these include heelpricks for blood sampling and injections, as well as minor and major surgery. When we see a baby crying, thrashing about and making facial grimaces in response to an injection, they are showing many of the same signals that we would call 'pain' if seen in older children and adults. Why then do some clinicians believe that infants do not feel pain, and that it is neither necessary nor desirable to use analgesics or anaesthetics during painful procedures? The problem is not just that evidence is required but that there are intrinsic difficulties with concepts of pain and the ability to measure it in infants. Furthermore pain in infants is a highly emotive issue and some researchers (on both sides of the argument) and parents have used emotional language in order to bring pressure to bear for change. For example:

> The present routine policy of ignoring pain in the very young and de-emphasising the occurrence of pain in all children, needs to be abandoned and replaced with routine measurement of pain in all age groups and the development of validated and widely accepted ways of preventing and treating pain.

> Anand and McGrath, 1993, p. 1

While such pleas are understandable, and many may argue laudable, there is a need for objectivity in the presentation and evaluation of the evidence. This approach, despite the difficulties involved, holds the best promise for improving treatment.

Pain

There are a number of definitions of pain, but one of the most used, for example by the influential International Association for the Study of Pain (IASP), is:

> . . . an unpleasant sensory or emotional experience associated with actual or potential tissue damage, or described in terms of such damage.
>
> Merskey, Albe-Fessard and Bonica, 1979, p. 25

Merskey et al. go on to note that pain is always subjective, which immediately raises the problem that subjective confirmation of pain is not possible in young infants (nor indeed in animals). For this reason some researchers have preferred to use the word 'distress' rather than 'pain' (e.g. Katz, 1977). However, Anand and McGrath (1993a) argue for specific use of the word 'pain' to refer to the experience that is associated with actual or potential tissue damage. It then becomes an empirical question as to whether the behavioural and physiological responses associated with this experience can be differentiated from those shown to other 'distressing' experiences such as hunger, cold, over-stimulation, etc.

It has been argued that as pain is a subjective experience, it is intimately tied to consciousness and the ability to think about events. Since neonates cannot do this, they are not actually *experiencing* pain. Cunningham (1993) has disputed this interpretation of subjectivity, pointing out that by 'subjective' we mean that we can only infer others' experiences and sensations; we cannot directly observe them. All we can observe directly are behavioural (including verbal) responses and physiological responses. Thus to doubt that infants experience pain is to refuse to use the analogies we use for older children and adults to infer that they have the same experiences of pain that we ourselves do.

Since self-reports are not possible for neonates and very young children, behavioural and physiological measurements are necessary. These may not reflect the subjective experience of pain but instead record some unconscious response. However, it can be noted that we do not require self-reports to believe in the perception of pain in animals where stringent controls are applied to control potentially painful procedures (ASAB, 1986).

The appearance of characteristic behavioural responses to noxious stimulation is seen from birth in premature babies from at least 28 weeks gestational age (Craig, Whitfield, Grunau et al., 1993), and may constitute an important social signal to caregivers (Darwin, 1872). Since it is crucial for the survival of the infant to be able to signal to caregivers that potentially tissue damaging stimulation is occurring in order that this can be removed, Darwin argued that this ability would have arisen through evolutionary pressures, and therefore would be present very early in development. For this reason pain would be one of the earliest emotions to be experienced. Anand (1996) supports this view and postulates that 'pain' need not be learned through early experience but may instead be an inherent quality of life itself, expressed in all living organisms as a defence against damage to the organism either from external or internal stimuli. Thus it would be counter-intuitive to believe that the perception of pain would need to be based on prior experiences: 'The first experience of tissue injury is painful, in much the same way that touch, smell, vision or hearing need not be learned in order to occur in the human organism' (Anand, 1996, p. 4).

An alternative view of pain is that it is a complex phenomenon involving biological, psychological and social factors, some of which are dependant on learning (Melzack and Wall, 1988). This view would not deny the possibility of pain in infants but would suggest that it is not the exact equivalent of pain in older children and in adults. However, whatever its nature, there are considerable methodological difficulties involved in studying pain and these are compounded by ethical and moral issues, all of which have an impact on the design of research studies.

The chapter concentrates on the study of pain in neonates, on the grounds that if the capacity to feel pain is present in premature babies (and indeed in the fetus by the end of the second trimester in utero; Anand and Hickey, 1987; Anand, 1988), then we must assume that all infants in the first year of life may experience pain.

Pain pathways and mechanisms

The perception of pain depends on the transmission of noxious stimulation from the site of tissue damage through the central nervous system (CNS) to the brain. By about 22 weeks gestation in utero, the pathways necessary for cutaneous sensory perception are complete. In the developing brain, EEG patterns are present but intermittent. The cortex is still developing, and myelinization is continuing in the nerve tracts of the spinal cord and brain stem. By 26 to 28 weeks gestation (an age when many premature babies are born and surviving), the pain systems are up and operating if at a slightly reduced level (Anand and Carr, 1989). Fitzgerald (1993) argues that if we are to correctly evaluate CNS maturity, a multidimensional approach looking at anatomical, neurochemical, neurophysiological, behavioural and clinical aspects, is necessary. In addition it is important to understand how pathways and mechanisms change pre- and post-natally.

The argument that incomplete myelination affects the infant's ability to perceive pain has been challenged. Melzack and Wall (1988) claim that it is simply wrong. They note that even in adults, nociceptive impulses (i.e. stimuli which are perceived as painful) are conducted primarily via unmyelinated and thinly myelinated fibres in peripheral nerves. Furthermore, Gilles, Shankle and Dooling (1983) have demonstrated complete myelination of nociceptive nerve tracts in the spinal cord and CNS during the second and third trimesters of gestation. Thus both peripheral receptors and nociceptive reflex arcs are developed and functional before birth. The latter are important, as the flexor reflex (i.e. the withdrawal of a limb from noxious stimulation) appears to be a useful measure of CNS nociceptive function; for example the threshold corresponds to perceived pain in adults, and this is also true when analgesics such as morphine are given. In neonates these reflexes are exaggerated compared to those in adults and have lower thresholds. Similar responses are seen in pre-terms where thresholds are much lower, particularly prior to 30 weeks gestation (Fitzgerald, Shaw and McIntosh, 1988). Furthermore neurotransmitters which enhance the perception of pain are being produced earlier than the production of endogenous opiates which moderate nociception (Anand, 1988). Pre-terms showed increased sensitization following repeated stimulation, and this was removed by local anaesthetic (Anand, 1993). Although not conclusive proof, this might imply that neonates are if anything more sensitive to noxious stimuli than are adults (a view previously propounded by Haslam (1969)).

In addition neurotransmitters necessary to signal pain are present from relatively early gestation (8 to 10 weeks), although the question of when they are present in sufficiently large quantities to signal pain has not yet been established (Fitzgerald, 1993).

Other pathways which may affect the perception of pain are descending inhibitory pathways from higher centres to the spinal cord. Wall and Melzack (1989) have studied these in depth, and these inhibitory pathways are central in their gate control theory of pain (Melzack and Wall, 1965, 1988). This theory revolutionized work on the assessment and management of pain, aiming to explain the processes underlying the experience of pain. With modifications, it remains the dominant theory influential today. In it, Melzack and Wall proposed that the synapses in the dorsal horn of the spinal cord act like a gate to increase or reduce the flow of nerve fibres to the spinal cord cells that project to the sensory cortex or the limbic system of the brain. These map the relative position of body sites and are involved in motivation and emotion. There are at least two pain transmission systems which have different processes and effects. The *lateral system* which transmits impulses very quickly from the small nerve fibres gives rise to sharp or acute pain. However, this is subject to efferent or downward flowing inhibition so that the sharp or acute pain may be quickly dampened down. The *medial system* transmits impulses slowly from the large myelinated and unmyelinated nerve fibres giving rise to tonic or more long lasting pain.

Melzack and Wall suggested that the 'gating mechanism' is operated when successive synapses, which transmit impulses to the brain, are stimulated and reach a critical level at which point pain occurs. The theory suggests that large fibre activation involving gentle touch and other forms of normal stimulation would close the 'gate', while small fibre activation caused by intense or tissue damaging stimulation would open the 'gate' causing an increase in pain. However, in neonates, due to their immature physiological development, even gentle rubbing may cause an increase in pain depending on their level of arousal. Once a neonate reaches a critical level of arousal (and this varies with each baby and for each baby according to state, illness, age, etc.), even stimulation which is usually soothing, such as touch or stroking, may be perceived as pain.

The descending inhibitory pathways may be lacking in neonates, producing the increased sensitivity to noxious stimulation seen in very young infants. However, Grunau and Craig (1987) found that infant responsivity to invasive stimulation was a function of ongoing behavioural state, rather than simply reflecting tissue damage. They concluded that underlying biological mechanisms for the moderation of pain expression are already functional in the new-born period but that their operation depends on complex factors.

It would also be logical to assume that as neonates have no way of conceptualizing what is happening to them, they may experience more pain, since understanding of the situation appears to lessen the pain reported by older children (Fradet, McGrath, Kay et al., 1990).

Measuring pain in infants

If we are to establish whether or not infants feel pain, there must be valid and reliable methods of assessment. Since they are incapable of verbal responses, other techniques for measuring their responses must be utilized, such as physiological and behavioural measures.

Physiological measures

A number of changes in cardiovascular responses have been found among neonates exposed to painful procedures. These include extreme variability in transcutaneous PO_2, increases in arterial blood pressure and in intracranial pressure. In studies of circumcision such changes were prevented by the use of local anaesthetic (e.g. Holve, Bromberger, Groveman et al., 1983; Friesen, Honda, Thiene, 1987).

Changes in circulating hormonal and metabolite concentrations characteristic of stress responses also occur in response to noxious stimulation. Thus Anand and Hickey (1992) showed that in neonates undergoing surgery, there were marked increases in plasma catecholamines, glucagon and glucocorticosteroids, and a suppression of insulin secretion. In addition Giannakoulopoulos, Sepulveda, Kourtis et al. (1994) reported sharp rises in hormones linked with the pain response in fetuses aged 23 to 34 weeks undergoing intrauterine transfusions into a vein in the abdomen.

Behavioural measures

While physiological measures have been used to study pain in infants and have provided evidence that even very premature babies respond adversely to noxious stimulation (McVey, Niven, Ibhanesebhor et al., 1995), the use of behavioural measures is more widespread. In part this may reflect our current knowledge of infant competencies. By using innovative experimental techniques and methodologies such as the habituation paradigm, this has increased exponentially in the last thirty years. Most of the work has demonstrated that neonates are much more competent in their monitoring of the environment than had previously been supposed. For example, from birth infants can discriminate between stimuli (Slater and Bremner, 1989) and habituation and learning in the fetus from gestational ages of 34 weeks has been demonstrated (Hepper and Shahidulla, 1992). Although there is virtually no work as yet on the perceptual and learning competencies of the pre-term infant, it is likely that they too are more competent perceptually than had been supposed. This area of research has utilized behavioural measures of response very successfully and has had a powerful influence on the methodologies used by other researchers working in the area of infancy.

Craig and Grunau (1993) argue that a vigorous means of signalling distressing states would be expected in infants since, as first emphasized by Darwin (1872) it is important for the infant's survival not to be exposed to noxious stimulation, and thus to be able to communicate states of pain to caregivers.

However, in studying such signals (and also of course in studying physiological responses), a number of methodological difficulties arise. The most pressing of these is to obtain control over variables which are likely to affect responding. It is necessary, therefore, to study routine clinical situations in which an infant is exposed to noxious stimulation. These might include routine heel pricks for blood sampling, intravenous cannulation, chest drain insertion, lumbar puncture, circumcision and major and minor surgery. In such situations precise experimental control is not possible, but real life relevance is high. Variables which may affect behaviour include such things as infant state (e.g. sleeping or waking), time since feeding, medication for various conditions and health status. It is not possible to control these, but it is possible to measure them, and given sufficient sample size to put them into a statistical analysis as co-variates (McVey, Niven, Ibhanesebhor et al., 1995).

The neonate's responses to noxious stimulation are similar to those of older children and adults. These include crying, facial expressions of pain, and body position and movement. However there are some differences, the most obvious of which is that no verbal behaviour occurs. The question is: are there non-verbal responses which are specific to the experience of pain, and distinguishable from the distress seen in situations of hunger, cold and over-stimulation? And at what gestational ages are these seen? The answers are not clear. Behaviour in response to noxious stimulation has been well described, but as yet there is a paucity of studies comparing these to those shown in non-noxious stimulation situations. In addition the large majority of studies investigate sudden acute pain situations (particularly heel pricks) with few on the perception of longer term pain likely to be associated with post-operative recovery.

Acute pain responses have been extensively studied in neonates by Craig and Grunau (e.g. 1993). They report the following behaviours as typical of responses to noxious stimulation.

1. **Cry**: There is a sudden onset of an initially high-pitched prolonged cry, followed by a protracted episode of respiratory inspiration and then a transition to further cycles of more standard crying for a protracted period of time. To date there is no strong evidence that a pain cry can be distinguished from crying for other reasons (Johnston and O'Shaugnessy, 1988).
2. **Body movement and posture**: Craig, McMahon, Morison and Zaskow, 1984 described a wide range of movements as signalling pain in older infants – from rigidity to thrashing. The capacity to reflexly withdraw from physical pain is present in full-term neonates.
3. **Facial movement**: Izard (1978) developed a system for scoring emotional expression seen in older infants. This scores movement in three regions of the face: forehead and brow, eyes and nose, and mouth. A typical pain expression is shown in Figure 12.1.

This system has been used with infants from gestational ages from 28 weeks by Martin, Glenn, Padden and Berry (1995). Identical facial expressions are seen in all gestational ages, with the exception of the mouth, where instead of the square mouth seen in older infants it was more common to see a stretched horizontal mouth in pre-term infants. In addition with increased gestational age all three areas of face were likely to show movement. A rather similar system was developed by Grunau and Craig (1987) called the Neonatal Coding System. Studies are needed to determine whether such facial expressions are specific to pain in the neonate or characteristic of all types of

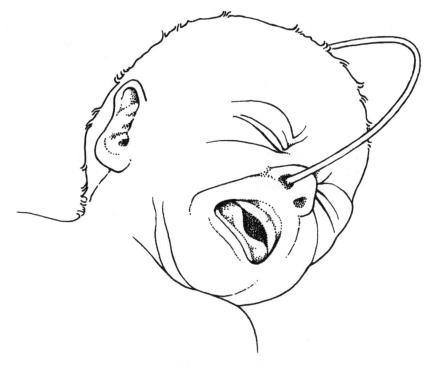

Figure 12.1 © Rebecca Freear

distress from whatever source. However, Craig and Grunau (1993) note that even in deep sleep a neonate will respond to a noxious stimulus with a characteristic facial grimace. Martin, Glenn, Padden and Berry (1995) have demonstrated that this is also true in pre-term infants of 28 weeks gestation.

There has been less work on post-operative pain, although this is an important aspect of clinical practice. Horgan, Choonara and Glenn (1995) and Horgan, Al-Waidh, Ashby et al., (1996) have studied the behavioural responses of neonates following surgery for a variety of conditions from minor (for example simple inguinal hernia repair) to major (involving invasive abdominal) surgery, in order to develop an objective scoring system for measuring post-operative pain. The system is based on eight behavioural categories, each quantified on a six-point scale. These are: spontaneous movement, spontaneous excitability, flexion of fingers and toes, muscle tone, facial expression, cry quality, cry quantity, sleep pattern and amount of sleep. To date it has demonstrated inter-rater reliability and validity in that the duration of pain behaviour is well related to type of surgery and the administration of analgesia. Further development is now taking place to simplify the scoring system and thus make it more suitable for clinical use.

Another system (CRIES) developed by Krechel and Bildner (1995) use five categories including two physiological ones: requires oxygen for saturation, and increased heart rate or blood pressure in comparison to that pre-operation. The same behavioural cues of crying, facial expression and sleeplessness are used as in Horgan et al.'s (1996) system, but movement patterns and muscle tone are not identified and monitored.

The assessment tools which have been devised for use in clinical settings have varying degrees of validity and usefulness. For a fuller discussion of assessment tools of neonatal pain, the reader is directed to the review paper by Bours, Abu-Saad, Hamers and Van Dongen (1996). Studies comparing different systems, not only for their ability to discriminate pain signals, but also for their ease (and therefore likelihood) of use in ward situations are needed.

Measures of behavioural responses are also important because they are the ones that caregivers can see. It can be argued from an evolutionary perspective that these behaviours are designed to elicit caregiver responses to remove the source of pain and prevent damage to the infant. However, many studies have shown that the caregiver's judgement of neonatal pain often underestimates its presence and intensity. This is especially true for premature babies (Shapiro, 1994; Hester and Foster, 1991; Briggs, 1995).

Neonates, whether full-term or premature, have a rich communicative repertoire involving vocalizations, behavioural indicators (which may be increased movements such as thrashing about or equally may be flaccid unresponsivity), facial expressions, changes in skin colour, together with physiological measures such as heart and respiration rate, blood pressure variation, saturated oxygen and carbon dioxide levels, cortisol levels, etc. To be sensitive and responsive to these vulnerable babies, caregivers must be open to 'hear' this rich and varied 'language' and respond to it. The assumption that experiences are only important when they can be conceptualized and expressed according to adult terms of reference and expression has to be avoided and the focus of care has to be 'neonate-centred'.

Long term effects of pain in infancy

The effect of painful experiences early in life on later development is extremely difficult to study, considering the large number of variables which might affect outcome. For the sick or pre-term infant it might be argued that distress from any source, including pain, produces undesirable imbalances in the infant's physiological and behavioural equilibrium, and hence may adversely affect development (Als, 1986). A recent study by Grunau, Whitfield, Petrie and Fryer (1994) showed that extremely low birthweight infants (ELBW) who had had lengthy stays in the neonatal intensive care unit in infancy (and by implication extreme early painful experiences), had significantly more somatic complaints of unknown origin than full-term healthy neonates at three and four-and-a-half years of age; there were no differences in actual medical problems. Low maternal sensitivity was also related to higher somatization. A previous study (Grunau, Whitfield, Petrie and Fryer, 1991) had shown less reaction to pain in ELBW toddlers at 18 months, with some parents reporting a need to teach the children to respond appropriately to common childhood hurts. This, although not conclusive, supports the notion of long term effects of early painful experiences interacting with low maternal sensitivity, to make children less likely to respond appropriately to bodily sensations. Several other recent studies (e.g. Coderre et al., 1993) suggest that it is theoretically possible that there is an anatomical alteration to 'pain gating' in response to peripheral tissue damage or nerve injury in early infancy. Andrews and Fitzgerald (1994) argue that there is increasing evidence that unrelieved pain in the neonatal period may affect future pain thresholds.

Investigations from a number of different perspectives have indicated that brain plasticity is highest during the last trimester of pregnancy and in the neonatal period. It is likely therefore, that experiences at this age will have a high potential for long term effects. Thus the neonate may not consciously remember painful experiences, but nonetheless these may affect the rest of the child's life. More positively however, Als, Lawhon, Brown et al. (1986) showed that minimizing stress through individual care plans in a neonatal intensive care unit produced better outcomes while the infants were in the NICU, and more optimal development up to five months of age in such infants than in infants receiving standard care, so it is possible that such adverse long term effects can be avoided.

The use of analgesics and anaesthetics

Given the evidence presented so far, and on the basis of a more extensive review by Anand (1993), it can be concluded that the pain system is highly developed in neonates, and that clinical, physiological and psychological sequelae can be a serious consequence of inadequately treated pain. This would seem to suggest that pain in infants should be moderated or prevented through the use of analgesics and anaesthetics.

The increased sophistication of modern neonatal intensive care has resulted in far larger numbers of neonates undergoing surgery in recent years. Kiely (1984) noted that the outcome in terms of postoperative morbidity and mortality was much worse than in older children and adults. Anand and McGrath (1993a) speculate that part of the reason for this may be the large hormonal and metabolic stress responses seen in neonates operated on with minimal anaesthesia; such stress responses are correlated with a poor clinical outcome. Again this would indicate that there should be an increased use of pain relieving drugs. However, a common argument against the use of anaesthetics and analgesics is that such drugs are dangerous, especially for sick infants.

For example, Guthrie (1894) reported the death of small children from delayed chloroform poisoning leading to hepatic failure. However, at this time the only clinical monitoring that was available was by observation. The increased risk of respiratory depression from opiates was also reported in neonates. This, together with a belief in the lack of pain perception in infants, was a major factor in subsequent suggestions that anaesthetics were not appropriate for neonates and infants so that, for example, Jackson-Rees (1960) advocated the use of muscle relaxants and minimal anaesthesia.

The introduction of halothane as an anaesthetic, apparently with potent and non-irritant effects on children produced interest in its use for neonates but early studies by Gregory, Eger and Munson (1969) for example, suggested that higher concentrations were needed in young infants, and these produced increased incidences of hypertension, bradycardia and cardiac arrest. However, more recent studies (e.g. Lerman, Robinson, Willis and Gregory, 1983) showed that neonates actually required smaller concentrations of halothane. In a randomized control study using halothane and fentanyl anaesthesia on full-terms and pre-terms, Anand (1986) found greater clinical stability during the operation, together with decreased incidence of post-operative complications. Burrows and Bede (1993) reviewed anaesthetic and analgesic use for very young infants, making several recommendations about which might be used. They suggested that for minor surgery peripheral nerve blockade might be used. For major surgery they note that epidural anaesthesia with local anaesthetics or opioids or both, give excellent analgesia with very good effects on post-operative recovery. They conclude:

> Pain is a complex multidimensional phenomenon and its historical under-treatment in children reflects both the nature of pain and the attitudes towards and values concerning pain and children. Unfortunately, this lack of treatment has allowed the persistence of unnecessary suffering in children, particularly in those most vulnerable – infants and critically ill children.

> Burrows and Bede, 1993, p. 816

Cunningham in an important paper on moral and ethical issues in clinical practice (Cunningham, 1993) has pointed out that many drugs, not just analgesics, are dangerous for unstable pre-terms. There seems to be, she suggests, a belief among clinicians that it would be worse to cause the death of an infant accidentally with pain relieving drugs, than with any other potentially helpful drug. She points out that it has never been demonstrated that infants are at risk of addiction to narcotic drugs used for pain control. Nonetheless this is a concern constantly cited by physicians to explain partially their unwillingness to prescribe such analgesics – she also argues that:

> If caregivers are not aware of research already completed about the use of analgesia, if they do not work hard to discover the possible serious consequences of pain, if they consider the only serious consequences to be short term medical ones, if they do not seriously compare the use of analgesic drugs with the use of paralytic drugs, for example, and if they ignore the infant experience of pain, then their current practice of choosing to under-treat rather than to over-treat is immoral.

> Cunningham, 1993, p. 263

She points out that the belief within professional ethical practice that saving lives takes precedence over reducing suffering is illogical since these need not be mutually exclusive and she goes on to speculate that physicians and nurses may find it difficult to carry out the necessary procedures on infants if they believe that infants are experiencing pain as a result. They may believe that a procedure is necessary to treat a neonate, and may therefore reduce their own distress at producing pain by a cognitive restructuring process which protects them by denying the experience of pain in infants and young children. They may argue that change in practice is unnecessary, as they have 'always done it that way' and their patients do well. Training on behavioural indices of pain and distress in very young pre-terms and full-terms should produce greater sensitivity in care staff. However, if such training interferes with some self-protective mechanism which denies the existance of pain in patients being treated, it may be ineffective or even counter-productive unless combined with strategies which are designed to reduce the pain induced by staff treatment.

The danger of analgesics is an argument repeatedly used; however this provides a case for research on safer anaesthetics and analgesics, together with research on administration procedures. Thus, for example, large, irregular doses of morphine may be ineffective, whereas smaller doses given through continuous infusion may be both safer and more effective. It is also argued that analgesics are dangerous as they may mask symptoms, and delay diagnosis; this may be so, but once a diagnosis is made this should not matter. The counter argument may be presented: that stress responses produced by noxious stimulation may in themselves be harmful to the infant and delay recovery.

There is also a trend to increase the use of sedation for neonates which gives the *appearance* of quietness and rest and therefore the assumption that they are not in pain. However, this is a dangerous assumption since sedatives such as the benzodiazepines (e.g. valium) only mask the behavioural indices of pain without relieving it. When used in addition to analgesics however, they have a significant role to play.

Such issues can also arise in the treatment of adults who present as a poor anaesthetic risk. However, in these cases, different or local anaesthetics are typically suggested. It would be extremely unlikely that there would even be a suggestion that anaesthetics were not used. Fortunately recent research and pressure by researchers and clinicians such as Anand and McGrath is now leading to more attention being paid to the development of safe anaesthetics for infants and children.

Modifications in practice can be influenced by education, by models of good practice, and by consumer (parent) pressure. Cunningham (1993) suggests a list of questions which might be used in producing a pain protocol:

- Is the procedure necessary?
- Is the painful part of it necessary?
- Can the pain be lessened through improved skill or improved technology?
- How will pain be assessed?
- What options for pain control have been available and are now available?
- When signing the consent form are parents made aware of the unit's policy on pain relief?
- What is the procedure for reviewing and updating this pain protocol?

The use of other techniques to reduce distress

All neonates nursed in hospital benefit from having their environment improved in terms of light, noise and aversive interactions. Reducing light, instigating 'rest periods' when no interventions are carried out, and providing positive calming interactions such as containing and wrapping, have all been shown to improve neonatal outcome (Philips, 1995). However, it is not clear whether some of these interventions have a specific effect with regard to pain relief. Questioning whether heel stabs and other invasive interventions are really necessary, and providing alternative methods for collecting blood will obviously reduce the potential for pain and should be considered on an individual basis. The use of EMLA cream (eutectic mixture of lignocaine and prilocaine) has revolutionized painful procedures for children older than six months by providing local anaesthesia prior to intravenous cannulae insertion, venous punctures, etc. Its use in neonates is debated, and further work on a safe local anaesthetic for neonates is needed. For full-term neonates, Campos (1994) reported that both the use of pacifiers and rocking reduced crying following a routine heelprick; however, pacifiers predominantly produced sleep states and rocking produced alert states. The use of sucrose as an analgesic has been investigated by Haouari, Wood, Griffiths and Levene (1995), and this decreased crying over time significantly more than water in babies having heel stab.

In the care of pre-terms in a neonatal intensive care unit there has been considerable debate as to whether stimulation is desirable or not (e.g. see Wolke, Chapter 13, this volume) with many contradictory results evident. This may be because insufficient attention has been paid to individual variation in such factors as infant state, gestational age, timing in relation to other procedures, etc. For example, Oehler, Eckerman and Wilson (1988) found that only talking produced desirable behavioural states in pre-terms (e.g. eye-opening when in low activity, and decreased activity when in highly active states). Stroking alone, or both talking and stroking either produced or maintained states suggestive of agitation. Other studies, however, do report positive effects from touching/stroking so care is necessary. It is probable that the type of touching is important (e.g. Adamson-Macedo, de Roiste, Wilson et al., 1994); furthermore, it is **vitally** important to monitor the individual infant's response and state, as infants may respond differently at different times, and at different stages of development. A pre-term infant is not like a fetus of the same gestational age. At birth, respiratory and digestive systems alter their modes of operation, and this may also be the case for the sensory systems. Thus a pre-term infant may require different types of stimulation from that received by a fetus in the womb, or by a full-term healthy baby.

Conclusion

Most evidence is now consistent with the view that from 28 weeks gestation, pain is experienced by neonates. In recent years research from a number of different perspectives has increased our understanding of the neurophysiological, biochemical and anatomical basis of pain, and work on its behavioural manifestations is now well established. Some of this research has been embraced by clinical practice; however, work still remains to be done. Attitudes are changing, but despite this some neonates and young infants continue to suffer pain. Successful pain management remains a challenge to carers, and more research is needed in the area of clinical practice using well-validated pain assessment tools.

As in any area of clinical practice there is always a danger that attitudes shift, and techniques become implemented without sufficient research. Anand and McGrath (1993a) comment:

> The history of neonatology is replete with the dangers of implementing well-meaning change without careful and controlled evaluation. . . . The excitement we all feel about the area of neonatal pain, and the emotional and moral commitment that we have to preventing and alleviating pain in new-borns, must not be allowed to lead us into well-meaning but disastrous interventions.
>
> Anand and McGrath, 1993a, p. 323

We do not yet have all the answers, and caution is necessary. However, this is a vitally important area of enquiry, as otherwise this vulnerable group of newly born babies are at risk of possible long term developmental problems as well as short term pain and distress.

Applications

1. Infants do feel pain
Assume that what is painful for the adult is also painful for the infant. While infants' perception of pain may be questioned because of their limited cognitive abilities, the counter argument may be presented that they may equally have no idea why they are experiencing pain, or when (or if) it may stop.

2. Be sensitive to the signals infants are providing
Behavioural indices such as cries, facial expressions and movements, as well as physiological indices and blood chemistry measures if available, should be assessed. Ongoing and regular assessment of pain is fundamental in providing effective analgesia. Be aware that there are many individual differences in pain cues.

3. Question the necessity for painful procedures
Are certain procedures critically important for clinical management, or are they simply being carried out under an outdated protocol, with no implications for change in management?

4. If painful procedures are necessary, question what analgesia is available and what is used
Analgesic procedures need evaluating in the clinical area, and complementary therapies need investigation for their efficacy in providing alternatives to drug therapy.

5. If working in a clinical area ensure that there are written records of pain management
These would include pain protocols, and records for individual infants.

Further reading

Anand, K. J. S. and McGrath, P. J. (eds) (1993). *Pain in Neonates*. Pain Research and Clinical Management Vol 5. Elsevier Science Publishers B.V.

Bours, G. J. J. W., Abu-Saad, H. H., Hamers, J. P. H. and Van Dongen, R. T. M. (1996). *The Assessment of Neonatal Pain*. University of Limburg, Department of Nursing Science, Maastricht, Netherlands.

Carter, B. (1994). Child and Infant Pain. *Principles of Nursing Care and Management*. London: Chapman and Hall.

Skevington, S. (1995). *The Psychology of Pain*. Bognor Regis: Wiley.

References

Adamson-Macedo, E. N., de Roiste, A., Wilson, A., de Carvalho, F. A. and Dattani, I. (1994). TAC-TIC therapy with high-risk, distressed, ventilated preterms. *Journal of Reproductive and Infant Psychology*, **12**, 249–52.

Als, H. (1986). A synactive model of neonatal behavioral organisation: framework for the assessment of neurobehavioral development in the premature infant and for support of infants and parents in the neonatal intensive care environment. In *The High-Risk Neonate: Developmental Therapy Perspectives* (J. K. Sweeney, ed.). New York: Haworth Press.

Als, H., Lawhon, G., Brown, E., Gibbs, R., Duffy, F., McAnulty, G. and Blickman, J. (1986). Individualised behavioral and environmental care for the very low birth weight preterm infant at high risk for bronchopulmonary dysplasia: neonatal intensive care unit and developmental outcome. *Pediatrics*, **78**, 1123–32.

Anand, K. J. S. (1986). Hormonal and metabolic functions of infants undergoing surgery. *Current Opinion in Cardiology*, **1**, 681–9.

Anand, K. J. S. (1988). Pain and its effects in the human neonate. 1st International Symposium on Pediatric Pain. Seattle, pp. 22–4.

Anand, K. J. S. (1993). The applied physiology of pain. In *Pain in Neonates*. Pain Research and Clinical Management Vol. 5 (K. J. S. Anand and P. J. McGrath, eds). Elsevier Science Publishers B.V.

Anand, K. J. S. (1996). Foreword. In Bours, G. J. J. W., Abu-Saad, H. H., Hamers, J. P. H. and Van Dongen, R. T. M. (1996). *The Assessment of Neonatal Pain*. University of Limburg, Department of Nursing Science, Maastricht, Netherlands.

Anand, K. J. S. and Carr, D. B. (1989). The neuroanatomy, neurophysiology, and neuro-chemistry of pain, stress, and analgesia in new-borns and children. *Pediatric Clinics of North America*, **36**, 795–822.

Anand, K. J. S. and Hickey, P. R. (1987). Pain and its effects in the neonate and fetus. *The New England Journal of Medicine*, **19**, 1321–9.

Anand, K. J. S. and Hickey, P. R. (1992). Pain and stress responses in neonatal cardiac surgery. *New England Journal of Medicine*, **326**, 126–7.

Anand, K. J. S. and McGrath, P. J. (eds) (1993a). *Pain in Neonates*. Pain Research and Clinical Management Vol. 5. Elsevier Science Publishers B.V.

Anand, K. J. S. and McGrath, P. J. (1993b). An overview of current issues and their historical background. In *Pain in Neonates*. Pain Research and Clinical Management Vol. 5 (K. J. S. Anand and P. J. McGrath, eds). Elsevier Science Publishers B.V., pp. 1–18.

Andrews, K. and Fitzgerald, M. (1994). The cutaneous withdrawal reflex in human neo-nates: sensitization, receptive fields, and the effect of contralateral stimulation. *Pain*, **56**, 95–101.

ASAB (Association for the Study of Animal Behaviour) (1986). Guidelines for the use of animals in research. *Animal Behaviour*, **34**, 315–18.

Bigelow, H. J. (1848). Anaesthetic agents, their mode of exhibition and physiological effects. *Transatlantic American Medical Association*, **1**, 197–214.

Bours, G. J. J. W., Abu-Saad, H. H., Hamers, J. P. H. and Van Dongen, R. T. M. (1996). *The Assessment of Neonatal Pain*. University of Limburg, Department of Nursing Science, Maastricht, Netherlands.

Briggs, M. (1995). Principles of acute pain assessment. *Nursing Standard*, **9** (19), 23–7.

Burrows, F. A. and Bede, C. B. (1993). Optimal pain relief in infants and children. *British Medical Journal*, **307**, 815–16.

Campos, R. G. (1994). Rocking and pacifiers: two comforting interventions for heelstick pain. *Research in Nursing and Health*, **17**, 321–31.

Coderre, T. J., Katz, J., Vaccarino, A. L. et al. (1993), Contribution of central neuroplasticity to pathological pain – review of clinical and experimental evidence. *Pain*. **52**, 259–85.

Craig, K. D. and Grunau, R. V. E. (1993). Neonatal pain perception and behavioral measurement. In *Pain in Neonates*. Pain Research and Clinical Management Vol. 5 (K. J. S. Anand and P. J. McGrath, eds). Elsevier Science Publishers B.V., pp. 67–105.

Craig, K. D., McMahon, R. G., Morison, J. D. and Zaskow, C. (1984). Developmental changes in infant pain expression during immunisation injections. *Social Science and Medicine*, **19**, 1331–7.

Craig, K. D., Whitfield, M. F., Grunau, R. V. E., Linton, J. and Hadjistavropoulos, H. D. (1993). Pain in the preterm neonate: behavioural and physiological indices. *Pain*, **52**, 287–99.

Cunningham, N. (1993). Moral and ethical issues in clinical practice. In *Pain in Neonates*. Pain Research and Clinical Management Vol. 5 (K. J. S. Anand and P. J. McGrath, eds). Elsevier Science Publishers B.V., pp. 255–73.

Darwin, C. (1872). *The Expression of Emotions in Man and Animals*. London: John Murray.

Fitzgerald, M. (1993). Development of pain pathways and mechanisms. In *Pain in Neonates*. Pain Research and Clinical Management Vol. 5 (K. J. S. Anand and P. J. McGrath, eds). Elsevier Science Publishers B.V., pp. 19–37.

Fitzgerald, M., Shaw, A. and McIntosh, N. (1988). The postnatal development of the cutaneous flexor reflex: a comparative study in premature infants and new-born rat pups. *Developmental Medical Child Neurology*, **30**, 520–26.

Fradet, C., McGrath, P. J., Kay, J., Adams, S. and Luke, B. (1990). A prospective study of reactions to blood tests by children and adolescents. *Pain*, **40**, 53–60.

Friesen, R. H., Honda, A. T. and Thiene, R. E. (1987). Changes in anterior fontanel pressure in preterm babies during tracheal intubation. *Anaesthesia and Analgesia*, **66**, 874–8.

Giannakoulopoulos, X., Sepulveda, W., Kourtis, P., Glover, V. and Fisk, N. M. (1994). Fetal plasma-cortisol and beta-endorphin response to intrauterine needling. *Lancet*, **344**, 77–81.

Gilles, F. H., Shankle, W. and Dooling, E. C. (1983). Myelinated tracts: growth patterns. In *The Developing Human Brain* (F. H. Gilles, A. Leviton and E. C. Dooling, eds). Boston: Wright and Co.

Gregory, G. A., Eger, E. I. and Munson, E. S. (1969). The relationship between age and halothane requirement in man. *Anaesthesiology*, **30**, 491–9.

Grunau, R. V. E. and Craig, K. D. (1987). Pain expression in neonates: facial action and cry. *Pain*, **28**, 395–410.

Grunau, R. V. E., Whitfield, M. F., Petrie, J. G. and Fryer, L. (1991). Pain sensitivity in toddlers of birthweight < 1000 grams compared with heavier pre-term and full birthweight toddlers. *Pediatric Research*, **29**, 256A.

Grunau, R. V. E., Whitfield, M. F., Petrie, J. H. and Fryer, E. L. (1994). Early pain experience, child and family factors, as precursors of somatization: a prospective study of extremely premature and full-term children. *Pain*, **56**, 353–9.

Guthrie, L. G. (1894). On some fatal after effects of chloroform on children. *Lancet*, **1**, 193–7, 257–61.

Haouari, N., Wood, C., Griffiths, G. and Levene, M. (1995). The analgesic effect of sucrose in full term infants: a randomised controlled trial. *British Medical Journal*, **310**, 1498–500.

Haslam, D. R. (1969). Age and the perception of pain. *Psychonomic Science*, **15**, 86–7.

Hepper, P. and Shahidulla, S. (1992). Habituation in normal and Down's Syndrome fetuses. *Quarterly Journal of Experimental Psychology*, **44**, 305–17.

Hester, N. O. and Foster, R. L. (1991). Critical dimensions of nurses' decisions about children's pain. *Journal of Pain and Symptom Management*, **63**, 148(A).

Holve, R. L., Bromberger, B. J., Groveman, H. D., Klauber, M. R., Dixon, S. D. and Snyder, J. M. (1983). Regional anaesthesia during new-born circumcision: effect on infant pain response. *Clinical Pediatrics*, **22**, 813–18.

Horgan, M., Choonara, I. and Glenn, S. M. (1995). The development of a scale to measure post-operative pain/distress in the neonate. *Journal of Reproductive and Infant Psychology*, **13**, 169(A).

Horgan, M., Al-Waidh, M., Ashby, D., Franklin, A., Hayes, A., Jones, M., McLoughlin, J., Bowhay, A., Lloyd, D. A., Morton, J., Sambrooks, J. and Choonara, I. (1996). The development of an objective scoring system for measuring post-operative pain in the neonate. *Paediatric Nursing*, **8**, 24–27.

Izard, C. E. (1978). On the ontogenesis of emotions and emotion-cognitive relationships in infancy. In *The Development of Affect* (M. Lewis and L. Rosenblum, eds). New York: Plenum Press.

Jackson-Rees, G. (1960). Paediatric anaesthesia. *British Journal of Anaesthetics*, **32**, 132–40.

Johnston, C. C. and O'Shaugnessy, D. O. (1988). Acoustical attributes of infant pain cries. Discriminating features. In Proceedings of the Vth World Congress on Pain (R. Dubner, G. F. Gebhart and M. R. Bond, eds). Amsterdam: Elsevier.

Katz, J. (1977). The question of circumcision. *Int. Surgery*, **62**, 490–92.

Kiely, E. (1984). Surgery in very low birth weight infants. *Archives of Disease in Childhood*, **59**, 707–8.

Krechel, S. W. and Bildner, J. (1995). CRIES: a new neonatal postoperative pain measurement score. Initial testing of validity and reliability. *Paediatric Anaesthesia*, **5**, 53–61.

Lawson, J. R. (1988). Standards of practice and the pain of premature infants. *Bulletin of National Center for Infant Programs*, **9** (2), 1–5.

Lerman, J., Robinson, S., Willis, M. M. and Gregory, G. A. (1983). Anaesthetic requirements for halothane in young children 0–1 month and 1–6 months of age. *Anaesthesiology*, **59**, 421–4.

Martin, R., Glenn, S. M., Padden, T. and Berry, N. (1995). The pain expression and its genesis in premature infants. *Journal of Reproductive and Infant Psychology*, **13**, 168–9(A).

McVey, C., Niven, C., Ibhanesebhor, S., Carroll, D. and Alroomi, L. (1995). The effect of touch intervention in the time taken by preterm babies to recover from behavioural and physio-logical distress in response to essential blood-sampling procedures. *Journal of Reproductive and Infant Psychology*, **13**, 170(A).

Melzack, R. and Wall, P. (1965). Pain mechanisms: a new theory. *Science*, **150**, 971–9.

Melzack, R. and Wall, P. (1988). *The Challenge of Pain* (2nd edition). Penguin Books, UK.

Merskey, H., Albe-Fessard, D. G. and Bonica, J. J. (1979). Pain terms: a list with definitions and notes on usage: recommended by the IASP subcommittee on taxonomy. *Pain*, **6**, 249–52.

Oehler, J. M., Eckerman, C. O. and Wilson, W. H. (1988). Social stimulation and the regulation of premature infants' state prior to term age. *Infant Behavior and Development*, **11**, 333–51.

Philips, P. (1995). Neonatal pain management: a call to action. *Pediatric Nursing*, **21**.

Shapiro, C. R. (1991). Nurses' judgements of pain intensity in term and preterm new-borns. *Journal of Pain and Symptom Management*, **63**, 148(A).

Slater, A. and Bremner, G. (eds) (1989). *Infant Development*. Lawrence Erlbaum Associates, UK.

Wall, P. D. and Melzack, R. (1989). *The Textbook of Pain* (2nd edition). Edinburgh: Churchill Livingstone.

Wolff, H. G. and Wolff, S. (1958). *Pain*. Springfield: H. Thomas.

13

Premature babies and the Special Care Baby Unit (SCBU)/Neonatal Intensive Care Unit (NICU): environmental, medical and developmental considerations

Dieter Wolke

A book on current issues in infancy would be incomplete without some discussion of pre-term babies, that is babies born before 37 weeks of gestation. Currently around 1 in 15 of the babies born in industrialized countries is pre-term. Almost all of these babies will experience SCBU or NICU care. In this chapter Dieter Wolke considers the physical and psychological development of pre-term and very pre-term (<32 weeks gestation) babies. Do these babies go on to have problems at school, for instance? Is the development of pre-term babies influenced by the type of care or the care environment in the early weeks? SCBU and NICU environments are generally bright and noisy, and babies are frequently disturbed for medical procedures, but have little opportunity for social interaction with adults. Does a 'gentler' approach to NICU care have long-term benefits? How best can care be organized to integrate both the medical and psychological needs of pre-term babies?

Introduction

There are both theoretical and practical reasons to consider the effect of being cared for in the NICU or SCBU. From a theoretical perspective it may provide insight into the influence of the early care environment on short- and long-term developmental progress. From a practical perspective, the efficacy and cost-effectiveness of different forms of care are critically important. For example, do particular care approaches have effects on the physiological or behavioural organization of the infant, lead to more or less induced complications (iatrogenic effects) or a shorter time on the SCBU, and are they associated with different developmental outcomes? From a health economist's perspective, earlier discharge from the NICU or SCBU and fewer long-term developmental problems mean cost savings for the health services and psychosocial after-services and gains in terms of later contribution of the infants to society.

NICU/SCBU care is a recent phenomenon. Prior to the middle of the nineteenth century, infants, whether full-term or pre-term, were rarely weighed at birth. The term 'premature infant' only entered the English language in 1870 (Helders, 1989). Prior to this date infants before term were referred to as 'weaklings' or 'congenitally debilitated' babies. Pre-term infants did not receive any special care but were allowed to 'pine away' and die (Budin, 1900). The first children's hospital was established in Halle in 1701 (Germany) and the first such facility in Britain was established in

Lamb's Conduit Street by Thomas Coram in 1741 near the present site of Great Ormond Street Children's Hospital in London. First attempts to provide some sort of special care were made during the eighteenth and nineteenth centuries. Alphonse Le Roy in 1775 in France recorded his method of providing direct suckling of foundling infants from goats. In 1835, the Czarina Theodorovna, the wife of Czar Paul the first, delivered a weak infant and von Ruehl, a physician working at the Moscow Foundling Hospital designed the first incubator to keep the infant warm. It consisted of a double walled metal bath to nurse infants: the space between the walls could be filled with warm water. In 1895 the first premature baby unit was established at the Hôpital Port Royale in Paris by Pierre Budin. He maintained a permanent staff of wet nurses at the hospital and also was the first to introduce audit to neonatal care following the growth of his discharged infants very carefully in his 'Consultations de Nourissons'. Subsequently, in the early twentieth century, the development of special care took off into an unexpected direction. Martin Couney, an American pupil of Budin with an enterprising mind, started exhibiting pre-term infants in their incubators to the public for an admission charge as part of world and regional exhibitions all around Europe and the United States (Silverman, 1979). Special care units started to appear in the United States from the 1930s (Blackfan and Yaglou, 1933; Silverman, 1979). In Great Britain, initial interest in providing special care facilities can be dated to the mid-1940s (Ministry of Health, 1944), although no clear guidelines or recommendations for widespread introduction of such facilities were given. It was not until 1961 that a memorandum recommended, as a national policy, the establishment of special care nurseries in the larger maternity units in Britain (Central Health Services Council, 1961). Neonatal intensive care providing full respiratory support including ventilation, monitoring and parenteral feeding was introduced in most central European countries at around the same time.

To evaluate whether current NICU/SCBU care is adaptive from a medical and psychological perspective, or whether improvements may be warranted, a range of issues need to be addressed. These include: the differences between SCBU, NICU and normal post-natal care; the changing population of infants cared for in NICUs and SCBUs; the long-term development of babies after being discharged from NICUs; the characteristics of the NICU environment and whether the NICU is adapted to the bio-psychological needs of the pre-term infant and his/her family; whether the reasons for being in NICU care (e.g. immaturity, illness) can be differentiated from the effects of the NICU environment; and how the NICU environment could be improved to benefit the pre-term infant. These are the issues which will be discussed in this chapter.

Definition of SCBU and NICU care

Special Care Baby Units, as the name implies, are facilities of post-natal care which provide specialized care for infants with increased care needs. These are full-term and pre-term infants who require special observation (e.g. monitoring of respiration, heart rate or oxygen by transcutaneous transducers) or have an increased dependency on medical and nursing care for their physiological regulation due to antenatally diagnosed medical conditions, unforeseen obstetric or neonatal complications or because the infants are immature. Special treatments include a whole range of medical or nursing interventions ranging from assistance with thermoregulation (e.g. incubator care), nutrition (parental glucose supplementation or naso-gastric feeding) or respiration (e.g. oxygen supplementation), phototherapy, etc. (Campbell and McIntosh, 1992). SCBUs are found in most district hospitals and have a recommended ratio of 1.25 nurses per cot to cover care for 24 hours. SCBU care is sufficient for the majority of infants who are born premature or have transient neonatal complications.

Neonatal Intensive Care Units differentiate themselves from SCBUs in the degree, i.e. the intensity, range and expertise of care they can provide beyond special care. NICUs have specially equipped intensive care places (cots) to allow continuous monitoring of all vital functions and to support physiological functions of the most immature and sick infants (e.g. continuous parenteral nutrition and continuous ventilation). NICUs are ideally located in hospital facilities integrating a variety of specialities. The care of high dependency patients requires specially trained staff such as neonatologists or neonatal intensive care nurses who in most hospitals almost exclusively work with this high dependency population. The NICU, according to recommendations of the British Paediatric Association, should be headed by a consultant neonatologist, include at least an experienced paediatric registrar and senior house officer for continuous 24 hour cover. The nursing ratio to allow for 24 hour cover and leave should be four trained nurses to one cot (Campbell and McIntosh, 1992).

The changing population of pre-term infants in SCBUs and NICUs

Pre-term infants are those born before 37 weeks of gestation. Around 6–8 per cent of infants in Britain or other industrialized countries are born prematurely (Hack, Horbar, Malloy et al., 1991; Pharoah, Cooke and Rosenbloom, 1990; Riegel, Ohrt, Wolke and Österlund, 1995) with some suggesting that the number is increasing (Williams, 1995). Most infants born just a few weeks premature are able to breathe for themselves, have few complications and will nowadays receive routine post-natal care after initial observation in the SCBU. In contrast, those born very pre-term (i.e. VPI more than 8 weeks early) or at very low birthweight (VLBW; < 1.500g) or those with respiratory problems or medical complications often diagnosed antenatally (e.g. hydrops) are most likely to receive neonatal intensive care (Alberman and Botting, 1991). VLBW and very pre-term infants (VPI) account for 0.7 to 1.1 per cent of all infants born (Bauchner, Brown and Peskin, 1988; Wolke, 1991a). While only 30 years ago, most VLBW infants would not have survived the neonatal period, advances in neonatal intensive care and medical technology mean that 90 per cent of these infants will now be discharged into the care of their parents. Extremely low birthweight (ELBW < 1000g) and extremely pre-term infants (<28 weeks gestation) are now routinely treated in the delivery wards and admitted for specialist neonatal care and are more likely to be discharged alive than not (Roberton, 1993). Medical innovation and changing attitudes of obstetricians and neonatologists have pushed the frontiers of viability even further and infants considered as non-viable only 15 years ago (i.e. infants born at 25 weeks or less and below 500 g birthweight) are now more or less routinely resuscitated and admitted to regional neonatal intensive care units (Williams, 1995). Although the survival rate of these incredibly tiny babies is still low (circa 10–40 per cent) (Roberton, 1993), more and more reports of 'miracle babies' are hitting the headlines (Allen, Donohue and Dunsman, 1993). Increasing numbers of neonatologists are optimistic that ever smaller babies with birthweights as little as 350 g can survive and grow up normally (Holtrop, Ertzbischoff, Roberts et al., 1994; Ginsberg, Goldsmith and Stedman, 1992).

Developmental outcomes for very pre-term infants

Neonatal mortality rates have reduced dramatically in most western countries mainly due to the increased survival of VLBW and VPI infants. Does a higher rate of survival lead to a higher rate of VLBW with major neurodevelopmental handicaps? It has been speculated that, while medical knowhow may secure survival of an increasing number of infants, it may also lead to a higher rate of infants with major handicaps. Infants who suffered neonatal complications (e.g. bleedings into the brain) or alternatively, those who have suffered antenatal complications or congenital problems now survive and add to the rate of major neurodevelopmental handicaps. The first task has been to document changing rates of cerebral palsy as related to birthweight and gestation. There is good evidence that the risk of cerebral palsy is 30–40 times higher in very pre-term than in full-term infants (Hagberg, Hagberg and Zetterström, 1989; Riegel, Ohrt, Wolke and Österlund, 1995; de Vonderweid, Spagnolo, Corchia et al., 1994; Escobar, Littenberg and Petitti, 1991). Monitoring the incidence of cerebral palsy in the whole population of children and progress in neonatal intensive care (i.e. survival rates) showed that cerebral palsy rates increased in the 1970s and 1980s. This was attributed to the increased survival of very pre-term infants (Hagberg, Hagberg and Zetterström, 1989; Hagberg and Hagberg, 1993; Pharoah, Cooke and Rosenbloom, 1990). Others have argued that even in the early years of NICU-care, the relative frequency of CP started to drop (Stewart, Reynolds and Lipscomb, 1981). However, as only around 50–70 per cent of CP cases are identified by two years of age, long-term follow-up is necessary for correct estimations which were not available in the early 1980s (Stanley and Blair, 1991). Independent of whether there has been a slight increase or decrease in CP rates for VLBW infants as more VLBW infants survive, a higher absolute number of VLBW infants with major neurodevelopmental handicaps is to be found in the population (Atkinson and Stanley, 1983; Emond, Golding and Peckham, 1989; Hagberg and Hagberg, 1993). There is furthermore a continuing debate about whether cerebral palsy is the result of obstetric or neonatal complications and treatment or due to the increased survival of neonates who have congenital disorders. These themselves may have led to pre-term labour in the first place. For the latter group, the major handicap is not preventable by neonatal care.

There have been more than 150 studies on the cognitive development of VLBW infants and children. The IQs of VLBW and very pre-term infants have been reported to be in the normal range, though roughly half a standard deviation below the mean in standardized tests (IQ around 92). Wolke, Ratschinski, Ohrt and Riegel (1994) and Wolke (1995a, 1997a) recently demonstrated that these conclusions underestimate the true rate of cognitive deficits. Most studies lacked control groups and relied on IQ-tests with out-moded norms, leading to a mistaken overestimation of true performance (Gross et al., 1992). Furthermore, IQ-deficits for VLBW children are under-estimated when the samples are small, drawn from one specialist rather than from epidemiological samples, or have a high dropout rate (Wolke, Söhne, Ohrt and Riegel, 1995). Recent findings from multi-centre or epidemiological samples indicate that the IQ-scores of VLBW children, as a group, are more likely to be one standard deviation below the mean. The risk of VLBW to have an IQ < 70 (i.e. a learning difficulty) is 10 to 33 times greater than full-term controls (Wolke, Ratschinski, Ohrt and Riegel, 1997; Wolke, 1997a).

More frequent deficits in language development, pre-reading, reading and writing skills have also been reported for VLBW children (e.g. Klein, Hack and Breslau, 1989; Vohr, Garcia-Coll and Oh, 1988) which may be due to specific developmental disorders or to general IQ differences (Hunt et al., 1988). There is some recent evidence which suggests that VLBW children more often have multiple cognitive problems rather than specific learning difficulties (Wolke, 1997a).

VLBW and very pre-term infants have been consistently reported by their parents to have more behaviour problems than full-term controls (Buka, Lipsitt and Tsuang, 1992). Separate analyses according to sex and sympto-matology have indicated that VLBW boys appear to be more frequently affected and that the major behaviour problems are difficulties with attention and hyperactivity (Breslau, Klein and Allen, 1988; Sykes, Hoy, Bill et al., 1997; Wolke and Meyer, 1994). More attention problems as well as inter-nalizing behaviour problems have been found among VLBW infants both at preschool and school age (McGormick, Gortmaker and Sobol, 1990; Weisglas-Kuperus, Koot, Baerts et al., 1993).

Observational studies of LBW infants have indicated that their mothers are more likely to be 'intrusive and controlling' or 'passive and withdrawing' than mothers of normal birthweight babies (Field, 1980b; Lester, Hoffman and Brazelton, 1985). LBW infants who had suffered more severe and long-term illness in the neonatal period are more likely to be passive and less socially engaging in interaction (Minde, Whitelaw, Brown and Fitzhardinge, 1983). Recent investigations of long-term influences on the mother–child relationship have been carried out. Wolke (1995a) found that at six years old VPIs were much less oriented towards a joint task to be carried out by child and mother than controls. Although differences in mater-nal and joint behaviour between mother and child were found, these were small, indicating that there are larger differences between the behaviour of very pre-term and full-term children at early school age than between the behaviour of their mothers. Paradoxically, the poorer synchrony in mother–infant interaction of LBW dyads (Lester, Hoffman and Brazelton, 1985) found in the first year of life has not been reflected in poorer attachment relationships with their mothers at one year as measured in the laboratory with the Ainsworth strange situation. LBW infants have been found to be as often securely attached to their mothers as full-term infants (Easterbrooks, 1989; Goldberg, 1988).

The rate of schooling problems (i.e. special schooling, repeating a class, special needs within the mainstream school) have been found to be between 2 to 9 times higher in VLBW than in control children. Those VLBW children of low gestation, from more socially disadvantaged backgrounds, those with low IQ, physical handicaps or behaviour problems, that is those with multiple problems, are more likely to experience schooling problems (Wolke, 1993, 1997b; Hille, Den Ouden, Bauer et al., 1994). Children with a schooling problem are much more likely to encounter later difficulties ranging from unemployment to lower social status and income.

Statistical comparisons elucidate differences between groups of children. This does not imply that all VLBW infants will encounter problems in their development. Our own work has indicated that roughly one in three VPI will develop major developmental problems (motor, cognitive or behavioural), one in three will have minor developmental problems and one in three will develop normally in comparison to full-term infants (Riegel, Ohrt, Wolke and Österlund, 1995; Wolke, Ratschinski, Ohrt and Riegel, 1994; Wolke, 1997a,b a). This information is important for planning health service delivery and provides guidelines for estimating outcome. It is of limited help for the clinican who has to predict the developmental outcome for a particular infant in his or her care in the neonatal period. Information on the associations between particular neonatal complications and outcome (pathogenesis) is partly available. For example, the lower the gestation of the infant (e.g. 26 weeks), the longer the infant requires intensive care (i.e. ventilation) and the more severe the bleedings into the brain the greater the likelihood of adverse outcome (Riegel, Ohrt, Wolke and Österlund, 1995; Skouteli, Dobuwitz, Levene and Miller, 1985). However, the prediction of the exact type of problem such as CP, cognitive or behaviour problems is still far from perfect. Two infants diagnosed with the same type of condition may have a quite different prognosis in terms of the type and severity of problems they experience.

Little has been said about the developmental outcome of the majority of infants admitted to SCBUs, pre-term (32–36 weeks gestation) and sick full-term infants. These infants usually remain in special care for much briefer periods. Riegel, Ohrt, Wolke and Österlund (1995) and Wolke, 1997b reported on a bi-national study on the developmental progress until 4.8 years of all infants who required special neonatal care in two geographical areas, south Germany and south Finland. The findings were compared to matched full-term controls and a representative cohort of children born in the same year. It is one of the largest studies of at-risk infants to date involving some 8421 infants in Germany and 2194 in Finland. Ex-SCBU infants whether pre-term (32–36 weeks gestation) or full-term (>36 weeks gestation) had only slightly more often performance IQ-deficits (more than 2 standard deviations below the mean) and major verbal IQ-deficits than controls matched for sociodemographic variables. Ex-SCBU pre-term and full-term infants in comparison to full-term routine care infants experienced these cognitive deficits about 2 to 4 times more often. No differences were found in the number of minor deficits for ex-SCBU children in comparison. The lower the length of gestation (and the higher the associated neonatal complications), the more behaviour problems were apparent. Looking at the IQ-mean scores over time (5, 20 and 56 months), excluding those with major congenital, motor or sensory handicap, it was apparent that the mean scores hardly differed between ex-SCBU pre-term and full-term infants and full-term infants who received normal post-natal care. In contrast, very pre-term infants did much more poorly across time.

There is thus increasing evidence that VLBW or ELBW infants are at the highest risk for long-term adverse developmental outcome, and would thus be the best target for enhancing outcome by improving treatment, implementing prevention and early intervention (McCormick, Brooks-Gunn, Workman-Daniels et al., 1992). SCBU pre-term and full-term infants, in contrast, are generally only at a slightly increased risk for long-term developmental problems.

SCBU/NICU environments

To develop concepts of how treatment and the NICU environment could be changed for the better, it is crucial to first describe and analyse the effects of the modern NICU environment on the very pre-term infant.

Two types of neonatal care environments have been distinguished (Wolke and Eldridge, 1992). First, the *physical environment* consists of the nursery design and factors such as noise and light levels, the placing of infant (e.g. cot versus incubator, the bedding, the distance between cots and incubators, etc.) and the objects which are close to the infants (e.g. monitors and mobiles etc.). Second, the *social environment* relates to the opportunities for social experience of the pre-term infant: this includes handling by staff and parents and the provision of auditory, visual, tactile and vestibular stimulation. In practice such a distinction is blurred and not particularly useful because factors in the physical environment partly determine social encounters with the infant.

There are two pathways by which the environment can exert effects on the newborn. *Direct* influences are those characteristics of the physical care or social environment which lead to immediate responses detectable in the physiological, motor and state organization of the infant. The assumption that if better care is provided for parents and staff then they are able to provide better care for the infant is based on *indirect* effects on promoting the infants' development (Redshaw, Rivers and Rosenblatt, 1985; Klaus and Kennell, 1970).

Pre-term infants are exposed to moderate noise levels for weeks and months without having any control over the noise exposure (Saunders, 1995). Noise in the NICU is also one of the greatest concerns of parents (Redshaw and Harris, 1995). The main noise levels outside the incubator are in the range of 55–75 db(A) which resembles the noise pollution found in a busy office environment (Gottfried, 1985). Incubators made in the 1990s comply with the British safety standards which require that the mean noise level inside an incubator should not exceed 60 db(A). This protection against continuous noise is not given in open thermo-controlled radiant heater cots.

Frequencies of less than 500 Hz easily penetrate the incubator but human voices which are in the 100–5000 Hz range are obscured or masked (Bess, Finlayson-Peek and Chapman, 1979). Tape recordings from inside an incubator pick up human speech but it is muffled and indistinct and it is difficult to make sense of the sound source and type (Gottfried, 1985). Impulse sound pressures of 114 db(SPL) can be reached by opening and closing the incubator portholes in older type incubators (Wolke, 1987a). Overall, noise pollution is mainly caused by staff talking and laughing, radios playing, abrupt porthole closing, the placing of bowls and other equipment on the incubator and inconsiderate placement of sound sources such as the telephone located near the incubator (Becker, Grunwald, Moorman and Stuhr, 1991; Wolke, 1987b). Noise levels are generally higher in intensive compared to special care nurseries (Becker, Grunwald, Moorman and Stuhr, 1991).

The risk of hearing loss due to SCBU noise levels in the absence of other severe complications is negligible (Abramowich, Gregory, Slemick and Stewart, 1979). In contrast, sudden loud noises often lead to adverse physiological and behavioural effects, including sleep disturbance, motor arousals such as startles and crying, hypoxaemia, tachycardia and increased intracranial pressure (Long, Lucey and Philip, 1980; Zahr and Balian, 1995). The latter could contribute to the development of intraventricular haemorrhage when associated with poor autoregulation of cerebral blood flow in the pre-term infant's brain (Friis-Hansen, 1985; Volpe, 1989). Meaningful sounds are masked by the incubator and make it unlikely that the infant will acquire recognition and integration of a particular sound (e.g. a voice) with a particular visual stimulus (i.e. a face). This cross-integration is acquired by full-term infants in the first month of life. Bushnell and Slater (1986) suggested that pre-term infants have problems in concept learning and recognition and this may be related to poor cross-integration in the period after birth. Philbin, Ballweg and Gray (1994) found that pre-term infants at 40 weeks postconceptual age habituate less reliably than full-term infants and have also demonstrated that atypical sound exposure can alter habituation in otherwise healthy neonates using an animal model.

The intensity of light in hospital neonatal intensive care units had increased five to tenfold over two decades until the mid-1980s (Glass, Avery, Subramaniou et al., 1985). Adverse effects were reported based on a randomized controlled trial which indicated that normal neonatal intensive care unit light levels may contribute to retinopathy of prematurity in vulnerable extremely low birthweight infants (Glass, Avery, Subramaniou et al., 1985). The effects were more severe when extremely low birthweight infants were nursed near the nursery window allowing long-term exposure to sunlight. Despite these findings and other reports in the 1980s pointing to possible hazards of high levels of lighting (Wolke, 1987b), few changes have been noted in nurseries (Glotzbach, Rowlett, Edgar et al., 1993; Lotas, 1992). While high constant exposure may harm the eyes, sudden increases in light levels are likely to lead to physiological stress. Shogan and Shumann (1993) found that rapidly increasing illumination was associated with adverse changes in oxygen saturation in the more premature neonates in their sample (26–37 weeks gestation).

The amount of handling received by the pre-term infant has increased drastically from about 32 episodes/day in the early 1970s (Speidel, 1976) to a mean of 132–234 handling procedures/day in the mid-1980s (Murdoch and Darlow, 1984). Very pre-term infants in intensive care are handled on average as often as every 5–10 minutes and handling accounts for 4 hours in a

24 hour period. The main 'disturbers' are nursing and support staff, then the paediatricians and only lastly the parents. The sickest and most fragile infants are handled most frequently; however, there is uncertainty whether they are also handled for the longest duration (Symon and Cunningham, 1995). Despite this evidence, staff often underestimate how often very pre-term infants are handled. Less aversive and less frequent handling by staff occurs as the infant's condition improves. Most handling happens during nursing and medical routine procedures and social contact such as talking, gentle touching or rocking occurs infrequently in both intensive and post-intensive care nurseries. Social activities have been found to account for no more than a quarter of the total contact of the infant in intensive care and only up to one-third in the post-intensive care nurseries (Becker, Grunwald, Moorman and Stuhr, 1991; Linn, Horowitz, Buddin et al., 1985).

Handling carried out by nursing and medical staff has been consistently found to disrupt the young infant's sleep pattern. It is also associated with a significantly higher incidence of hypoxaemia, bradycardia, apnoea and behavioural distress with between 40 to 93 per cent of these episodes accounted for by handling only (Murdoch and Darlow, 1984; Long, Philip and Lucey, 1980; Gorski, Huntington and Lewkowicz, 1990; Zahr and Balian, 1995). Handling most frequently precipitates adverse physiological consequences, with the most uncomfortable and adverse procedures (endotracheal suctioning and chest physiotherapy) leading to a marked increase in cerebral blood flow and intracranial pressure. Lagercrantz, Nilsson, Redham and Hjemdal (1986) showed that handling also leads to increased release of catecholamines which in the reported levels are only found in the stressed human organism. Handling and high impulse sounds are also likely to increase the time the infant is spending in REM sleep and the incidence of apnoea has been reported as higher during REM compared to deep non-REM sleep (Hanson and Okken, 1980).

In contrast to the handling by the nursing and paediatric staff, parental handling has been found to be mostly benign (Murdoch and Darlow, 1984). Parents often intuitively talk to and gently stroke their infants (Wolke, 1991b). The indiscriminate encouragement of parents by nursing staff and paediatricians to hold even the very sick and ventilated pre-term infant has arisen from false interpretations of the concept of bonding and it is possible that a 'too pushy' approach may interfere with intuitive parenting, i.e. gentle stroking and minimal handling of the sick infant and with the natural acquisition of a close relationship (Richards, 1985). Offering close contact (i.e. kangaroo-ing) in a selective manner, depending on infant and parent state has no adverse and usually beneficial effects (Anderson, 1994).

Diurnal rhythms are characteristic features of human behaviour and day/night rhythms in sleeping and waking are acquired in the early months of human life (Wolke, 1994). Ultradian rhythms in temperature, heart rate and hormonal cycles are detected in the early weeks of life (Glotzbach, Edgar and Ariagno, 1995). However, pre-term infants in many intensive care units are reared in constant lighting (Shimada, Segawa and Higurashi, 1993; Wolke, Meyer, Ohrt and Riegel, 1995). Glotzbach, Edgar and Ariagno (1995) found very low amplitude circadian rhythms for rectal and skin temperatures, heart rate and activity which did not differ over the day in pre-term infants at 35 weeks of postconceptual age. Any indicators of rhythmicity were masked by caregiving events, in particular feeding, where the largest physiological changes were observed. There is increased evidence that quiet periods and a clear diurnal rhythm of activities are beneficial for very pre-term infants (Strauch, Brandt and Edwards-Beckett, 1993). The introduction of reduced noise, light and handling at night in intensive care units has been found to reduce staff interventions, support longer periods of deep sleep and fewer state changes in vulnerable pre-term infants while in the nursery (Fajardo, Browning, Fisher and Paton, 1990). Longer-term positive influences such as more rapid post discharge weight gain have also been reported (Mann, Haddow, Stokes and Goodley, 1986). However, the lack of day/night cycle before 35 weeks gestation has little long-term consequences for night sleeping behaviour (Wolke, Meyer, Ohrt and Riegel, 1995) in the early years of life. Wolke, Meyer, Ohrt and Riegel (1995) even found that very pre-term infants were less likely to wake at night at five months of age.

Young infants have no verbal language apart from crying and they acquire concepts about the world through sensorimotor experiences and by making associations between stimuli. During the early stages of development the function and structure of the brain are particularly dependent on interaction with the environment (Greenough, Black and Wallace, 1987); motor skills and perceptual and intellectual performances are consolidated by learning in early infancy (Slater, 1989) and the resilience and plasticity of the central nervous system allows recovery from moderately adverse early influences (Sameroff and Chandler, 1975; Wolke, 1993). The description of the intensive and special care baby unit environment indicates that there is little opportunity or support for early constructive learning (Wolke, 1991b). Many of the sensory motor experiences are unpleasant and during incubator nursing there are few opportunities for cross-modal integration and concept learning. Most of the handling and human sounds are non-contingent to the infant's state and the pre-term infant can exert little control over stimuli in the environment. Furthermore, although the pre-term infant's capacities for social interaction increase as the infant recovers and graduates to the post-intensive care nursery, the staff-to-patient ratio changes equally dramatically. There are fewer nurses to look after the more alert infant who is now potentially more often able to invite and cope with increased social action.

The findings to date reinforce the conclusions reached in the mid-1980s by Als, Lawhon, Gibes et al. (1985), Gottfried (1985) and Wolke (1987a, b; 1989) that there is a bad fit between the NICU and SCBU environment and the infant's behavioural organization and developmental needs. The review indicates that current, often 'too-intensive care' for small babies can have adverse effects on their physiological and behavioural organization. Changes in the physical and caretaking environment have mostly been determined by accommodating equipment and staff needs rather than the needs of the identified patient, the small newborn infant. Considerations for the infant have often only been afterthoughts (Hodgman, 1985). There is, however, some evidence that being housed in the neonatal unit contributes to subsequent development in ways not directly related to the reasons for being on such a unit (Lawson, Turkewitz, Platt and McCarton, 1985; Als, Lawhon, Duffy et al., 1994). Direct effects for the occurrence of retinopathy of prematurity have been described and adverse physiological variations, for example, in oxygen saturation due to handling or noise, may possibly contribute to bleedings into the brain. If it could be demonstrated that less invasive care is safe, cheaper and leads to the same or improved developmental outcome, then urgency for change might increase.

Longer-term effects of 'gentler' care

Does a 'gentler' approach to care in the NICU have benefits for infants? There are two ways of answering this question. First, differences in developmental outcome in different NICUs using care approaches which vary in intensity can be studied. Second, controlled intervention studies of the developmental effects of changing to a 'gentler' nursery are required.

Comparisons of the mortality and neonatal morbidity between different NICUs in the USA indicates large differences, for example, in respiratory distress and ventilation rates (Avery, Tooley and Keller, 1987; Hack, Horbar, Malloy et al., 1991). Wolke (1995a, 1997b) compared the complication rates and neonatal treatment approaches and developmental outcome at four to five years of age of very pre-term infants in south Germany (SG) and south Finland (SF). Mortality rates until five years were 29.3 per cent in SG and 33.3 per cent in SF and major neurodevelopmental sequelae (SG: 11.7 per cent; SF: 12.5 per cent) did not differ. To identify whether treatment approaches differed and affected development outcome, analyses of the developmental progress of infants without major neurological handicap (no MND) were carried out. The infants were born at the same birthweight, gestation, and had experienced the same number of complications during pregnancy and birth and neonatally. However, very pre-term infants had different experiences during their neonatal stay in the NICUs in SG and SF. Very pre-term SG-infants were more frequently mechanically ventilated, remained on the respirator significantly longer and received parenteral nutrition more often and for longer. The SF-infants received intensive care for shorter periods and they were discharged home more than two weeks earlier at a lower weight. The findings show that the decision to intubate and ventilate has a whole range of consequences for subsequent treatment. Invasive treatment in SG did not reduce mortality or neonatal morbidity and had no positive effects on later performance IQ. Rather, early routine respiratory treatment had a range of negative consequences: longer intensive treatment (more handling, more noise, less parental contact) and longer hospital stay. The Finnish infants, who received less invasive treatment, also had significantly higher verbal IQ scores.

Two recent studies with historical controls (i.e. changing the type of treatment and comparing the results to those for infants treated under the previous care regime) evaluated the effects of reducing routine interventions and using a minimal handling and invasiveness procedure. Jacobsen, Gronvall, Petersen and Andersen (1993) introduced a 'minitouch' regime which differed from routine treatment in that VLBW infants were not routinely intubated, only nasal CPAP or oxygen supplementation was initially given and the infants were left for two hours after birth without invasive investigations (i.e. blood sampling, X-rays, etc.). During this period the infant was non-invasively monitored. Jacobsen et al. (1993) found that the mechanical ventilation rate was reduced from 76 to 35 per cent. However, those who were judged to need ventilation received it for similar periods in the minitouch regime as before. The incidence of intracranial haemorrhage was reduced from 49 to 25 per cent. They concluded from these findings that the minitouch regime can prevent the progression of respiratory distress, reduce the need for ventilator treatment and is a safe and convenient alternative to routine mechanical ventilation in pre-term infants with mild respiratory distress. Porz et al. (1995) introduced an individualized approach to medical care avoiding invasive procedures as much as possible. He reported that the need for ventilation could be reduced from 95 to 63 per cent for ELBW infants and from 82 to 46 per cent for VLBW infants. Surfactant treatment could be halved. No increases in mortality or intracranial bleedings were found. However, neither of these studies followed the babies to report on developmental progress or rehospitalization rates, for example. In Wolke's study (1995a), more of the infants who received the less intensive form of care needed rehospitalization early in life. This was mainly for upper respiratory infections in Finland but for chronic illnesses (neurological problems) in Germany, indicating different referral patterns (Riegel, Ohrt, Wolke and Österlund, 1995). Brooten, Kumar, Brown et al. (1986) conducted a randomized controlled trial to determine the safety, efficacy and cost savings of early hospital discharge of VLBW infants. Early discharge may decrease the chances of contracting infections in hospital and counteract parents' feelings of inadequacy in caring in hospital. The infants in the early discharge group, who had to fulfil a certain set of criteria, were discharged a mean of 11 days earlier, weighed 200 g less and were two weeks younger at discharge than control infants. All early discharge infants received specially implemented regular nursing home care in the community. The net cost saving (in 1986) was US$18,560 per VLBW infant (and 36,000 VLBW infants are born per year in the USA alone). The findings of Brooten, Kumar, Brown et al. (1986) indicate that, if combined with community nursing care, earlier discharge has no negative effects and saves money.

Three studies so far have investigated an integrated individualized developmental approach to care, as advocated by Als (1992) and Wolke (1987a). In the first study, using historical controls, Als, Lawhon, Brown et al. (1986) found that longer-term complications (bronchopulmonary dysplasia) could be reduced by preventing inappropriate sensory input and providing individualized care depending on the developmental and behavioural status of the very pre-term infant. Infants in the experimental group had significantly shorter stays on the respirator, their feeding behaviour was normalized earlier, behavioural regulation was more efficient in infancy and they obtained higher scores in the Bayley Developmental Test. Becker, Grunwald, Moorman and Stuhr (1991) replicated this study, training nurses according to a modified version of Als' programme, and investigating whether individualized care actually led to reduced noise and light levels. They found tHat the physical changes (reduction of noise and light) in the environment were successfully implemented; however, a clear daily rhythm was not achieved in either the experimental or the control condition. Experimental infants had lower morbidity levels, were introduced to oral feeding sooner and had shorter stays in the hospital. Their overall behavioural organization at discharge was also better, as assessed by the Brazelton NBAS total score (Brazelton and Nugent, 1995). Similar positive effects on motor organization were reported by Mouradian and Als (1994). The findings indicate that the beneficial effects of developmental care can be achieved with the resources available in most nurseries. However, it is important to point out that the findings in this study with a larger sample were less dramatic and clear cut than in the previous study by Als, Lawhon, Brown et al. (1986).

Recently, Als, Lawhon, Duffy et al. (1994) reported on a second study designed to test the impact of individualized developmental care using random assignment of babies and initiation of the intervention at the time of admission. Subjects weighing less than 1250 g, born before 30 weeks gestation and mechanically ventilated within 3 hours of delivery were assigned randomly either to a control group (normal NICU care) or an experimental group (individualized developmental care; Als, 1992). The experimental infants did not receive continuous experimental treatment but at least one shift in a 24 hour cycle was staffed by a nurse specially educated in this approach. The groups did not differ according to medical variables at birth or sociodemographic indicators. Experimental infants developed intra-ventricular haemorrhage less often, had bronchopulmonary dysplasia (chronic lung disease) less frequently, were ventilated or required oxygen for shorter periods and had a shorter stay in the NICU and in hospital. The cost savings were large with the average cost of treatment for the control infants amounting to US$189,000 versus US$98,000 for the experi-mental group. Neurobehavioural assessment two weeks after discharge indicated more optimal autonomic and motor system control and better behavioural self-regulation. Furthermore, electrophysiological differences in brain functioning were demonstrated between the groups and developmental outcome assessed with the Bayley scales was significantly better for the experimental group at nine months of age. The positive developmental effects were only partly explained by fewer complications due to 'gentle' care. Individualized care appears to have further effects on promoting develop-ment and behavioural organization beyond the avoidance of complications.

This review clearly indicates that less invasive but medically closely monitored treatment is beneficial in reducing distress for infants, improving development and saving costs. Although the findings so far are impressive they were obtained in small studies and there is a need for further controlled research. Als' (1992) approach focuses on nursing and involves a lengthy and expensive training (i.e. NIDCAP, Als, 1992), making no reference to integrated changes in early medical care. For example, all infants in the Als, Lawhon, Duffy et al. (1994) study were routinely ventilated. The findings by Wolke (1995a), Jacobsen, Gronvall, Petersen and Andersen (1993) and Porz et al. (1995), however, show that invasive medical treatments can be reduced in the initial hours and this alone is putting NICU infants on track for less invasive subsequent care. Further studies are needed to investigate the rela-tive efficacy of changes in nursing and/or early medical care.

An integrated, individualized and developmental care approach (IIDCA)

The evidence of naturalistic studies of NICU environments suggests that there is not a good fit between the NICU and SCBU environment and the infants' behavioural organization. The intervention studies which reduce the invasiveness and stress during initial medical care, change the physical and caretaking environment to reduce behavioural disorganization and support the development of the infant while in NICU care, indicate the success of this approach. However, a whole range of other developmental support programmes guided by different theoretical models have been tried. Nurcombe, Howell, Rauh et al. (1984) and Wolke (1991a) distinguished between five major theoretical approaches:

1. programmes that aim to counteract neonatal sensory deprivation or overload;
2. programmes that aim to prevent faulty mother–infant bonding;
3. programmes that aim to help parents resolve the emotional crisis of premature delivery;
4. programmes that aim to help parents to be more sensitive and responsive to their baby's cues and improve mother–child interaction; and
5. compensatory programmes which are aimed at infants identified in the first year of life as having developmental problems (rehabilitation).

Programmes 1 to 3 are usually hospital based (NICU/SCBU; see Lacy and Ohlsson, 1993); 4 and 5 are usually community based (Wolke, 1991a; Brooks-Gunn, McCarton, Casey et al., 1994). Newborn sensory stimulation programmes (type 1 programmes) assume that the infant is deprived from his/her final weeks in utero (e.g. of mother's heartbeat sounds, vestibular stimulation) or may be deprived of appropriate extra-uterine stimulation (Field, 1980a; understimulation model). Others, in contrast, have suggested that the LBW infant is overstimulated in the NICU and needs protection from these stimuli (Cornell and Gottfried, 1976). Intervention modes have been extra-sensory stimulation using extra sucking, stroking, massages, nursing in hammocks, oscillating water beds, music playing, etc. (see Wolke, 1991a; Lacy and Ohlsson, 1993). Programmes in category 2 assume that 'if you want to improve the lives of children, improve the situation of the caregivers' (Klaus and Kennel, 1982, p. 189). Intervention methods include 'open' visiting policies, early holding of the baby and the 'kangaroo' method. These programmes assume that premature delivery represents a severe life stress for many parents (Minde, 1984; Redshaw and Harris, 1995) interfering with their potential for appropriate caretaking (Crnic, Ragozin, Greenberg et al., 1983). It has been argued that helping parents to resolve the emotional crisis will indirectly benefit the relationship with the infant and lead to developmental gains (Boukydis, 1986; Dammers and Harpin, 1982). Interventions usually involve guided self-help groups or individual counselling of the parents (e.g., Minde, Shosenberg, Thompson and Marton, 1983).

As Wolke (1991a) and Lacy and Ohlsson (1993) point out, not only are many of the intervention studies flawed, but they also offer only limited evidence of short- or long-term benefits for the pre-term infants. Nearly all interventions show some sort of improvement (e.g. weight gain or sleeping, etc.); however, the results may be due to unspecified effects, such as giving attention to particular babies or parents. Providing extra stimulation to fragile infants without regard to their ability to cope with that stimulation does not appear sensible. Nor does reducing stimulation for all infants find support in any developmental theory. It is now known that bonding is not a magical process initiated by immediate handling and holding. In a fragile infant may result in severe distress for both baby and parent (Wolke and Eldridge, 1992). Furthermore, there is little evidence that helping parents to cope with the emotional crisis leads automatically to better caretaking (Minde, Shosenberg, Thompson and Marton, 1983). Parents need not only to feel emotionally better but they need the skills to understand and interact with the small infant appropriately (Helfer, 1987). Thus others have employed the Neonatal Behavioural Assessment Scale (NBAS; Brazelton and Nugent, 1995) to demonstrate to parents the newborn's competences and weaknesses. When applied before discharge of pre-term infants from the SCBU, demonstrating and explaining the pre-term newborn's behaviour to parents and discussing its implications for caretaking and interaction has been found to have some small to moderate short-term effects on the pre-term infant's development (e.g. Widmayer and Field, 1980, 1981; Nugent, 1985; Culp, Culp and Harmon, 1989; Cole, 1995; Wolke, 1995b).

Other intervention approaches for LBW infants are home or community based (Wolke, 1991a). A range of studies have evaluated the effect of providing a wide range of social and practical support, additional early learning curricula (e.g. center-based day-care programmes), structured interaction and developmental coaching (e.g. Barrera, Rosenbaum and Cunningham, 1986; Barnard, Hammond, Sumner et al., 1987; Affleck, Tennen, Rowe et al., 1989; Brooks-Gunn, McCarton, Casey et al., 1994; Richmond, 1990; The Infant Health and Development Program, 1990). The underlying notion is that providing enrichment experiences in the first few years of life can protect children against biological disadvantages over extended periods of time. While the short-term effects of home or centre based interventions have been encouraging (see Wolke, 1991a), recent findings in multi-centre trials combining specialized centre care (from year 1 to year 3) and home visiting (hospital discharge to year 3) have been disappointing. Brooks-Gunn, McCarton, Casey et al. (1994), in the largest randomized trial so far, found that while gains of intervention were found at three years of age in terms of increased IQ and receptive language scores and fewer behavioural problems, these effects were mostly not sustained at five years of age, two years after the intervention ceased. The results were most dissappointing for infants below 2000 g birthweight with no sustained effects of the intervention programme detected at all at five years of age. Wolke's findings from the Bavarian Longitudinal Study indicated that biological risk and associated intensive care have persistent effects for the smaller pre-term infants (< 32 weeks gestation) with social factors making an additional contribution (Wolke, 1993; Riegel, Ohrt, Wolke and Österlund, 1995; Wolke, 1997b).

Finally, a number of studies have been carried out to test the effectiveness of integrated intervention, that is combining individualized sensory stimulation in the NICU with parent-centred interventions in hospital and continuing support at home (Rauh, Achenbach, Howell and Teti, 1988; Achenbach et al., 1993; Resnick, Davis Eyler, Nelson et al., 1987; Scarr-Salapatek and Williams, 1973). These studies have found highly significant and often long-term gains (e.g. eight years of age; Achenbach et al., 1993) in IQ scores. Achenbach et al. (1993) found that the pre-term intervention group had, on average, identical IQ scores to those of full-term children at four and eight years, while the pre-term children who did not receive intervention were significantly delayed (10–13 IQ points; Achenbach et al., 1993).

Developmental tasks of pre-term newborns: developmental neonatology

Most models of intervention have adopted ideas which originated from simple comparisons between the pre-term infant and the fetus, or have adapted approaches designed for other populations, such as socially disadvantaged families. These models often lack a clear theoretical basis – they are not rooted in developmental theory and are only loosely based on empirical studies of the 'natural' course of development of LBW and VLBW infants. Wolke (1987a), comparing the environmental experiences of full-term newborns (extra-uterine), pre-term infants (extra-uterine) and the fetus (intra-uterine) concluded that the premature newborn is neither similar to the fetus nor a deficient full-term infant, but a unique organism. The very premature baby is a cultural evolutionary product with special needs. S/he has irreversibly left the intra-uterine environment, with all that entails (nutrition, oxygenation, infection protection, etc.), yet her/his nervous system is geared to many more weeks of the intra-uterine environment's input and control. Very pre-term newborns are a new group of humans which did not exist decades ago and they have special developmental needs, addressed by a new sub-discipline, *developmental neonatology* (the study of developmental changes and progress of the pre-term or sick infant while in special care; see Wolke, 1987a; 1989; 1991b).

Als (1992), Wolke (1987a; 1989) and others (e.g. White-Traut, Nelson, Burns and Cunningham, 1994) thus argue that specific developmental models of adaptation are needed for very pre-term infants. From a developmental neonatology perspective (Wolke, 1987a), four developmental tasks need to be accomplished for behavioural integration by newborns (Figure 13.1):

- physiological and autonomic control (e.g. breathing, temperature control, skin diffusion, etc.),
- motor organization (from jerky, flacid, floppy tone and movements to smooth, well-toned movements),
- state organization (the development of six distinct behavioural states and controlled movement between them), and
- sustained alertness for interaction with the environment.

A fifth mechanism is responsible for the overall integrative control of the four partly hierarchically organized levels.

Healthy full-term infants are usually able to regulate their basic physiological functions such as breathing or temperature control. In contrast, very immature or sick newborns often need external support for these physiological functions (respirator, oxygen, incubator care, etc.). There are differences in the quality of motor organization in healthy full-term neonates (St. James-Roberts and Wolke, 1989; Wolke and St. James-Roberts, 1987) while pre-term infants are often very flacid, have low tone and jerky movements. Furthermore, very pre-term infants have a less differentiated state

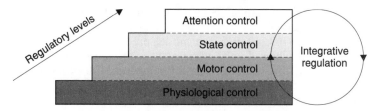

Figure 13.1

organization with more frequent changes in a less ordered and smooth fashion (transient states; Als, 1992). The development of differentiations of light and deep sleep are partly dependent on neurological development (Challamel, 1988; Wolke, 1994; Wolke, Meyer, Ohrt and Riegel, 1995) as are differentiations between drowsiness and alert state. Only when the infant has reasonable autonomic, motor and state control is s/he available for social interaction. Pre-term infants are more frequently hypoalert or when distressed hyperalert; they can only fleetingly attend, and too active interaction by a caretaker can have consequences ranging from gaze aversion to vomiting (Gorski, 1984). The final control system, the overall regulation, is concerned with integration of the different subsystems for homeostatic functioning. Overall control is self-regulation and coping, i.e. behaviours to maintain a balanced state. The full-term infant's efforts for self-regulation are, for example, sucking the fist or changing posture to maintain a balanced state. Pre-term infants when overloaded with input may use less constructive, defensive strategies such as avoiding eye contact to maintain a stable organization (Widmayer and Field, 1981).

This chapter has described the NICU/SCBU environment in which pre-term infants are reared, and a conceptual model of internal bio-behavioural organization and self-regulation of newborns has been introduced. Development of the pre-term newborn itself is the continuous process of adaptation of the internal and external system. Development is progressing well if there is a good fit between the physical and caretaking environment and the behavioural organization, at each point of time of the evolving system. However, development may be deviant if the fit between external and internal systems is unsatisfactory. Fortunately, due to the plasticity of the central nervous system and adaptability of the infant's internal system, the infant can deal with a number of reproductive or environmental hazards (Sameroff and Chandler, 1975). However, if the internal regulation system is impaired (dysfunctional), adaptation to the environment is difficult. Similarly, misfit may occur if the external system, the caretaking or home environment is impaired. Wolke, Brothwood, Gamsu and Cooper (1989) argued that a distinction needs to be drawn between impairments of internal control due to 'hardware' damage (i.e. structural CNS damage) and 'software' damage, i.e. learned patterns of responding which are dysfunctional. Hardware impairment (e.g. cerebral palsy, severe neuro-sensory problems, etc.) is reasonably well predicted by an accumulation of reproductive insults (Skouteli, Doubwitz, Levene and Miller, 1985; Wolke, Brothwood, Gamsu and Cooper, 1989). In contrast, long-term software problems (learning difficulties, behaviour problems, etc.) require transactional models which consider complex interchanges between the internal (infant) and external (environmental) factors.

Applied to the NICU/SCBU, the model predicts that if environmental demands are made which do not adapt or fit with the internal organization level of the infant, this leads to internal behavioural disorganization. For example, repeated (unnecessary) handling, noise or vigorous interaction attempts for a ventilated infant, still struggling to gain physiological control, are inappropriate and lead to disorganization at all levels (autonomic, e.g. hypoxaemia; motor, agitation, flaccidity; state, large state fluctuations; interaction, no preparedness, avoidance). Disorganization in behaviour is thus an indicator of the effects of the environment. Similarly, infants who are not on the respirator may be thrown into severe disorganization by apparently simple caretaking acts such as feeding. The infant may just be able to cope with oral feeding, but if talking and looking at the infant occurs at the same time, his/her organizational efforts may fall apart. Disorganization, if persistent at the physiological level, can affect the CNS of the infant (e.g. periventricular haemorrhages) due to poor blood flow autoregulation problems (Volpe, 1989). This is known to all neonatologists; however, the idea that the effects may be induced by a maladapted NICU environment (iatrogenic environmental effects) is new.

Improving the NICU environment

There are no easy recipes for optimal psychological development of the infant in hospital. However, there are three principles of care (see full recommendations in Wolke, 1987a,b; Wolke and Eldridge, 1992; Wolke, 1997b,c):

1. **Observe the baby.** How does s/he react to noises, light, handling and attempts at social interaction and show his/her distress or pleasure?
2. **Design an individual care plan.** Provide a caregiving and a nursery environment which reinforces the emerging abilities of the maturing infant.
3. **Grow up with the patient.** The pre-term infant develops during his/her time in the hospital. It is important that the care adapts adequately to these changes (Wolke, 1987a,b, 1991b).

Final comments

To date 'many of the different aspects of perinatal (medical) intensive care have never been and probably never will be validated' (Ens-Dokkum, Schreuder, Veen et al., 1992, p. 439). Many traditional medical or nursing routines in the NICU have never been subjected to empirical scrutiny. Gentle care approaches are increasingly subject to empirical validation, and Als, Lawhon, Duffy et al. (1994, p. 858) concluded on basis of their findings that 'provision of expert intensive medical care within an individualized, developmental framework is not only feasible but necessary to enhance the effectiveness of NICU care'. It is often difficult to change 'old' ways, to break the routine and start observing, monitoring and implementing new approaches of care. Higher standards of evidence including larger samples, better controls, reduced programme components, longer follow-up, etc., are (rightly) requested from this new approach which challenges traditional medical treatment and nursing. It may, however, take more than science to persuade more neonatologists and nursing staff that there is a strong link between NICU environment, infant physiology and development outcome and that proposed changes are safe. Critically ill newborns can be harmed not only by undertreatment but also by overtreatment. It will not be long before this could be reflected in legal proceedings against NICU carers (Silverman, 1992; Stahlman, 1990; Harrison, 1993). I hope that empirical evidence rather than legal ruling will lead to a more humane nursery in future, although for future NICU patients the care rather than the means by which it was implemented is of relevance.

Applications

1. Prevention of invasive treatment

- Transport (i.e. by in-utero transferral) and thus ventilation of the VLBW infant needs to be avoided.
- The routine use of intubation for VLBW/ELBW infants needs to be abandoned. Nasal CPAP and 'minitouch' treatment are proven alternatives (Jacobson, Gronvall, Petersen and Andersen, 1993).

2. Reduction of noise and light pollution and routine handling

- Reduction of noise by changing staff behaviour (e.g. no radio playing, no placing of bowls on incubator, use of noise absorbent flooring, shoes, etc.).
- Reduce lighting by flexible point lighting and introducing a clear day-night rhythm in illumination.
- Minimal handling of fragile infants; and calm infants after any handling.

3. Strengthen the role of parents and siblings

Recognize that parents are the primary caregivers and have rights for open and honest communication, need to be welcomed and have access to their infant. They also have responsibilities: to visit, to take over increasing amounts of are, to be involved, etc. Parents want to be involved but sometimes feel they cannot be.

4. Staff also have needs

Medical and nursing staff work under conditions of high emotional stress – they need regular formal supervision and meetings and informal means of communicating (e.g. coffee room, trusted person, counsellor).

Acknowledgements

I would like to thank Tina Gutbrod, Katherine Stanford, Cerian Hughes, Jörg Schulz, Renate Meyer and Brigitte Söhne for assistance in producing the reference list.

The reported research (BLS) was supported by the German Federal Government Ministry of Science (BMBF) (Jug 14) to K. Riegel, D. Wolke and B. Ohrt.

References

Achenbach, T. M., Howell, C. T., Aoki, M. F. and Rauh, V. A. (1993). Nine-year outcome of the Vermont Intervention Program for low birth weight infants. *Pediatrics*, **91**, 45–55.

Affleck, G., Tennen, H., Rowe, J., Roscher, B. and Walker, L. (1989). Effects of formal support on mothers' adaptation to the hospital-to-home transition of high-risk infants: the benefits and costs of helping. *Child Development*, **60**, 488–501.

Alberman, E. and Botting, B. (1991). Trends in prevalence and survival of very low birth weight infants, England and Wales 1983–1987. *Archives of Disabled Children*, **66**, 1304–8.

Allen, M., Donohue, P. and Dusman, A. (1993). The limit of viability: neonatal outcome of infants born at 22 to 25 weeks of gestation. *New England Journal of Medicine*, **329**, 1597–601.

Als, H. (1984). Manual for the naturalistic observation of the newborn (preterm and full-term). The Children's Hospital, Boston, MA.

Als, H. (1992). Individualized, family-focused developmental care for the very low birthweight preterm infant in the NICU. In *The Psychological Development of Low Birthweight Children* (S. L. Friedman and M. D. Sigman, eds). New Jersey: Ablex.

Als, H. and Duffy, S. H. (1982). The behavior of the fetal newborn: theoretical considerations and practical suggestions for the use of the APIB. *Issues in Neonatal Care*. Boston: Westar.

Als, H., Lawhon, G., Brown, E., Gibes, R., Duffy, F. H., McAnulty, G. and Blickman, J. G. (1986). Individualized behavioral and environmental care for the very low birth weight preterm infant at high risk for bronchopulmonary dysplasia: neonatal intensive care unit and developmental outcome. *Pediatrics*, **78**, 1123–32.

Als, H., Lawhon, G., Duffy, F. H., McAnulty, G. B., Gibes-Grossman, R. and Blickman, J. G. (1994). Individualized developmental care for the very low-birth-weight preterm infant. *Journal of the American Medical Association*, **272**, 853–8.

Als, H., Lawhon, G., Gibes, R., Brown, E. and Duffy, F. H. (1985). Individualized behavioral and environmental care for the VLBW preterm at high risk for chronic lung disease. Presentation at the Biennial Meeting of the Society for Research in Child Development Conference, Toronto, Canada, April 25–28.

Ambramowich, S. J., Gregory, S., Slemick, M. and Stewart, A. (1979). Hearing loss in very low birthweight infants treated with neonatal intensive care. *Archives of Disease in Childhood*, **54**, 421–5.

Anand, K. J. S. and Hickey, P. R. (1987). Pain and its effects in the human neonate and fetus. *New England Journal of Medicine*, **317**, 1321–9.

Anderson, G. C. (1994). Current knowledge about skin-to-skin (kangaroo) care for preterm infants. Paper presented at the International Conference on Infant Studies, Paris.

Atkinson, S. and Stanley, F. J. (1983). Spastic diplegia among children of low and normal birthweight. *Developmental Medicine and Child Neurology*, **25**, 693–708.

Avery, M. E., Tooley, W. H. and Keller, J. B. (1987). Chronic lung disease preventable? A survey of eight centers. *Pediatrics*, **79**, 26–30.

Barnard, K. E., Hammond, M. A., Sumner, G. A., Kang, R., Johnson-Crowley, N., Snyder, C., Spietz, A., Blackburn, S., Brandt, P. and Magyary, D. (1987). Helping parents with preterm infants: field test of a protocol. *Early Child Development and Care*, **27**, 255–90.

Barrera, M. E., Rosenbaum, P. L. and Cunningham, C. E. (1986). Early home intervention with low-birth-weight infants and their parents. *Child Development*, **57**, 20–33.

276 Current Issues in Infancy and Parenthood

Culp, R. E., Culp, A. M. and Harmon, R. J. (1989). A tool for educating parents about their premature infants. *Birth*, **16**, 23–6.

Dammers, A. and Harpin, V. (1982). Parents' meetings in two neonatal units: a way of increasing support for parents. *British Medical Journal*, **285**, 863–5.

Darlington, R. B., Royce, J. M., Snipper, A. S., Murray, H. W. and Lazar, I. (1980). Preschool programs and later school competence of children from low-income families. *Science*, **208**, 202–4.

de Vonderweid, U., Spagnolo, A., Corchia, Chiandotto, V., Chiappe, S., Chiappe, F., Colarizi, DeLuca, T., Didato, M. and Fertz, F. C. (1994). Italian multicentre study on very low birth weight babies. Neonatal mortality and two year outcome. *Acta Paediatrica*, **83** (4), 391–6.

Easterbrooks, M. A. (1989). Quality of attachment to mother and to father: effects of perinatal risk status. *Child Development*, **60**, 825–30.

Emond, A., Golding, J. and Peckham, C. (1989). Cerebral palsy in two national cohort studies. *Archives of Disease in Childhood*, **64**, 848–52.

Ens-Dokkum, M. H., Schreuder, A. M., Veen, S., Verloove-Vanhorick, S. P., Brand, R. and Ruys, J. H. (1992). Evaluation of care for the preterm infant: review of literature on follow-up of preterm and low birthweight infants. *Pediatric and Perinatal Epidemiology*, **6**, 434–59.

Escobar, G. J., Littenberg, B. and Petitti, D. B. (1991). Outcome among surviving very low birthweight infants: a meta-analysis. *Archives of Disease in Childhood*, **66**, 204–11.

Fajardo, B., Browning, M., Fisher, D. and Paton, J. (1990). Effect of nursery environment on state regulation in very-low-birth-weight premature infants. *Infant Behaviour and Development*, **13**, 287–303.

Field, T. (1980a). Supplemental stimulation of preterm neonates. *Early Human Development*, **4**, 301–14.

Field, T. (1980b). Interactions of high-risk infants: quantitative and qualitative differences. In *Exceptional Infant*, **4**, 299–312 (D. B. Sawin, R. C. Hawkins, L. Olszewski Walker and J. H. Penticuff, eds). London: Academic Press.

Fitzgerald, M., Millard, C. and MacIntosh, N. (1988a). Hyperalgesia in premature infants. *Lancet*, **1**, 292.

Friss-Hansen, B. (1985). Perinatal brain injury and cerebral flow in newborn infants. *Acta Paediatrica Scandinavica*, **74**, 323–31.

Ginsberg, H. G., Goldsmith, J. P. and Stedman, C. M. (1992). Hospital care techniques resulting in intact survival of a 380g infant. *Acta Paediatrica Supplement*, **382**, 13–15.

Glass, E., Avery, G. B., Subramaniou, K. N. S., Keys, M. P., Sostek, A. M. and Friendly, D. S. (1985). Effect of bright light in the hospital nursery on the incidence of retinopathy of prematurity. *New England Journal of Medicine*, **313**, 401–4.

Glotzbach, S. F., Edgar, D. M. and Ariagno, R. L. (1995). Biological rhythmicity in preterm infants prior to discharge from neonatal intensive care. *Pediatrics*, **95** (2), 231–7.

Glotzbach, S. F., Rowlett, E. A., Edgar, D. M., Moffat, R. J. and Artiagno, R. L. (1993). Light variability in the modern neonatal nursery: chronobiologic issues. *Medical Hypotheses*, **41** (3), 217–24.

Goldberg, S. (1988). Risk factors in infant–mother attachment. *Canadian Journal of Psychology*, **42** (2), 173–88.

Gorski, P. A. (1984). Premature infant behavioural and physiological responses to caregiving intervention in the intensive care nursery. In *Frontiers of Infant Psychiatry* (J. D. Call, E. Galenson and R. L. Tyson, eds). New York: Basic Books.

Gorski, P. A., Huntington, L. and Lewkowicz, D. J. (1990). Handling preterm infants in hospitals. *Clinics in Perinatology*, **17**, 103–12.

Gottfried, A. W. (1985). Environment of newborn infants in special care units. In *Infant Stress Under Intensive Care: Environmental Neonatology* (A. W. Gottfried and J. L. Gaiter, eds). University Park Press.

Greenough, W. T., Black, J. E. and Wallace, C. S. (1987). Experience and brain development. *Child Development*, **58**, 539–59.

Batton, D. G., Holtrop, P., DeWitte, D., Pryce, C. and Roberts, C. (1994). Current gestational age-related incidence of major intraventricular hemorrhage. *The Journal of Pediatrics*, **125**, 623–5.

Bauchner, H., Brown, E. and Peskin, J. (1988). Premature graduates of the newborn intensive care unit: a guide to follow-up. *The Pediatrics Clinics of North America*, **35**, 1207–25.

Becker, P., Grunwald, P. C., Moorman, J. and Stuhr, S. (1991). Outcomes of developmentally supportive nursing care for very low birth weight infants. *Nursing Research*, **40**, 150–55.

Bess, F. H., Finlayson-Peek and Chapman, J. J. (1979). Further observations on noise levels and infant incubators. *Pediatrics*, **63**, 100–106.

Blackfan, K. and Yaglou, C. (1933). The premature infant: a study of the effects of atmospheric conditions on growth and development. *American Journal of Diseases of Childhood*, **46**, 1175–84.

Bogdan, R., Brown, M. A. and Foster, S. B. (1982). Be honest but not cruel: staff/parent communication on a neonatal unit. *Human Organisation*, **41**, 6–16.

Boukydis, C. F. Z. (1986). *Support for Parents and Infants*. London: Routledge and Kegan Paul.

Bozzette, M. (1993). Observation of pain behaviour in the NICU: an exploratory study. *Journal of Perinatal and Neonatal Nursing*, **7**, 76–87.

Brazelton, T. B. and Nugent, K. (1995). *Manual of the Neonatal Behavioral Assessment Scale*. (3rd edition). Oxford: McKeith Press.

Breslau, N., Klein, N. and Allen, L. (1988). Very low birthweight: behavioral sequelae at nine years of age. *Journal of the American Academy of Child and Adolescent Psychiatry*, **27**, 605–12.

Brimblecombe, F. S. W. (1983). Evolution of special care baby units. In *Parent–Baby Attachment in Premature Infants* (J. A. Davis, M. P. M. Richards and N. R. C. Roberton, eds). Beckenham: Croom Helm.

Brooks-Gunn, J., McCarton, C. M., Casey, P. H., McCormick, M. C., Bauer, C. R., Bernbaum, J. C., Tyson, J., Swanson, M., Bennett, F. C., Scott, D. T., Tonascia, J. and Meinert, C. L. (1994). Early intervention in low-birth-weight premature infants: results through age 5 years from the Infant Health and Development Program. *Journal of the American Medical Association*, **272** (16), 1257–62.

Brooten, D., Kumar, S., Brown, L. P., Butts, P., Finkler, S. A., Bakewell-Sachs, S., Gibbons, A. and Delivoria-Papadopoulos, M. (1986). A randomized clinical trial of early hospital discharge and home follow-up of very-low-birth-weight infants. *New England Journal of Medicine*, **315**, 934–9.

Budin, P. (1990). *Le Nourisson*. Paris: Octave Dion. (English translation by W. J. Maloney, 1907, *The Nursling*). London: Caxton.

Buka, S. L., Lipsitt, L. P. and Tsuang, M. T. (1992). Emotional and behavioural development of low birthweight infants. In *The Psychological Development of Low Birthweight Children* (S. L. Friedman and M. D. Sigman, eds). New Jersey: Ablex.

Bushnell, I. W. R. and Slater, P. C. (1986). Concept formation in the preterm infant. Presentation at the Annual Conference of the British Psychological Society Developmental Section, Exeter, September 17–20.

Campbell, A. G. M. and McIntosh, N. (1992). *Forfar and Arneill's Textbook of Paediatrics* (4th edition). Edinburgh: Churchill Livingstone.

Central Health Services Council (1961). Report of the subcommittee on the prevention of prematurity and the care of premature infants. London: HMSO.

Challamel, M.-J. (1988). Development of sleep and wakefulness. In *Handbook of Human Growth and Developmental Biology* (E. Meisam and P. S. Timera, eds). Paris: CRC Press Inc.

Cole, J. G. (1995). Using the NBAS with high-risk infants. In *Neonatal Behavioral Assessment Scale* (T. B. Brazelton and J. K. Nugent, eds.), 3rd edn, London: Mac Keith Press, pp. 126–132.

Cornell, E. H. and Gottfried, A. W. (1976). Intervention with premature human infants. *Child Development*, **47**, 32–9.

Crnic, K. A., Ragozin, A. S., Greenberg, M. T., Robinson, N. M. and Basham, R. B. (1983). Social interaction and developmental competence of preterm and full-term infants during the first year of life. *Child Development*, **54**, 1199–210.

Gross, S. J., Slagle, T. A., D'Eugenio, D. and Mettelman, B. B. (1992). Impact of a matched term control group on interpretation of developmental performance in preterm infants. *Pediatrics*, **90**, 681–87.

Grunau, R. V., Whitfield, M. F., Petrie, J. H. and Fryer, E. L. (1994). Early pain experience, child and family factors, as precursors of somatization: a prospective study of extremely premature and fullterm children. *Pain*, **56** (3), 353–9.

Hack, M., Horbar, J. D., Malloy, M. H., Tyson, K. J. E., Wright, E. and Wright, L. (1991). Very low birth weight outcomes of the National Institute of Child Health and human development neonatal network. *Pediatrics*, **87**, 587–97.

Hagberg, B. and Hagberg, G. (1993). The changing panoramal of cerebral palsy in Sweden IV. *Acta Pediatrica Scandinavia*, **82**, 387–93.

Hagberg, B., Hagberg, G. and Zetterström, R. (1989). Decreasing perinatal mortality — increase in cerebral palsy morbidity? *Acta Paediatrica Scandinavia*, **78**, 664–70.

Hanson, N. and Okken, A. (1980). Transcutaneous oxygen tension of newborn infants in different behavioural states. *Pediatric Research*, **14**, 911–15.

Harrison, H. (1993). The principles for family-centered neonatal care. *Pediatrics*, **92**, 643–50.

Helders, P. J. M. (1989). *The Effects of A Sensory Stimulation/Range-Finding Program on The Development of Very Low Birthweight Infants*. Duurstede: ADDIX.

Helders, P. J. M. (1989). The effects of a sensory/range-finding program on the development of very low birthweight infants. Unpublished PhD thesis, University of Utrecht, Utrecht, Netherlands.

Helfer, R. E. (1987). The perinatal period, a window of opportunity for enhancing parent–infant communication: an approach to prevention. *Child Abuse and Neglect*, **11**, 565–79.

Hille, E. T. M., Den Ouden, A. L., Bauer, L., van den Oudenrijn, C., Brand, R. and Verloove-Vanhorik, S. P. (1994). School performance at nine years of age in very premature and very low birthweight infants: perinatal risk factors and predictors at five years of age. *Journal of Pediatrics*, **125**, 426–34.

Hodgman, J. E. (1985). Introduction. In *Infant Stress Under Intensive Care: Environmental Neonatology* (A. W. Gottfried and J. L. Gaiter, eds). Baltimore: University Park Press.

Holtrop, P. C., Ertzbischoff, L. M., Roberts, C. L., Batton, D. G. and Lorenz, R. P. (1994). Survival and short term outcome in newborns of 23 to 25 weeks' gestation. *American Journal of Obstetrics and Gynaecology*, **170** (1), 1266–70.

Hunt, J. M. (1961). Environment and experiences. New York, NY: Roland Press.

Hunt, J. V., Cooper, B. A. B. and Tooley, W. H. (1988). Very low birth weight infants at 8 and 11 years of age: role of neonatal illness and family status. *Pediatrics*, **82**, 596–603.

Jacobsen, T., Gronvall, J., Petersen, S., Andersen, G. E. (1993). 'Minitouch' treatment of very low-birth-weight infants. *Acta Paediatrica*, **82** (11), 934–8.

Jeffcoate, J., Humphrey, M. and Loyd, J. (1979). Disturbance in parent–child relationship following preterm delivery. *Developmental Medicine and Child Neurology*, **21**, 344–52.

Klaus, M. H. and Kennel, J. H. (1970). Mothers separated from their newborn infants. *Pediatric Clinics of North America*, **17** (4), 1015–37.

Klaus, M. H. and Kennell, J. H. (1982). Parent–infant bonding. St Louis: C.V. Mosby.

Klein, M. and Stern, L. (1971). Low birth weight and the battered child syndrome. *American Journal of Disabled Children*, **22**, 15–18.

Klein, N. K., Hack, M. and Breslau, N. (1989). Children who were very low birthweight. Development and academic achievement at 9 years of age. *Developmental and Behavioural Pediatrics*, **10**, 32–7.

Lacy, J. B. and Ohlsson, A. (1993). Behavioural outcomes of environmental or care-giving hospital-based interventions for preterm infants: a critical overview. *Acta Paediatrica*, **82**, 408–15.

Lagercrantz, H., Nilsson, F., Redham, I. and Hjemdal, P. (1986). Plasma catecholamines following nursing procedures in a neonatal ward. *Early Human Development*, **14**, 61–5.

Lawson, K. R., Turkewitz, G., Platt, M. and McCarton, C. (1985). Infant state in relation to its environmental context. *Infant Behaviour and Development*, **8**, 269–81.

Lee, V. E., Brooks-Gunn, J., Schnur, E. and Liaw, F. R. (1990). Are head start effects sustained? A longitudinal follow-up comparison of disadvantaged children attending head start, no preschool, and other preschool programs. *Child Development*, **61**, 495–507.

Lester, B. M., Hoffman, J. and Brazelton, B. (1985). The rhythmic structure of mother–infant interaction in term and preterm infants. *Child Development*, **56**, 15–27.

Linn, P. L., Horowitz, F. D., Buddin, B. J., Leake, J. C. and Fox, H. A. (1985). An ecological description of a neonatal intensive care unit. In *Infant Stress Under Intensive Care: Environmental Neonatology* (A. W. Gottfried and J. L. Gaiter, eds). University Park Press.

Long, G. J., Lucey, J. F. and Philip, A. G. S. (1980). Noise and hypoxaemia in the intensive care nursery. *Pediatrics*, **65**, 143–5.

Long, J. G., Philip, A. G. S. and Lucey, J. F. (1980). Excessive handling as a cause of hypoxaemia. *Pediatrics*, **65**, 203–7.

Lotas, M. J. (1992). Effects of light and sound in the neonatal intensive care unit environment on the low birth weight infant. *Clinical Issues of Perinatology, Women's Health and Nursing*, **3** (1), 34–44.

Mann, N. P., Haddow, R., Stokes, L. and Goodley, S. R. N. (1986). Effect of night and day on preterm infants in a newborn nursery: randomised trial. *British Medical Journal*, **293**, 1265–7.

McCormick, M. C., Brooks-Gunn, J., Workman-Daniels, K., Turner, J. A. and Peckham, G. J. (1992). The health and developmental status of very low-birth-weight children at school age. *Journal of the American Medical Association*, **267**, 2204–8.

McCormick, M. C., Gortmaker, S. L. and Sobol, A. M. (1990). Very low birth weight children: behavior problems and school difficulty in a national sample. *The Journal of Pediatrics*, **117**, 687–93.

Minde, K. K. (1984). The impact of prematurity on the later behaviour of children and on their families. *Clinics in Perinatology*, **11**, 227–44.

Minde, K., Shosenberg, N., Thompson, J. and Marton, P. (1983). Self-help groups in a premature nursery – follow-up at one year. In *Frontiers of Psychiatry* (J. D. Call, E. Galenson and R. L. Tyson, eds). New York: Basic Books.

Minde, K., Whitelaw, A., Brown, J. and Fitzhardinge, P. (1983). Neonatal complications and parent–infant interactions. *Developmental Medicine and Child Neurology*, **25**, 763–77.

Ministry of Health (1944). Care of premature infants (Circular 20/44). London: Ministry of Health.

Mouradian, L. E. and Als, H. (1994). The influence of neonatal intensive care unit caregiving practices on motor functioning of preterm infants. *American Journal of Occupational Therapy*, **48** (6), 527–33.

Murdoch, D. R. and Darlow, B. A. (1984). Handling during neonatal intensive care. *Archives of Disease in Childhood*, **59**, 957–61.

Nugent, J. M. (1985). Using the NBAS with infants and their families: guidelines for intervention. New York: March of Dimes Defects Foundation.

Nurcombe, B., Howell, D. C., Rauh, V. A., Teti, D. M., Ruoff, P. and Brennan, J. (1984). An intervention program for mothers of low-birthweight infants: preliminary results. *Journal of the American Academy of Child Psychiatry*, **23**, 319–25.

Pharoah, P. O. D., Cooke, R. W. I. and Rosenbloom, L. (1990). Birthweight specific trends in cerebral palsy. *Archives of Disease in Childhood*, **65**, 602–6.

Pharoah, P. O. D. (1986). Perspectives and patterns. *British Medical Bulletin*, **42**, 119–26.

Philbin, M. K., Ballweg, D. D. and Gray, L. (1994). The effect of an intensive care unit sound environment on the development of habituation in healthy avian neonates. *Developmental Psychobiology*, **27** (1), 11–21.

Porz, F., von Schoenach, P. and Bernsau, U. (1995). *Auswirkungen eines neuen Erstversorgungskonzepts der "individuellen Pflege" auf die Morbidität kleiner Frühgeborener*. Paper presented at the Symposium der Deutsch-Österreichischen Gesellschaft für Neonatologie und Pädiatrische Intensivmedizin. Proceedings: Munich: Alete Wissenschaftlicher Dienst, pp. 214–15.

Ramey, C. and Campbell, F. (1991). Poverty, early childhood education, and academic competence: the Abecedarian experiment. In *Children in Poverty* (A. Huston, ed.). Cambridge, Mass: Cambridge University Press.

Rauh, V., Achenbach, T., Nurcombe, B., Howell, C. and Teti, D. (1988). Minimizing adverse effects of low birthweight: Four-year results of an early intervention. *Child Development*, **59**, 544–53.

Redshaw, M. E. and Harris, A. (1995). Maternal perceptions of neonatal care. *Acta Paediatrica*, **84**, 593–8.

Redshaw, M. E., Rivers, R. P. A. and Rosenblatt, D. B. (1985). *Born too Early*. Oxford: Oxford University Press.

Resnick, M. B., Davis Eyler, F., Nelson, R. M., Eitzman, D. V. and Bucciarelli, R. L. (1987). Developmental intervention for low birth weight infants: improved early developmental outcome. *Pediatrics*, **80**, 68–74.

Reynolds, E. O. E. and Taghizadeh, A. (1974). Improved prognosis of infants mechanically ventilated for hyaline membrane disease. *Archives of Disease in Childhood*, **49**, 505–10.

Richards, M. P. M. (1985). Bonding babies. *Archives of Disease in Childhood*, **60**, 293–4.

Richmond, J. (1990). Low-birth-weight babies: can we enhance their development? *Journal of the American Medical Association*, **262**, 3069–70.

Riegel, K., Ohrt, B., Wolke, D. and Österlund, K. (1995). Die Entwicklung gefährdet geborener Kinder bis zum fünften Lebensjahr. Die ARVO-YLLPÖ Neugeborenen-Nachfolge Studie in Südbayern und Südfinnland. Stuttgart: Enke Verlag.

Roberton, N. R. C. (1993). Should we look after babies less than 800 g? *Archives of Disabled Children*, **68**, 326–9.

Sameroff, A. J. and Chandler, M. J. (1975). Reproductive risk and the continuum of caretaking casualty. In *Review of Child Development Research* (F. D. Horowitz, J. Hetherington, S. Scarr-Salapatek and G. Siegel, eds), **4**, 187–243.

Saunders, A. N. (1995). Incubator noise: a method to decrease decibels. *Paediatric Nursing*, **21** (3), 265–8.

Scarr-Salapatek, S. and Williams, M. L. (1973). The effects of early stimulation on low-birth-weight infants. *Child Development*, **44**, 94–101.

Shimada, M., Segawa, M. and Higurashi, M. A. H. (1993). Development of the sleep and wakefulness rhythm in preterm infants discharged from a neonatal care unit. *Pediatric Research*, **33**, 159–63.

Shogan, M. G. and Schumann, L. L. (1993). The effect of environmental lighting on the oxygen saturation of preterm infants in the NICU. *Neonatal Networks*, **12** (5), 7–13.

Silverman, W. A. (1979). Incubator-baby side shows. *Pediatrics*, **64**, 127–41.

Silverman, W. A. (1992). Overtreatment of neonates? A personal retrospective. *Pediatrics*, **90** (6), 971–6.

Skouteli, H. N., Dubowitz, L. M. S., Levene, M. I. and Miller, G. (1985). Predictors for survial and normal neurodevelopmental outcome of infants weighing less than 1001 grams at birth. *Developmental Medicine and Child Neurology*, **27**, 588–95.

Slater, A. (1989). Visual memory and perception in early infancy. In *Infant Development* (A. Slater and G. Bremner, eds). Hillsdale, NJ: Lawrence Erlbaum.

Speidel, B. D. (1976). Adverse effects of routine procedures on preterm infants. *Lancet*, **1**, 864–6.

St. James-Roberts, I. and Wolke, D. (1989). Do obstetric factors affect the mother's perception of her newborn's behaviour? *British Journal of Developmental Psychology*, **7**, 141–58.

Stahlman, M. T. (1984). Newborn intensive care: success or failure? *The Journal of Pediatrics*, **105**, 162–7.

Stahlman, M. T. (1990). Ethical issues in the nursery: priorities versus limits. *The Journal of Pediatrics*, **116**, 167–70.

Stanley, F. J. and Blair, E. (1991). Why have we failed to reduce the frequency of cerebral palsy? *The Medical Journal of Australia*, **154**, 623–6.

Stewart, A. (1985). Early prediction of neurological outcome when the very preterm infant is discharged from the intensive care unit. *Annual of Pediatrics*, **32**, 27–38.

Stewart, A. L., Reynolds, E. O. R. and Lipscomb, A. P. (1981). Outcome for infants of very low birthweight. Survey of World Literature. *Lancet*, **1**, 1038–40.

Strauch, C., Brandt, S., Edwards-Beckett, J. (1993). Implementation of a quiet hour: effect on noise levels and infant sleep states. *Neonatal Networks*, **12** (2), 31–5.

Sykes, D. H., Hoy, E. A., Bill, J. M., Halliday, H. L., McClure, B. G. and Reid, M. M. (1997). Behavioural adjustment in school of very low birthweight children. *Journal of Child Psychology and Psychiatry*, **38**, (3), 315–26.

Symon, A. and Cunningham, S. (1995). Handling premature neonates: a study using time-lapse video. *Nursing Times*, **91** (17), 35–7.

The Infant Health and Development Program (1990). Enhancing the outcomes of low-birthweight, premature infants: a multi-site, randomized trial. *Journal of the American Medical Association*, **263**, 3035–42.

Vohr, B. R., Garcia-Coll, C. and Oh, W. (1988). Language development of low-birthweight infants at two years. *Developmental Medicine and Child Neurology*, **30**, 608–15.

Volpe, J. J. (1989). Intraventricular hemorrhage in the premature infant: current concepts, part 1. *Annual of Neurology*, **25** (3), 3–11.

Weisglas-Kuperus, N., Koot, H. M., Baerts, W., Fetter, W. P. F. and Sauer, P. J. J. (1993). Behaviour problems of very low-birthweight children. *Developmental Medicine and Child Neurology*, **35**, 406–16.

White-Traut, R. C., Nelson, M. N., Burns, K. and Cunningham, N. (1994). Environmental influences on the developing premature infant: theoretical issues and applications to practice. *Journal of Obstetrics and Gynaecological Neonatal Nursing*, **23** (5), 393–401.

Whitelaw, A. and Sleath, K. (1985). Myth of the marsupial mother: home care of very low birth weight babies in Bogota, Columbia. *Lancet*, **25**, 1206–8.

Widmayer, S. M. and Field, T. M. (1980). Effects of Brazelton demonstrations on early interactions of preterm infants and their teenage mothers. *Infant Behaviour and Development*, **3**, 79–89.

Widmayer, S. M. and Field, T. M. (1981). Effects of Brazelton demonstrations for mothers on the development of preterm infants. *Pediatrics*, **67**, 711–14.

Williams, L. (1995). Is the money well spent? Use of resources in neonatal intensive care. *Child Health*, **3** (2), 68–72.

Wolke, D. (1987a). Environmental and developmental neonatology. *Journal of Reproductive and Infant Psychology*, **5**, 17–42.

Wolke, D. (1987b). Environmental neonatology (Annotation). *Archives of Disease in Childhood*, **62**, 987–8.

Wolke, D. (1989). The neonatal intensive care unit environment: effects on the baby and possible interventions. In *Biopsychology of Early Mother–Infant Communication* (J. Gomes-Pedro, ed.). Lisbon: Fundacao Calouste Gulbenkian.

Wolke, D. (1991a). Supporting the development of low-birthweight infants (Annotation). *Journal of Child Psychology and Psychiatry*, **32**, 723–41.

Wolke, D. (1991b). Psycho-biologische Aspekte der Pflege von Frühgeborenen. *Deutsche Krankenpflege-Zeitschrift (Schwerpunktthema Perinatalmedizin)*, **44**, 478–83.

Wolke, D. (1993). Langzeitprognose von Frühgeborenen: was wir wissen und was wir wissen sollten (longterm prognosis of pretern infants: what we know and what we should know). In *Aktuelle Neuropädiatrie 1992* (A. Lischka and G. Bernert, hrsg). Wehr/Baden: Verlag Ciba Geigy.

Wolke, D. (1994). Feeding and sleeping across the lifespan. In *Development through Life: A Handbook for Clinicians* (M. Rutter and D. Hay, eds). Oxford: Blackwell Scientific Publications.

Wolke, D. (1995a). Verhaltensprobleme und soziale Beziehungen ehemals sehr kleiner Früehgeborener: Einfluesse des intensivmedizinischen handlings. *Zeitschrift fuer Geburtshilfe und Neonatologie*, **199**, 208.

Wolke, D. (1995b). Parent's perceptions as guides for conducting Brazelton clinical sessions. In *Manual of the Neonatal Behavioral Assessment Scale* (3rd edition) (T. B. Brazelton and K. Nugent, eds). Oxford: McKeith Press.

Wolke, D. 1997a). Entwicklung Sehr Fruhgeborener bis zum 7. Lebensjahr (development of very preterm infants until the seventh year of life). In *Frühforderung und Frühbehandlung — Wissenschaftliche Grundlagen, Praxisorientierte Ansätze und Perspektiven Interdisziplinärer*

Zusammenarbeit (T. Horstmann and C. Leyendecker, eds). Heidelberg: Universitätsverlag C. Winter.

Wolke, D. (1997 b). The environment of care. In *Forfar and Arneill's Textbook of Paediatrics* (5th edition) (A. G. M. Campbell and N. McIntosh, eds). Edinburgh: Churchill Livingstone.

Wolke, D. (1997c). The preterm responses to the environment — long term effects? In *Advances in Perinatal Medicine*, (F. Cockburn, ed.), Carnforth: Parthenon Publishing, pp. 305–14.

Wolke, D. and Eldridge, T. (1992). The environment of care. In *Forfar and Arneill's Textbook of Paediatrics* (4th edition) (A. G. M. Campbell and N. McIntosh, eds). Edinburgh: Churchill Livingstone.

Wolke, D. and St. James-Roberts, I. (1987). Multi-method measurement of the early parent–infant system with easy and difficult newborns. In *Psychobiology and Early Development* (H. Rauh and H. C. Steinhausen, eds). Amsterdam: North-Holland/Elsevier.

Wolke, D. and Meyer, R. (1994). Psychologische langzeitbefunde bei sehr frühgeborenen. *PerinatalMedizin*, **6**, 121–3.

Wolke, D., Brothwood, M., Gamsu, H. and Cooper, D. (1989). Prediction of neurodevelopmental sequelae outcome in VLBW infants: implications for developmental theories. In *Biopsychology of Early Mother–Infant Communication* (J. Gomes-Pedro, ed.). Lisbon: Fundacao Calouste Gulbenkian.

Wolke, D., Ratschinski, G., Ohrt, B. and Riegel, K. (1994a). The cognitive outcome of very preterm infants may be poorer than often reported: an empirical investigation of how methodological issues make a big difference. *European Journal of Pediatrics*, **153**, 906–15.

Wolke, D., Gray, P. and Meyer, R. (1994b). Excessive infant crying: a controlled study of mothers helping mothers. *Pediatrics*, **94**, 322–32.

Wolke, D., Söhne, B., Ohrt, B. and Riegel, K. (1995). Follow-up of preterm children: important to document dropouts. *Lancet*, **345** (No. 8947), 447.

Wolke, D., Meyer, R., Ohrt, B. and Riegel, K. (1995). The incidence of sleeping problems in preterm and full-term infants discharged from special neonatal care units: an epidemiological longitudinal study. *Journal of Child Psychology and Psychiatry*, **36** (2), 203–23.

Zahr, L. K. and Balian, S. (1995). Responses of preterm infants to routine nursing interventions and noise in the NICU. *Nursing in Research*, **44** (3), 179–85.

Index